Progress in Inflammation Research

Series Editor

Prof. Dr. Michael J. Parnham
PLIVA
Research Institute
Prilaz baruna Filipovica 25
10000 Zagreb
Croatia

Published titles:
T Cells in Arthritis, P. Miossec, W. van den Berg, G. Firestein (Editors), 1998
Chemokines and Skin, E. Kownatzki, J. Norgauer (Editors), 1998
Medicinal Fatty Acids, J. Kremer (Editor), 1998
Inducible Enzymes in the Inflammatory Response, D.A. Willoughby, A. Tomlinson (Editors),
1999
Cytokines in Severe Sepsis and Septic Shock, H. Redl, G. Schlag (Editors), 1999
Fatty Acids and Inflammatory Skin Diseases, J.-M. Schröder (Editor), 1999
Immunomodulatory Agents from Plants, H. Wagner (Editor), 1999
Cytokines and Pain, L. Watkins, S. Maier (Editors), 1999
In Vivo Models of Inflammation, D. Morgan, L. Marshall (Editors), 1999
Pain and Neurogenic Inflammation, S.D. Brain, P. Moore (Editors), 1999
Anti-Inflammatory Drugs in Asthma, A.P. Sampson, M.K. Church (Editors), 1999
Novel Inhibitors of Leukotrienes, G. Folco, B. Samuelsson, R.C. Murphy (Editors), 1999
Vascular Adhesion Molecules and Inflammation, J.D. Pearson (Editor), 1999
Metalloproteinases as Targets for Anti-Inflammatory Drugs, K.M.K. Bottomley, D. Brad-
shaw, J.S. Nixon (Editors), 1999

Forthcoming titles:
Gene Therapy in Inflammatory Diseases, Ch. Evans, P. Robbins (Editors), 1999
New Cytokines as Potential Drugs, S.K. Narula, R. Coffman (Editors), 2000
High-Throughput Screening for Novel Antiinflammatories, M. Kahn (Editor), 2000

Free Radicals and Inflammation

Paul G. Winyard
David R. Blake
Christopher H. Evans

Editors

Springer Basel AG

Editors

Dr. Paul G. Winyard
St. Bartholomew's and
The Royal London School of Medicine and Dentistry
Queen Mary and Westfield College
25–29 Ashfield Street
London E1 1AD
UK

Prof. Christopher H. Evans
University of Pittsburgh School of Medicine
Musculoskeletal Institute
986 Scaife Hall
Pittsburgh, PA 15261
USA

Prof. David R. Blake
School of Postgraduate Medicine
University of Bath
Claverton Down
Bath BA2 7AY
UK

A CIP catalogue record for this book is available from the Library of Congress, Washington D.C., USA

Deutsche Bibliothek Cataloging-in-Publication Data
Free radicals and inflammation / ed. by Paul G. Winyard ... - Basel
; Boston ; Berlin : Birkhäuser, 2000
  (Progress in inflammation research)
  ISBN 978-3-0348-9586-6   ISBN 978-3-0348-8482-2 (eBook)
  DOI 10.1007/978-3-0348-8482-2

© 2000 Springer Basel AG
Originally published by Birkhäuser Verlag in 2002
Softcover reprint of the hardcover 1st edition 2000
Printed on acid-free paper produced from chlorine-free pulp. TCF ∞
Cover design: Markus Etterich, Basel
Cover illustration: Macrophage-like cells within the rheumatoid synovium staining positive for activated NF-κB. With the friendly permission of Dr. Paul G. Winyard, St. Bartholomew's and The Royal London School of Medicine and Dentistry, London, UK

ISBN 978-3-0348-9586-6

9 8 7 6 5 4 3 2 1

Contents

List of contributors

Nigel Benjamin, Department of Clinical Pharmacology, St. Bartholomew's and The Royal London School of Medicine and Dentistry, Charterhouse Square, London EC1, UK; e-mail: n.benjamin@qmw.ac.uk

Timothy R. Billiar, Department of Surgery, A1010 Presbyterian University Hospital, 200 Lothrop Street, University of Pittsburgh, Pittsburgh, PA 15261, USA

David R. Blake, School of Postgraduate Medicine, University of Bath, Claverton Down, Bath BA2 7AY, UK; e-mail: BLAKED@rhnrd-tr.swest.nhs.uk

Tulin Bodamyali, School of Postgraduate Medicine, University of Bath, Claverton Down, Bath BA2 7AY, UK; e-mail: mpsts@bath.ac.uk

Christopher A. Bombeck, Department of Surgery, University of California, Davis-East Bay, 1411 East 31st St., Oakland, CA 94602, USA; e-mail: bombeck@pop.pitt.edu

Wing-Fai Cheung, Connective Tissue Research Group, Samuel Lunenfeld Research Institute, Mount Sinai Hospital, Toronto, Ontario M5G 1X5 and Department of Cellular and Molecular Pathology, University of Toronto, Ontario M5S 1A8, Canada

Tony F. Cruz, Connective Tissue Research Group, Samuel Lunenfeld Research Institute, Mount Sinai Hospital, Toronto, Ontario M5G 1X5 and Department of Cellular and Molecular Pathology, University of Toronto, Ontario M5S 1A8, Canada

Sally E. Edmonds, Oxford Regional Rheumatic Diseases Research Centre, Stoke Mandeville Hospital NHS Trust, Mandeville Road, Aylesbury, Bucks HP21 8AL, UK

Chris H. Evans, Center for Molecular Orthopaedics, Harvard Medical School, 221 Longwood Avenue, Boston, MA 02115, USA

Vanessa Gilston, Bone and Joint Research Unit, St. Bartholomew's and The Royal London School of Medicine and Dentistry, Queen Mary and Westfield College, University of London, 25–29 Ashfield Street, London E1 2AD, UK

Helen R. Griffiths, University of Leicester, Division of Chemical Pathology, Hodgkin Building, MRC Centre for Mechanisms in Human Toxicity, Lancaster Road, Leicester, LE1 9HN, UK

Matthew B. Grisham, Ph.D., Department of Molecular and Cellular Physiology, Louisiana State University Medical Center, 1501 Kings Highway, Shreveport, LA 71130, USA; e-mail: mgrish@lsumc.edu

Barry Halliwell, Department of Biochemistry, National University of Singapore, 10 Kent Ridge Crescent, Singapore 119260; e-mail: bchbh@nus.edu.sg

John T. Hancock, Department of Biological and Biomedical Sciences, University of the West of England, Coldharbour Lane, Bristol, BS16 1QY, UK; e-mail: john.hancock@uwe.ac.uk

Roger Harrison, Department of Biology and Biochemistry, University of Bath, Bath BA2 7AY, UK; e-mail: bssrh@bath.ac.uk

Owen T.G. Jones, Department of Biochemistry, University of Bristol, School of Medical Sciences, University Walk, Bristol, BS8 1TD, UK

Harparkash Kaur, Northwick Park Institute of Medical Research, Department of Surgical Research, Watford Road, Harrow, Middlesex HA1 3UJ, UK; e-mail: h.kaur@ic.ac.uk

Jianrong Li, Department of Surgery, A1010 Presbyterian University Hospital, 200 Lothrop Street, University of Pittsburgh, Pittsburgh, PA 15261, USA

Yvonne Y.C. Lo, Connective Tissue Research Group, Samuel Lunenfeld Research Institute, Mount Sinai Hospital, Toronto, Ontario M5G 1X5 and Department of Cellular and Molecular Pathology, University of Toronto, Ontario M5S 1A8, Canada

Joseph Lunec, University of Leicester, Division of Chemical Pathology, Hodgkin Building, MRC Centre for Mechanisms in Human Toxicity, Lancaster Road, Leicester, LE1 9HN, UK

Heather MacPherson, Department of Medicine and Therapeutics, Foresterhill, Aberdeen AB25 2ZD, Scotland, UK; e-mail: h.macpherson@abdu.ac.uk

George A.C. Murrell, Department of Orthopaedic Surgery, University of New South Wales, St. George Hospital Campus, Sydney 2217, Australia;
e-mail: admin@ori.org.au

Takashi Okamoto, Department of Molecular Genetics, Nagoya City University Medical School, 1 Kawasumi Mizuho-cho, Mizuho-ku, Nagoya 467, Japan;
e-mail: tokamoto@med.nagoya-cu.ac.jp

Stuart H. Ralston, Department of Medicine and Therapeutics, Foresterhill, Aberdeen AB25 2ZD, Scotland, UK; e-mail: s.ralston@abdu.ac.uk

Maja Stefanovic-Racic, Department of Orthopaedic Surgery, University of Pittsburgh School of Medicine, Room C313 PUH, 200 Lothrop Street, Pittsburgh, PA 15213, USA

Cliff R. Stevens, School of Postgraduate Medicine, University of Bath, Claverton Down, Bath BA2 7AY, UK; e-mail: mpscrs@bath.ac.uk

Toshifumi Tetsuka, Department of Molecular Genetics, Nagoya City University Medical School, 1 Kawasumi, Mizuho-cho, Mizuho-ku, Nagoya 467, Japan;
e-mail: tetsuka@med.nagoya-cu.ac.jp

Paul G. Winyard, Bone and Joint Research Unit, St. Bartholomew's and The Royal London School of Medicine and Dentistry, 25–29 Ashfield Street, London E1 2AD, UK; e-mail: P.G.Winyard@mds.qmw.ac.uk

Robert E. Wolf, Division of Rheumatology, Louisiana State University Medical Center, 1501 Kings Highway, P.O. Box 33932, Shreveport, LA 71130-3932, USA

Johnson M.S. Wong, Banting and Best Department of Medical Research and Department of Molecular and Medical Genetics, University of Toronto, Toronto, Ontario M5G 1L6, Canada

Preface

As in so many fields of scientific endeavour following the molecular biology revolution, our knowledge of the role of radicals not only in pathological states, but in basic physiology has developed exponentially. Indeed, our evolving concepts have, like so many political parties, been forced into dramatic "U-turns" and contortions. Within our working lives, we have had to debate whether radicals made any contribution to any pathology, whilst now it is difficult not to entertain the view that every physiological process is pivotally controlled by exquisitely sensitive radical reactions.

Inflammation is, of course, an example of pathology evolving from physiology, and in this book we have called upon both scientists and clinicians who have research interests in the complex switching mechanisms that sustain these transitions. The book as a whole explores, from a physiological standpoint, how deterministic radical systems sensitive to their initial conditions can interdigitate, iterate and feed back to control diverse cellular processes that create the inflammatory response.

Whilst systems such as these to a mathematician would provide the basis for a chaotic response, one is forced to marvel how, for all stages of an inflammatory reaction, this system appears exquisitely controlled, making therapeutic manipulation both possible and, to some extent, predictable.

July 1999

Paul G. Winyard
David R. Blake
Chris H. Evans

Introduction

David R. Blake[1], Tulin Bodamyali[1], Cliff R. Stevens[1] and Paul G. Winyard[2]

[1]School of Postgraduate Medicine, University of Bath, Claverton Down, Bath BA2 7AY, UK;
[2]Bone and Joint Research Unit, St. Bartholomew's and The Royal London School of Medicine and Dentistry, 25–29 Ashfield Street, London E1 2AD, UK

What is inflammation?

Inflammation, in the broadest sense, is a physiological, protective response to injury or tissue destruction. It is a complex network of co-ordinated cellular responses designed to destroy, dilute, or "wall-off" both the noxious stimuli and the injured tissue. Such cellular activity controls critical events which lead to repair and resolution of the tissue injury.

It is beyond doubt that, as a physiologically controlled self-limiting phenomenon, inflammation plays a central role in mediating immune mechanisms of host defence and wound healing. Disruption of the physiological control mechanisms of this defence system, however, forms the basis of the pathology of many diseases. In this setting, a physiological defence mechanism either mediates pathology or contributes to it.

The inflammatory response is often categorised according to the duration and the kinetics of the reaction as acute and chronic. Chronicity of the inflammatory response does not directly infer pathology. This reaction, whether acute or chronic, is self-limiting and will eventually resolve. We argue that acute inflammation can be considered as a rapid physiological defence mechanism and chronic inflammation as an organised repair system.

Mechanisms of the inflammatory response

Several theories have been put forward with respect to the initiation of the inflammatory response. Firstly, "humoral theory" argues for the initial response arising from the blood and tissue fluids. The alternative view to humoral inflammation, is the "cellular theory" which supports the idea that the cells, which appear during the inflammatory process, are the main protection of the body against microbial infection. Detailed research to date has indicated that the two theories cannot be mutually exclusive. Later, the role of the immune system (immune complexes and immune cells) in inflammation was examined in detail and several observations led to the classification of different types of immune reactions, leading to inflammation. It was recognised that antibody/antigen interactions (immune complexes) were not the only component of an inflammatory reaction, but polymorphonuclear leucocytes (PMN) were also involved. Phagocytosis of immune complexes by PMN is accompanied by degranulation of lysosomes and release of hydrolytic enzymes, which can break down the connective tissue matrix. Macrophages are mononuclear cells that are also phagocytic. Immune complexes induce these cells to secrete lysosomal enzymes, including neutral proteases capable of degrading connective tissue components such as collagen.

Other types of antigen-induced inflammatory responses such as anaphylactic shock, the immediate-hypersensitivity reaction or allergy, immune complex disease, and delayed hypersensitivity have also been described. Then came the recognition of the role for lymphoid cells and the identification of T lymphocytes (antigen recognition) and B lymphocytes (antibody synthesis), which led to the term "cell-mediated immunity". The interaction of T lymphocytes with antigen or mitogen leads to the activation of metabolic processes of the cell, increased DNA synthesis, mitosis and the synthesis of small proteins or polypeptides called lymphokines, cytokines and many other proinflammatory factors. It is now recognised that the production of such factors is not exclusive to the immunomodulatory cells but such mediators/modulators of the inflammatory response are also released by different cell types including fibroblasts and endothelial cells. These products provide a system of communication between cells by means of molecular signals. These signals, we argue, are probably responsible for many cellular interactions, as well as surveillance against infectious organisms, malignancies and grafts.

Mediators of inflammation

A vast array of factors mediate the inflammatory process. The following is a summary of some of the "key players" in the process.

1. *Plasma enzyme cascades and inhibitors/acute phase proteins* including the coagulation system, the fibrinolytic system, the kallikrein-kinin system, and the complement system: The coagulation system stems the initial bleeding and forms a barrier which limits the spread of the noxious stimulus and of inflammation itself (fibrin deposition). The fibrinolytic system controls excessive intravascular thrombosis and removes formed thrombi (fibrin breakdown to soluble products). The kallikrein-kinin system (mainly bradykinin) initiates the vascular changes of inflammation in concert with other systems or factors. The complement system maintains the vascular changes and initiates cellular infiltration, neutralising, killing or lysing the provoking agent. The inflammatory effects of the components of the four enzyme cascades are summarised in Scheme 1.

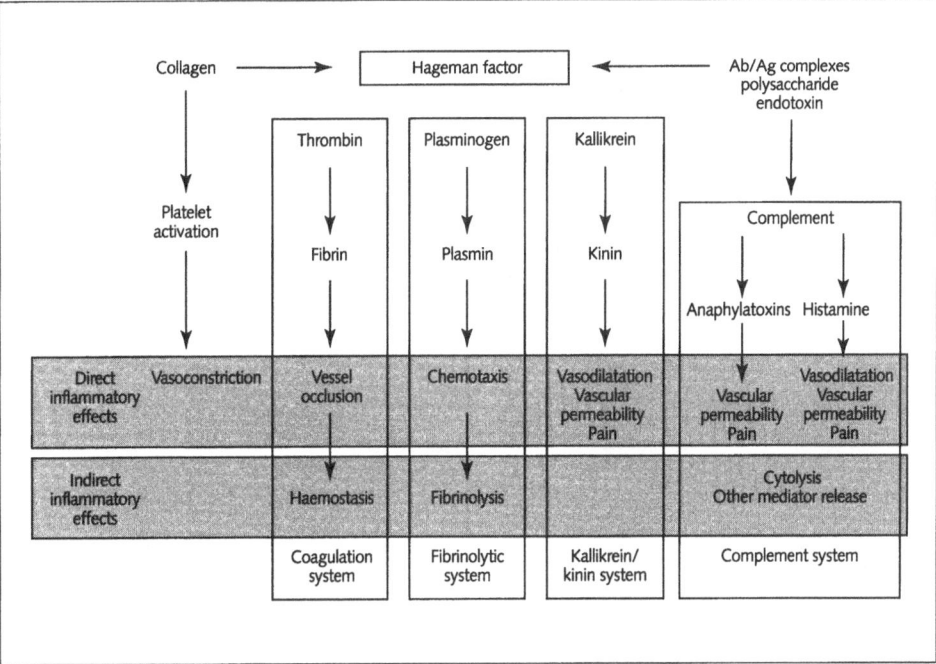

Scheme 1
Proteolytic enzyme cascades

In addition to these proteolytic enzyme cascades which mediate several stages of the inflammatory process, aerobic cells have an intrinsic system of inhibitors which "neutralise" the activities of the cascades. These inhibitors, listed in Table 1, play an important role in the dynamic equilibrium required for limiting the inflammatory process when injury is resolved.

2. *Acute phase proteins*: Similar to the functions of the proteolytic enzyme cascades, the acute phase proteins also help to restore disturbed homeostasis by stopping bleeding; by demarcation and resorption of the necrotic tissue; lysis of foreign cells and bacteria; by binding and removal of excessive amounts of proteases and exogenous substances and by preparing conditions for repair processes and wound healing.

3. *Arachidonic acid products*: The main phospholipid-derived arachidonic acid products are prostaglandins and leukotrienes. The role of these products in the inflammatory reaction are summarised in Schemes 2a and 2b.

Table 1

Inhibitor	Principal enzyme	Function
C1-inactivator	C1s	Activation control of blood coagulation,
	C1r	fibrinolysis, kallikrein and complement
	Kallikrein	
Antithrombin III	Thrombin	Local limitation of coagulation
α_2-Macroglobulin	Kallikrein	
	Elastase	
	Collagenase	
α_2-Macroglobulin	Thrombin	Limitation of fibrinolysis to the pathological
C1-inactivator	Kallikrein	substrates
	Elastase	
	Collagenase	
α_2-Macroglobulin	As above	Control of infections and inflammation by
α_1-Antitrypsin	Plasma trypsin	inhibition of proteinases involved, their
		neutralisation and clearance. Prevention of
		autodigestive processes and side reactions to
		the coagulation system.

4. *Platelet-derived mediators*: Platelets contain a vast array of potent intracellular mediators which play an important role in certain types of inflammation (indicated in Table 2). They carry preformed mediators which are rapidly available to counteract vascular injury. They also possess an armamentarium which can regulate the alteration of many other systems involved in the inflammatory response. They are believed to play a role in the very early phase of this process.

5. *Mediators derived from mast cells, PMN leucocytes, monocytes/macrophages, and lymphocytes*: Cells recruited from circulation to sites of injury, where an inflammatory reaction is triggered also generate a plethora of inflammatory mediators. The main mediators released from each cell type are listed in Table 3.

6. *Other mediators*: Along with the humoral factors and immune cell-derived mediators of inflammation, differentiated cells of diverse functionality and phenotype (as resident components of various tissues and organs), play significant parts as mediators of inflammation. A vast array of lymphokines, monokines and cytokines originally identified as immune-cell derived mediators of inflammation, as well as other mediators such as proteinases, are now known to be also

4

Scheme 2a - Actions of prostaglandins

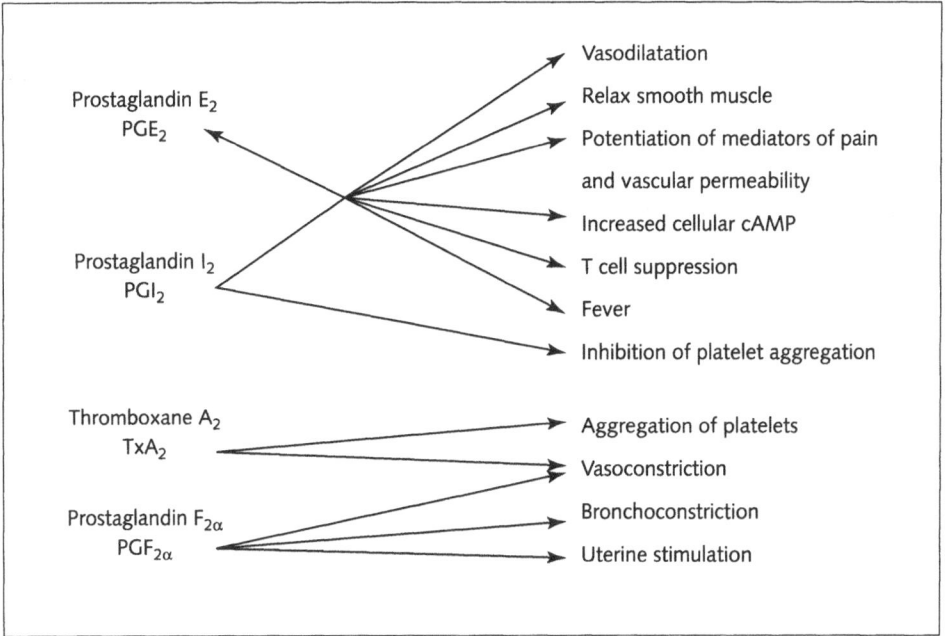

Scheme 2b - Actions of leukotrienes

Peptidolipids	Leukotriene C_4 (LTC$_4$)	Smooth muscle contraction Bronchoconstriction
	Leukotriene D_4 (LTD$_4$)	Release of cyclo-oxygenase products Vasoconstriction
Dihydroxy-derivatives	Leukotriene B_4 (LTB$_4$)	Microvascular permeability Chemotaxis Immunosuppression

produced and released by additional cell types including endothelial cells, fibroblasts, chondrocytes, and osteoblasts. One significant feature of many of these inflammatory mediators, however, is that reactive oxygen species (ROS) and reactive nitrogen species (RNS) may be involved in their mechanism of action. Many of the cell types regulating the inflammatory response can, under defined microenvironmental conditions, be induced to generate ROS and RNS, which

Table 2 - Platelet-derived mediators

Mediator	Aspect of inflammation affected
Prothrombinase	Clotting via fibrinogen to fibrin conversion
Adenosine diphosphate (ADP)	
Platelet activating factor (PAF)	
Thrombin	Aggregation
Thromboxane A_2 (TxA_2)	
Prostaglandin G_2 (PGG_2)	
Prostaglandin H_2 (PGH_2)	Vasoconstriction
5-Hydroxytryptamine (5-HT)	
PGG_2	
Prostaglandin E_2 (PGE_2)	Vasodilation
PAF	
12-Hydroxy-eicosatetraenoic acid (12-HETE)	Activation of PMNs and increase in
Activated complement (C5a)	vascular permeability
Lysosomal enzymes (acid and neutral protease)	Tissue degradation
Platelet-derived growth factor (PDGF)	Intimal thickening

include a number of free radical species (see chapter by Bodamyali et al., this volume). Such capacity infers a potential for cells to utilise ROS/RNS as a means of rapid bactericidal or antimicrobial defence and/or to employ them as efficient signalling molecules in the communication and relay of messages. There is no doubt that aerobic cells utilise these species as a bactericidal defence system via the neutrophil "respiratory burst" during acute inflammation. In chronic and/or persistent inflammation, ROS/RNS may have an even more significant role via their signalling characteristics. Many of the following chapters of this book discuss, in detail, the pivotal role of these species in the modulation of the inflammatory response.

Almost all of these inflammatory factors, in some way, alter the activities of the others. This inter-relationship varies from a many-fold amplification to suppression of one system by another. Within these mediator-producing systems are also important moderating factors which ensure that the inflammatory response is self-limiting.

Table 3 – Mediators from other inflammatory cells

Cell type	Mediator(s)	
Mast cells/basophils	Stored:	Histamine
		Heparin
		Neutral protease
		Acid hydrolase
		Eosinophil chemotactic factor (ECF)
	Newly formed:	Phospholipids
		PAF
		Arachidonic acid (lipoxygenase
		and cyclo-oxygenase products)
Leukocytes/PMN	Myeloperoxidase	
	Lysozyme	
	Elastase	
	Cathepsins G, B and D	
	Proteolytic enzymes (degranulation) and	
	ROS (respiratory burst)	
Monocytes/macrophages	Interferons	
	Cytotoxic and cytostatic factors	
	Antigen presentation	
T lymphocytes	Interleukins (IL-2, IL-1, etc.)	
	Macrophage activating factor (MAF)	
	Chemotactic factors	
B lymphocytes	Antibody production	

Chronic, persistent inflammation – A basis for pathology

In some cases, the chronicity of an inflammatory reaction, combined with disruption of its physiological control, leads to persistent inflammation which never resolves. Several arguments exist with relevance to the persistent nature of some inflammatory conditions.

One of these theories is based on "inappropriate" triggering or persistent recruitment of the immunomodulatory cells, mainly T lymphocytes, which are believed to be responsible for the continual production of proinflammatory mediators (mainly cytokines). The role of T lymphocytes in persistent inflammation is discussed later in this volume by Lunec and Griffiths, as well as elsewhere [1].

Other arguments are based on the role of iron in persistent inflammation. We have previously reviewed the role of iron [2] as well as chronic hypoxia, hypoxia/reperfusion cycles and reactive oxygen species [3].

Inflammatory disease states – Examples

A wide range of disease states involve a persistent, non-resolving or re-occurring inflammatory component. Such diseases include rheumatoid arthritis (RA), atherosclerosis, inflammatory bowel disease (IBD) and Alzheimer's disease. Atherosclerosis causes the thickening and hardening of the arteries. Monocyte recruitment is a key event in the formation of the earliest vascular lesion, the fatty streak. Macrophage uptake of oxidatively modified LDLs gives rise to foam cells in the atheroma.

At later stages of disease more macrophage-derived foam cells are found in the lesions of the arteries and macrophages release lipids into the intima. Growth factors released by macrophages in the plaque cause proliferation of smooth muscle cells and the plaque becomes fibrotic. Recruited macrophages in atherosclerotic lesions are important in the pathophysiology of atherosclerosis. In addition to the uptake of modified LDLs via scavenger receptors, macrophages in lesions contribute to the disease process by producing free radicals, bioreactive lipids, complement components, coagulation cascade components, proteases and protease inhibitors, cytokines and chemokines. The major involvement of these mediators in the pathology of atherosclerosis points out the inflammatory reaction as the initiating event. Reactive oxygen species have been implicated in the formation of oxidised LDL and development of foam cells.

Such characteristics have also been described in rheumatoid synovitis, pointing out inflammation and reactive oxygen species as a common element in the pathology of such diseases [4]. Similarly, oxidatively modified proteins (through ROS activity) are believed to play a significant role in the pathology of Alzheimer's disease, which has been described as "arthritis of the brain". The pathology of inflammatory bowel disease (IBD) is often related to oxidative activity attributable to ROS. On this basis, several therapeutic approaches for such inflammatory conditions involve the use of antioxidants and radical scavengers ([5]; see also Edmonds, this volume).

Acknowledgements
The School of Postgraduate Medicine, University of Bath receives Programme Grant support from the Arthritis Research Campaign (ARC) for The United Kingdom. Bone and Joint Research Unit, St. Bartholomew's and The Royal London School of Medicine and Dentistry also receive support from ARC.

References

1 Panayi GS, Lanchbury JA, Kingsby GH (1992) The importance of the T cell in initiating and maintaining the chronic synovitis of rheumatoid arthritis. *Arthritis Rheum* 35: 729–735

2 Trenam CW, Winyard PG, Morris CJ, Blake DR (1992) Iron promoted oxidative damage in rheumatic diseases. In: RB Lauffer (ed): *Iron and human disease*. CRC Press, Boca Raton, 395–417

3 Bodamyali T, Stevens CR, Billingham MEJ, Ohta S, Blake DR (1998) The influence of hypoxia in inflammatory synovitis. *Ann Rheum Dis* 57: 703–710

4 Winyard PG, Tatzber F, Esterbauer H, Kus ML, Blake DR, Morris CJ (1993) Presence of foam cells containing oxidised low density lipoprotein in the synovial membrane from patients with rheumatoid arthritis. *Ann Rheum Dis* 52: 677–680

5 Halliwell B (1994) Free radicals, antioxidants, and human disease: curiosity, cause or consequence? Lancet 344: 721–724

Suggestions for further reading

JI Gallin, IM Goldstein, R Snyderman (eds): *Inflammation: Basic principles and clinical correlates*. Raven Press, 1988

GP Lewis (ed): *Mediators of inflammation*. IOP Publishing Ltd., 1986

HZ Movat: *The inflammatory reaction*. Elsevier Science Publishers, New York 1985

Reactive oxygen/nitrogen species and acute inflammation: A physiological process

Tulin Bodamyali[1], Cliff R. Stevens[1], David R. Blake[1] and Paul G. Winyard[2]

[1]School of Postgraduate Medicine, University of Bath, Claverton Down, Bath BA2 7AY, UK;
[2]Bone and Joint Research Unit, St. Bartholomew's and The Royal London School of Medicine and Dentistry, 25–29 Ashfield Street, London E1 2AD, UK

Introduction

There is an increasing body of experimental evidence implicating partially reduced forms of oxygen in a wide variety of pathological states and xenobiotic metabolism and associated toxicity. What is often dismissed, however, is the role of such species in physiology. Relatively recent evidence showing the signalling capacity of many forms of "reactive oxygen species" (ROS) has strengthened the view that they are not only associated with toxicity and pathology but have significant controlling influences in many physiological processes such as the acute inflammatory response. Recently, the biological signalling functions of nitric oxide, a "reactive nitrogen species" (RNS) have come to the fore. In this chapter, we summarise the characteristics of well known ROS and RNS, discuss the endogenous sources of such species in different environmental settings and describe how such species can bring about a physiological defence mechanism such as the acute inflammatory response.

What are reactive oxygen and nitrogen species?

Oxygen is well recognised as the major biological oxidising agent and having two electrons orbiting alone, in separate orbitals with parallel spins (spin restriction), makes it well suited for receiving electrons, one at a time, in an ordered fashion. In the respiratory pathway of aerobic organisms, the "electron transport chain" eventually adds four electrons to two oxygen molecules to make two water molecules, but the electrons are added singly. Several endogenous enzymes and enzyme systems present in aerobic cells can also catalyse this reduction by using molecular oxygen as their substrate. This sequential univalent reduction of dioxygen generates a number of ROS, which include, amongst others, superoxide, hydrogen peroxide and hydroxyl radical (see Fig. 1). A free radical may be defined as any atom or molecule which possesses one or more unpaired electrons. The term ROS encompasses both the free radicals which are formed by the reduction of oxygen, such as superoxide

Free Radicals and Inflammation, edited by P. G. Winyard, D. R. Blake and C. H. Evans
© 2000 Birkhäuser Verlag Basel/Switzerland

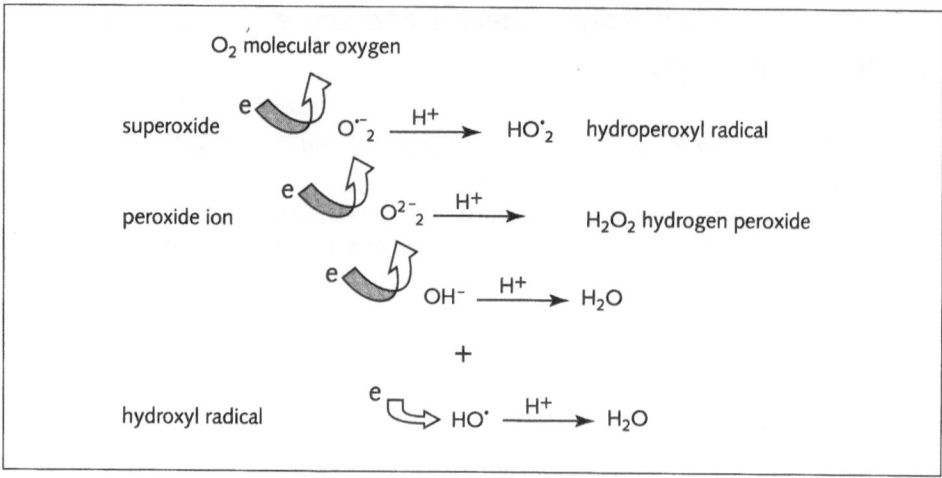

Figure 1
Univalent reduction of molecular oxygen leading to superoxide, hydrogen peroxide and hydroxyl radical formation.

and hydroxyl radical, and the related reactive species such as hydrogen peroxide which are not free radicals.

A whole range of nitrogen based reactive species also exist and specific ones are implicated in many biological processes. Such species include nitric oxide (NO$^{\bullet}$) and peroxynitrite.

Biological sources of ROS and RNS

All aerobic lifeforms use oxygen through the stepwise enzymatic reductions of the molecule, employing transition metals to overcome the spin restrictions. The sources of ROS thus generated may be a result of an accidental leakage or intentionally produced substrates for further reactions. Mitochondrial respiration is one of the main sources of ROS in normal metabolism. Apart from leakage from respiration, mitochondria generate superoxide through an NADH oxidase that may exist on the mitochondrial outer membrane. Many other sources exist which are highly relevant to the inflammatory reaction. Peroxisomal β-oxidation is also a source of hydrogen peroxide. Prostaglandins and leukotrienes are important local hormones generated by the oxidation of arachidonic acid through the cyclooxygenase or lipoxygenase pathways, respectively (see Blake et al., this volume). These pathways are both stimulated by and are sources of ROS.

Activation of granulocytes, as an integral part of an acute inflammatory reaction, leads to a sudden increase in oxygen consumption and of the hexose monophosphate shunt. More than 90% of the oxygen consumed in this "respiratory burst" is converted to superoxide through cellular NAD(P)H oxidase (see Jones and Hancock, this volume). Superoxide is converted to hydrogen peroxide that is utilised by the enzyme myeloperoxidase with the production of the highly bactericidal ROS, hypochlorous acid.

Endothelium derived relaxing factor (EDRF) is NO˙, a reactive nitrogen species, which is generated from both the constitutive and inducible forms of the enzyme nitric oxide synthase (cNOS and iNOS respectively) (see Benjamin, this volume).

Xanthine oxidase, another enzyme physiologically involved in purine and pyrimidine metabolic pathways, is also capable of generating both superoxide and hydrogen peroxide (see Harrison, this volume). Recent findings have revealed novel functions for this enzyme under hypoxic conditions, where other enzymes discussed above are functionally restricted because of limited substrate availability. This function of xanthine oxidase relates to its capacity to effectively utilise NADH as the substrate, resulting in superoxide generation. Similarly, even more recent data reveals that this enzyme is also capable of utilising endogenous nitrates and nitrites, producing nitric oxide and possibly peroxynitrite (see Blake et al. and Harrison, this volume). These characteristics present xanthine oxidase as a pivotal enzyme in inflammatory conditions where transient and chronic hypoxia is an established feature.

Role of ROS/RNS in acute inflammation

The inflammatory reaction is a very complex, but extremely orchestrated series of physiological cellular reactions designed to limit damage and initiate repair following potentially infective trauma. Increasing evidence indicates a role for ROS at virtually every stage of this physiological defence process. Historically, early interest in the role of ROS in inflammation was driven by their bactericidal properties at high concentration. However, once the initial, localised defence mechanism is activated, it appears that low levels of ROS may act as signalling molecules that initiate reparative responses leading to resolution of the inflammatory response and re-establishment of tissue integrity.

The acutely generated bacteriostatic/bactericidal environment created by the activity of ROS generating enzymes is designed to compartmentalise the inflammatory process and minimise spread systemically. In compartmentalising the inflammatory process, healthy tissue is damaged, but this has the benefit of creating a localised cavity in which a repair process can take place. In doing so, this cavity is "walled off" from surrounding healthy tissues protecting the latter from the noxious bactericidal gases. Damage and response can then occur almost simultaneously. Radical gases, such as $O_2^{\cdot-}$ and $NO^{\cdot}$, as well as hydrogen peroxide, can influence all these processes as redox-based mediators and the cellular responses to ROS are diverse (see Gilston et al.; Grisham; Okamoto and Tetsuka; Lo et al.; Evans and Stefanovic-Racic; MacPherson and Ralston; Lunec and Griffiths; Murrell; Bombeck et al., all this volume).

The initiation of an acute inflammatory response to a potentially infective trauma involves rapid vasoconstriction, leading to transient, localised hypoxia. In this setting, hypoxia, change in shear stress, the local release of bradykinin and the activation of nociceptive neuropeptide-containing nerves will all act upon endothelial cells to raise the intracellular calcium which, in turn, will activate the constitutive form of NOS to release $NO^{\cdot}$. The released $NO^{\cdot}$, acting upon local smooth muscle cells, functions as EDRF, opening the vessel and aiding the reperfusion process. The reperfusion phase will increase the local concentrations of superoxide which, in turn, will react with $NO^{\cdot}$, forming peroxynitrite and other secondary toxic bactericidal radicals including the hydroxyl radical. As well as being directly bactericidal, ROS, such as superoxide and hydrogen peroxide have been reported to show chemoattractant properties. This aids in the recruitment of phagocytic cells from the circulation, which in turn enhance bactericidal activity via the "respiratory burst".

Both recruited and resident cells, under the direct influence of the injurious insult, lose their capacity to channel electrons effectively through the mitochondrial electron transport chain in a controlled way and "leak" electrons, often termed "uncoupling" of the electron transport chain. Molecular oxygen readily accepts these electrons, leading to the generation of ROS from this oxidatively stressed, focally hypoxic, necrosing tissue. The cell population surrounding the focally necrotic area is under the influence of decreasing levels of oxidative stress. A gradient of oxidative influences therefore exists between the site of direct injury and the distant cells within the tissue. Differential and diverse cellular responses to ROS are thus observed. The nature of these responses is not only dependent on the extent of oxidative stress the cells are exposed to, but also to the intrinsic antioxidant status of different cell types. These characteristics may be the major determinants of the "sensitivity" of different cell populations within the injured tissue. The cells that show highest sensitivity to oxidant stress die by necrosis. In the cell populations which are more resistant to oxidative stress, the responses are controlled by the activation of specific genes and transcription factors (see Gilston et al., this volume) that aid in the repair and resolution of injury. The role of radicals in modulating gene transcription, particularly in relation to inflammatory cytokine production, adhesion molecule expression (see Grisham et al., this volume), matrix metalloproteinase expression (see Lo et al., this volume) and apoptosis (see Bombeck et al., this volume) is discussed in detail later. The redox-regulated protein, thioredoxin, appears to play a critical part in many of these processes (see Okamoto and Tetsuka, this volume).

Antioxidant systems

High reactivity and thus potential toxicity of ROS are controlled by an extensive range of antioxidant systems intrinsic to aerobic cells. The spontaneous dismutation reaction rate of superoxide is greatly enhanced by superoxide dismutase (SOD), yielding hydrogen peroxide and molecular oxygen. The hydrogen peroxide is broken down by catalase, resulting in the formation of water and oxygen.

Superoxide dismutase:

$$O_2^{\cdot-} + O_2^{\cdot-} \xrightarrow{2\,H^+} H_2O_2 + O_2$$

Catalase:

$$H_2O_2 + H_2O_2 \longrightarrow 2\,H_2O + O_2$$

A third enzymic system, glutathione peroxidase, coupled with reduced glutathione, removes hydrogen peroxide. This line of defence therefore, relies heavily on the availability of GSH. Thus all systems involved in the reduction of GSSG are essential, including NADPH formation, GSSG reductase and GSSG transport from the cell. Total thiol status of the cell, for this reason, is an important modulator of its redox status, since it dictates the net effects of ROS on cellular biomolecules.

Glutathione peroxidases:
$$ROOH + 2\,GSH \longrightarrow ROH + GSSG + H_2O$$

Additional to these enzymic systems, non-enzymic antioxidant systems also exist. These include α-tocopherol (vitamin E), ascorbate (vitamin C) and urate as direct scavengers and chain breaking antioxidants.

$$RO^{\cdot}O + VitE\text{-}OH \longrightarrow ROOH + VitE\text{-}^{\cdot}O$$
$$VitE\text{-}^{\cdot}O + VitC\text{-}H \longrightarrow VitE\text{-}OH + VitC^{\cdot-}$$
$$VitC^{\cdot-} + 2H^+ \longrightarrow VitC\text{-}H + DHA$$

The product of the reaction between α-tocopherol (VitE-OH) and lipid peroxyl radicals (ROO$^{\cdot}$), itself a less reactive radical (VitE-O$^{\cdot}$), is removed by its reaction with ascorbic acid and formation of dehydroascorbic acid (DHA).

It has also been proposed that radicals directly react with oxygen in a cyclic manner to yield superoxide or with GSH to generate superoxide and GSSG. On this basis, it is argued that in the absence of SOD, superoxide would continue to cycle with GSH to yield hydrogen peroxide and GSSG. It follows that the removal of superoxide from the cycle by SOD would reduce the production of hydrogen peroxide and GSSG and thus only one enzyme would be necessary to remove a whole range of ROS. In support of this, it has been relatively recently discovered that endothelial cells, a cell type most exposed to extracellular pO_2 changes, possess a form of SOD, extracellular SOD (EC-SOD), on their surface.

In addition to these antioxidant/scavenger systems, storage and transport proteins limit the availability of catalytic transition metals, which facilitate generation of hydroxyl radicals (see Kaur and Halliwell, this volume). Copper is stored and transported by caeruloplasmin. Similarly, iron is transported by transferrin and stored by the intracellular protein ferritin.

It appears that ROS-generating capacity is a universal cellular phenomenon which provides aerobic cells with the armamentarium to combat extracellular changes. Thus, so long as homeostasis between the rate of ROS generation and their dissipation is maintained, cellular ROS production is not damaging. However, a significant increase in ROS generation or a decrease in cellular antioxidant/scavenger defences will disrupt this balance, resulting in a state of oxidative stress (see Blake et al., this volume). The cumulative effects of such ROS-initiated events may be either immediate, resulting in cytotoxicity and tissue necrosis, or subtle and delayed resulting in more chronic disorders, such as rheumatoid arthritis.

Acknowledgements

The School of Postgraduate Medicine, University of Bath receives Programme Grant support from the Arthritis Research Campaign (ARC) for The United Kingdom. Bone and Joint Research Unit, St. Bartholomew's and The Royal London School of Medicine and Dentistry also receive support from ARC.

General references

Sies H (ed) (1997) *Antioxidants in disease mechanisms and therapy*, Advances in pharmacology, vol. 38. Academic Press, San Diego

Halliwell B, Gutteridge JMC (1999) Free radicals in biology and medicine, 3rd ed, Clarendon Press, Oxford

Sahinoglu T, Stevens CR, Blake DR (1995) The joint, a redox sensitive microenvironment? An hypothesis. *Scand J Rheumatol* 24 (Suppl 101): 131–136

Bodamyali T, Stevens CR, Billingham MEJ, Ohta S, Blake DR (1998) Influence of hypoxia in inflammatory synovitis. *Ann Rheum Dis* 57: 703–710

Free radicals and pathology: current concepts

David R. Blake[1], Tulin Bodamyali[1], Cliff R. Stevens[1] and Paul G. Winyard[2]

[1]School of Postgraduate Medicine, University of Bath, Claverton Down, Bath BA2 7AY, UK;
[2]Bone and Joint Research Unit, St. Bartholomew's and The Royal London School of Medicine and Dentistry, 25–29 Ashfield Street, London E1 2AD, UK

Historically, free radicals, by virtue of their high reactivity, have been extensively studied and described in chemical reactions. Initial descriptions of free radical-mediated "bacterial killing" by Babior led way to a "biological era of radical chemistry" [1].

Over the years, better understanding of free radical interactions within biological systems facilitated a progressive move towards recognition of radicals as intrinsic defence systems.

Relatively recent evidence identified free radicals, specifically reactive oxygen and nitrogen species (ROS and RNS) with free radical characteristics, as signalling molecules. Such species are now widely recognised as physiological intra-/extracellular mediators of an entire spectrum of cellular responses (see Gilston et al.; Grisham; Okamoto and Tetsuka; Lo et al.; Evans and Stefanovic-Racic; MacPherson and Ralston; Lunec and Griffiths; Murrell; Bombeck et al., all this volume).

We now understand that the microenvironment within which radical generation occurs dictates the outcome of radical-mediated responses.

We discuss the pathological condition "familial amyotrophic lateral sclerosis" (ALS), in order to emphasise the significance of uncoupling of this oxidant/antioxidant balance within the tissue microenvironment. It is now established that the pathology associated with this condition is strongly linked with a single amino acid mutation in the gene for the antioxidant Cu/Zn superoxide dismutase (SOD). Although this mutation does not appear to affect the dismutase activity of SOD, it is observed to alter the peroxidase activity of the enzyme, enhancing an unknown toxic reaction that leads to the selective degeneration of motor neurones. This toxicity is believed to be associated with enhanced catalysis of protein nitration. Two possible mechanisms have been put forward for this enhanced protein nitration. One argument is the catalysis of the nitration of tyrosines by imperfectly folded mutant SOD [2]. The alternative proposal involves nitration through the use of peroxynitrite or from peroxidation arising from elevated production of hydroxyl radicals through use of hydrogen peroxide as a substrate [3]. It appears therefore that the interaction of ROS and RNS within a compartmentalised tissue microenvironment may play a significant role in the pathology of ALS.

We argue that the pathology observed in synovitis parallels the situation described above in that it also displays another example of a microenvironment where the oxidant/antioxidant balance is compromised and ROS play a significant role ([4]; see also Edmonds, this volume). We have reviewed the evidence that the inflamed rheumatoid synovium is chronically hypoxic and that movement simulates intermittent hypoxia/reperfusion cycles [5]. During hypoxia, a complex series of events contribute to the creation of an environment where a functional compartmentalisation of the sub-synovium and the "invasive" surface lining, or pannus, occurs. Due to the differential vascular distribution of these two compartments, it seems likely that sub-synovium is more prone to oxidative influences during reperfusion of the joint, leading to the persistence of the inflammatory reaction. In contrast, hypoxia-driven events play a greater role in the development of the pathology involving the pannus tissue, which abuts bare bone. This functional compartmentalisation due to chronic hypoxia with intermittent cycles of hypoxia/reperfusion leads to the creation of a microenvironment where uncoupling of the redox balance (oxidant stress) occurs.

Our earlier observations of lack of measurable SOD within inflamed joints were thought to underlie the observed effects of ROS and the associated oxidant stress. Reports on the presence of an extracellular-SOD (EC-SOD) bound to endothelial cell surface glycosaminoglycans [6] altered the way we perceived the characteristics of the inflamed synovial microenvironment. Subsequent findings revealed that the ROS-generating enzyme xanthine oxidase also has high affinity for surface GAGs such as heparan sulphate. In addition, we have recently discovered that xanthine oxidase, in a hypoxic microenvironment is capable of generating nitric oxide from inorganic nitrates and nitrites [7, 8].

These observations predict that ROS and RNS generated via XO activity within the hypoxic microenvironment of inflamed synovium may play a significant role in the pathology observed. In support of this, we have previously shown that *ex vivo* simulated hypoxia/reperfusion results in the generation of ESR-detectable ROS, which were inhibited by XO inhibitors [9]. We and others (see Evans and Stefanovic-Racic, this volume) have also reported enhanced nitrite levels in rheumatoid synovial fluid [10], indicating the availability of substrates for NO˙ generation via XO under hypoxia. Furthermore, analysis of inflamed synovial fluid [11] revealed enhanced nitration of tyrosine residues (nitrotyrosine formation), indicating ROS and RNS influences via peroxynitrite formation (see also Evans and Stefanovic-Racic, this volume). Our current studies are designed to ascertain the extent of XO involvement in these events.

In conclusion, redox homeostasis (oxidant/antioxidant balance) is well maintained physiologically. Uncoupling of this balance due to alterations within the microenvironment, we believe, is the underlying basis for pathology.

Acknowledgements

The School of Postgraduate Medicine, University of Bath receives Programme Grant support from the Arthritis Research Campaign (ARC) for The United Kingdom. Bone and Joint Research Unit, St. Bartholomew's and The Royal London School of Medicine and Dentistry also receive support from ARC.

References

1   Babior BM (1978) Oxygen dependent microbial killing by phagocytes (in two parts). *N Engl J Med* 298: 659–668, 721–725

2   Beckman JS, Caeson M, Smith CD, Koppenol WH (1993) *Nature* 364: 584

3   Wiedau-Pazos M, Goto JJ, Rabizadeh S, Gralla ED, Roe JA, Valentine JS, Bredesen DE (1996) *Science* 271: 515–518

4   Sahinoglu T, Stevens CR, Blake DR (1995) The joint, a redox sensitive microenvironment? An hypothesis. *Scand J Rheum* 24 (Suppl 101): 131–136

5   Bodamyali T, Stevens CR, Billingham MEJ, Ohta S, Blake DR (1998) Influence of hypoxia in inflammatory synovitis. *Ann Rheum Dis* 57: 703–710

6   Karlsson K, Marklund SL (1988) Extracellular superoxide dismutase in the vascular system of mammals. *Biochem J* 255: 223–228

7   Millar TM, Stevens CR, Benjamin N, Eisenthal R, Harrison R, Blake DR (1998) Xanthine oxidoreductase catalyses the reduction of nitrates and nitrite to nitric oxide under hypoxic conditions. *FEBS Lett* 427: 225–228

8   Zhang Z, Naughton D, Winyard PG, Benjamin N, Blake DR, Symons MCR (1998) Generation of nitric oxide by a nitrite reductase activity of xanthine oxidase: a potential pathway for nitric oxide formation in the absence of nitric oxide synthase activity. *Biochem Biophys Res Comm* 249: 767–772

9   Singh D, Nazhat NB, Fairburn K, Sahinoglu T, Blake DR, Jones P (1995) Electron spin resonance spectroscopic demonstration of the generation of reactive oxygen species by diseased human synovial tissue following *ex vivo* hypoxia reoxygenation. *Ann Rheum Dis* 54: 94–99

10 Farrell AJ, Blake DR, Palmer RM, Moncada S (1992) Increased concentrations of nitrite in synovial fluid and serum samples suggest increased nitric oxide synthesis in rheumatic diseases. *Ann Rheum Dis* 51: 1219–1222

11 Kaur H, Halliwell B (1994) Evidence for nitric oxide-mediated oxidative damage in chronic inflammation.Nitrotyrosine in serum and synovial fluid from rheumatoid patients. *FEBS Lett* 350: 9–12

The NADPH oxidase of neutrophils and other cells

Owen T.G. Jones[1] and John T. Hancock[2]

[1]Department of Biochemistry, University of Bristol, School of Medical Sciences, University Walk, Bristol, BS8 1TD, UK; [2]Department of Biological and Biomedical Sciences, University of the West of England, Coldharbour Lane, Bristol, BS16 1QY, UK

Introduction

Neutrophils and other "professional" phagocytes (including monocytes, macrophages and eosinophils) have an important role in the response of the immune system to microbial infections. They are attracted to infection sites by chemoattractants secreted by the excited cells of the immune system, by tissue cells such as endothelial cells and fibroblasts, and by peptides derived from disrupted bacteria. Complement activation generates fragment C5a which is an important attractant for phagocytes. There are receptors on the neutrophil plasma membrane for these attractants and activation of the receptors initiates a complex series of events which prepare the neutrophil for its cytocidal role [1]. The primed neutrophils move to the target opsonised microbes, phagocytose, kill and digest them. The killing process involves the release of an array of granule proteins into the developing phagosome as the neutrophil degranulates and the activation of a plasma membrane NADPH oxidase which forms superoxide radicals and directs these into the phagocytic vacuole. Superoxide is unstable and reactive and is the progenitor of a family of reactive oxygen species (ROS). These are themselves microbicidal and can also act in concert with the granule-derived proteins to increase their cytotoxicity. The importance of the production of superoxide by NADPH oxidase is clearly demonstrated in the rare genetic condition of chronic granulomatous disease (CGD). The patients with this defect have neutrophils lacking in NADPH oxidase which are unable to form superoxide, with the consequence that the patients suffer chronic infections because they are unable to mount an effective attack on the pathogen.

It is possible for the NADPH oxidase to be activated in circumstances which lead to damage to the host tissues. Neutrophil-generated reactive oxygen species have been reported to cause damage in a number of inflammatory diseases, such as rheumatoid arthritis, adult respiratory distress syndrome, emphysema and nephritis and ischaemia-reperfusion injury [2]. This chapter will describe the properties of this oxidase and its activation and will discuss the superoxide generating processes of other cell types.

Free Radicals and Inflammation, edited by P. G. Winyard, D. R. Blake and C. H. Evans
© 2000 Birkhäuser Verlag Basel/Switzerland

Components of NADPH oxidase

It was noted in 1933 that as neutrophils phagocytosed there was a great increase in their oxygen consumption [3]. This respiratory burst was not inhibited by cyanide and was later found to be due to the activity of a plasma membrane NADPH oxidase which converted all the additional oxygen of the respiratory burst to superoxide. This oxidase catalyses the following reaction:

$$NADPH + 2\ O_2 \longrightarrow 2\ O_2^{\cdot-} + NADP^+ + H^+$$

The NADPH consumed by the oxidase is replaced by the activity of the neutrophil pentose phosphate pathway [4].

The superoxide produced by the oxidase undergoes a series of reactions many of which have products that are potentially damaging to cellular components. These products are called reactive oxygen species (ROS). Examples of such reactions are shown below:

$$O_2^{\cdot-} + O_2^{\cdot-} + 2\ H^+ \longrightarrow O_2 + H_2O_2 \text{ (hydrogen peroxide)}$$
$$H_2O_2 + O_2^{\cdot-} \longrightarrow O_2 + OH^- + OH^{\cdot} \text{ (hydroxyl radical)}$$

This latter reaction, yielding the highly reactive $OH^{\cdot}$, is catalysed by iron (Fe^{3+}) in the well known Fenton reaction.

The granules of neutrophils contain an abundance of the enzyme myeloperoxidase which catalyses the production of another cytotoxic oxidant, the hypochlorite ion:

$$H_2O_2 + Cl^- \longrightarrow H_2O + OCl^- \text{ (hypochlorite)}$$

Since the NADPH oxidase initiates the release of such an array of reactive oxygen species, capable of damaging the host tissues as well as the target microbe, it is important that the activity of the oxidase is carefully controlled. It is a well regulated enzyme complex assembled from components derived from both the cytosol and the membrane. These components are brought together only when the resting neutrophil is stimulated by interaction with a microbe or some other stimulus. The cytosolic components translocate to the membrane and form the active complex. A scheme which represents this process is shown in Figure 1. The properties of the components are discussed below.

Cytochrome b$_{558}$

This cytochrome catalyses the electron transfer activities of the oxidase. It can be clearly seen in oxidised-minus-reduced spectra of neutrophils [5]. This cytochrome

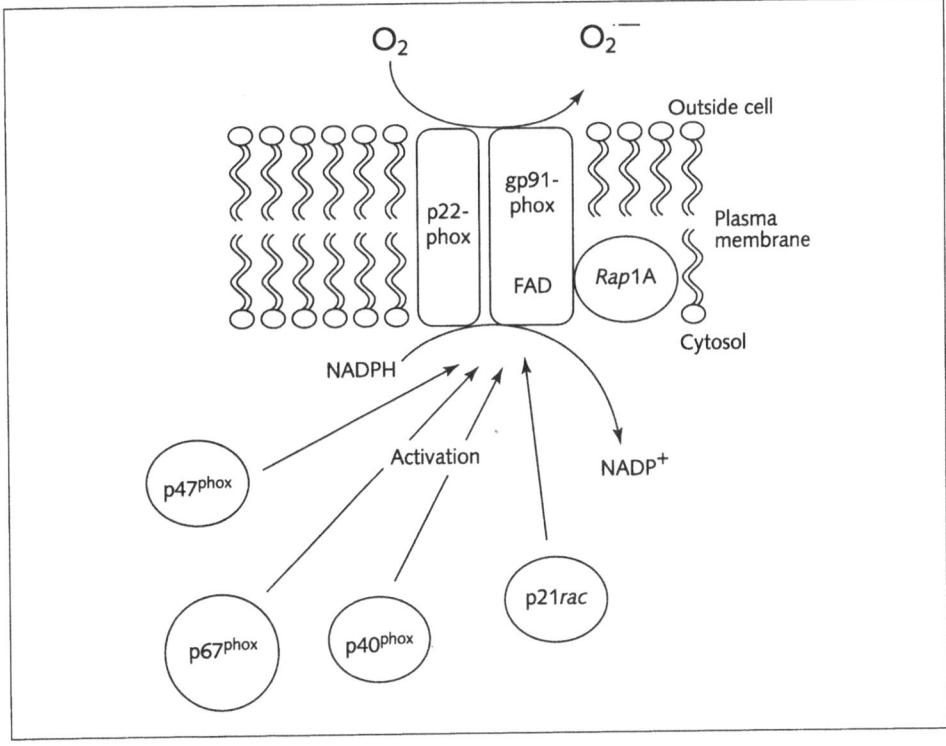

Figure 1
A schematic representation of the components of the NADPH oxidase of neutrophils and of the translocation of cytosolic factors to the plasma membrane components. Electron transfer from NADPH to oxygen through the flavocytochrome dimer does not occur until the cytosolic factors have docked on the membrane.

was absent from neutrophils of patients with the X-linked form of CGD [6] (with some very few exceptions discussed later) and was present in diminished amounts in neutrophils from the maternal carriers. This genetic information was very important in helping to understand the mechanism of the oxidase. CGD, although rare, continues to provide information about the nature of NADPH oxidase and its regulation. The mid-point oxidation-reduction potential for this cytochrome was reported to be unusually low at -245 mV [7], which is important if it is involved in the rapid transfer of electrons to the $O_2/O_2^{\cdot-}$ couple, which has an $E_{m,7.0} = -160$ mV. This picture, of a simple cytochrome b with a single haem prosthetic group involved in transfer of electrons to O_2, has been altered by the observation of a case of X-linked CGD where cytochrome b was present but with an Arg/Ser mutation in its sequence. Two haem groups could be resolved with differing mid-point potentials of

–220 mV and –300 mV[8]. Re-examination of redox data from normal neutrophils showed that there were two haems present with close but different mid-points of –225 mV and –265 mV. The presence of two haem groups has significance in considering mechanisms for the oxidase and the orientation of the cytochrome in the membrane.

Cytochrome b_{558} is believed to have its protohaem prosthetic group(s) in the low spin hexacoordinate state with bis axial histidine ligands[9]. This requires ligand displacement if the haem iron is to transfer electrons to oxygen by an inner sphere mechanism and there is some evidence from CO-binding studies that such a mechanism is possible. Alternatively, electrons could be passed to O_2 from the edge of the haem plane.

Purification of the cytochrome showed that it was a dimer with a large 91 kDa subunit which is extensively glycosylated [10, 11] and is often called gp91[phox] (from phagocyte oxidase) together with a smaller subunit of 22 kDa called p22[phox]. The stoichiometry of the subunits is slightly uncertain but is likely to be 1:1 [12]. The gene for gp91[phox] is located on the X chromosome and is missing or defective in X-linked CGD. The gene for p22[phox] is located quite separately on chromosome 16 [13]. The presence of both subunits is necessary for the stable expression of the protein of either subunit [14]. Neutrophils from CGD patients lacking gp91[phox] do not express the protein p22[phox], similarly patients lacking the p22[phox] subunit do not express the protein gp91[phox]. The cytochrome is distributed between the plasma membrane (about 10–20%) and the specific granule membranes (80–90%) in resting neutrophils [5].

Another protein, rap1A, is closely associated [15, 16] with the cytochrome b. This 22 kDa GTP-binding protein may have a role in modulating the activity of the oxidase (see later).

The full sequences of both subunits of the cytochrome are known and have been used in constructing hydropathy plots which show that the 570 residue gp91[phox] has six potential membrane spanning regions and that the 195 amino acid residue p22[phox] has two such regions [17, 18] (Fig. 2) These membrane spanning regions may have a functional role in haem binding or the formation of proton conducting channels (see below). The sequence of gp91[phox] showed that it had regions of homology with the NADPH-binding region of the flavin nucleotide reductase (FNR) family of oxidoreductases [19, 20]. There was also homology with the FAD-binding region of these enzymes. The concentration of FAD in the plasma membrane of neutrophils from X-linked CGD patients is diminished which also indicates an association of FAD with the cytochrome and suggests that cytochrome b_{558} is a flavocytochrome, like the closely related ferric reductase of yeast. Of particular note is the presence in ferric reductase (FRE I) of a haem binding motif which has two haem groups coordinated to four histidines located in two helices, predicted to span the membrane. Each helix has two histidines located 12–14 residues apart. In each helix one histidine would lie towards the inner face and the other to the outer face of the

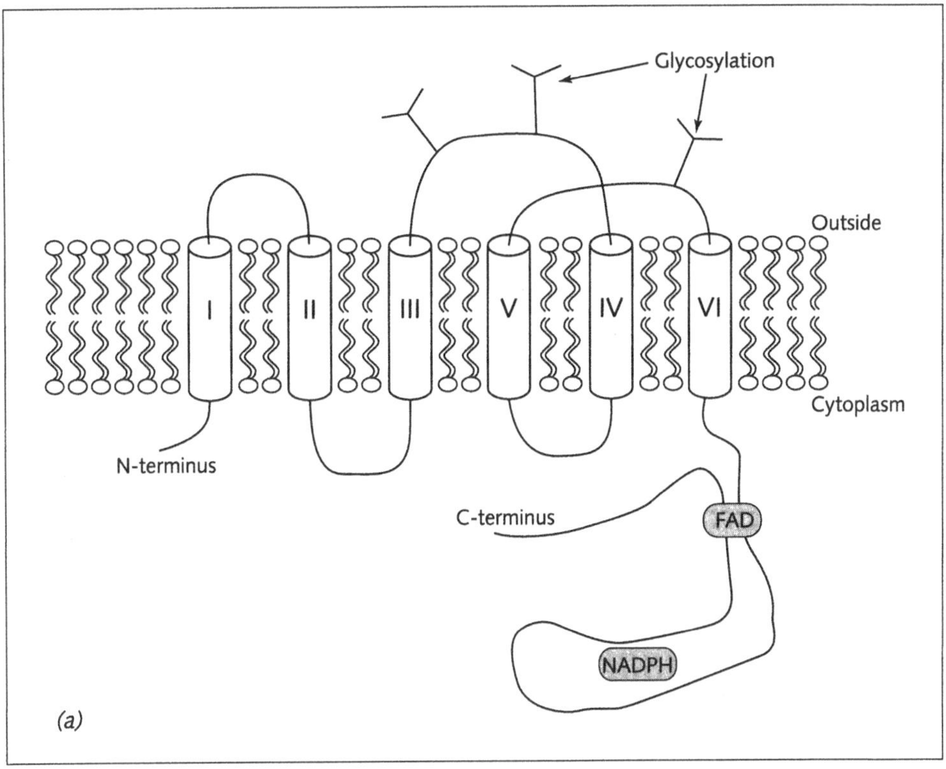

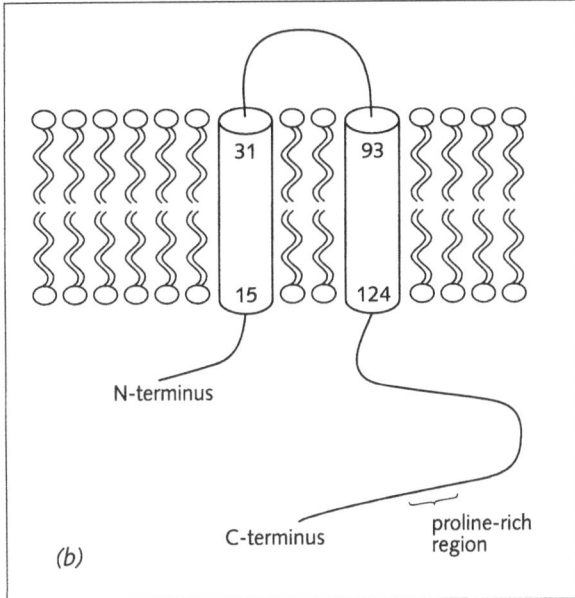

(a)

(b)

Figure 2
Representation of the predicted membrane spanning regions of gp91phox (a) and p22phox (b). The likely NADPH and FAD binding sites are indicated [20], together with the proline-rich region of p22phox.

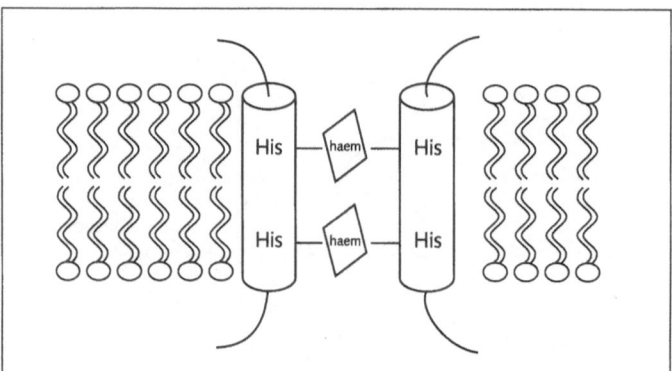

Figure 3
Possible haem-binding region of gp91^phox. Redrawn from [22].

membrane bilayer with the haems coordinated between the two helices [21, 22] (Fig. 3). Very similar organisation can be predicted for a haem binding region in gp91^phox, which has a group of four conserved histidines appropriately located in two of the predicted membrane spanning helical regions (Fig. 2). Loss of His101, His209, or His222 leads to CGD, loss of the characteristic cytochrome spectrum and instability of the protein [23]. A representation of the structures of gp91^phox and p22^phox is given in Figure 2, which also illustrates the proposed cytosolic loops of these proteins which are so important in the activation of the oxidase. An alternative view, that one haem is associated with p22^phox is rather less persuasive. Of its two potential coordinating histidines, only one is invariant, the other being polymorphic [24], and a model would require that one haem was located in gp91^phox and one haem was suspended between the two subunits. Attempts to clarify the issue by looking at the distribution of haem in purified subunits do not yield compelling results because the detergents used in solubilising the membrane proteins tend to decrease the affinity of the haem for its usual ligands. The same problem has prevented the purification of a gp91^phox subunit with FAD bound to it and so the most convincing evidence that it is a bis-haem flavocytochrome remains that of comparison with the FNR proteins and with FRE1. Affinity labelling with FAD analogues supports this association of FAD with gp91^phox and so does the appearance of CGD in patients where there are mutations in the putative binding sites for FAD [23, 25].

It is likely that the prosthetic groups of gp91^phox are sufficient to catalyse the electron transfer function of NADPH oxidase, as shown below:

$$NADPH \xrightarrow{e} FAD \xrightarrow{e} haem1 \xrightarrow{e} haem2 \xrightarrow{e} O_2/O_2^{\cdot -}$$

The bis-haem motif is found in cytochromes of the b-type which are involved in the transfer of electrons from the inner face of membranes to the outer face, as in the $b/c1$ complexes of mitochondria, chloroplasts and microbes. Such vectorial movement of electrons is a necessary feature of the function of NADPH oxidase.

Cytosolic factors and activation of NADPH oxidase

Soon after the observation that cytochrome b was absent from the neutrophils of patients with X-linked CGD, other groups of patients were found where CGD was present and the cytochrome was also present. It was found that neutrophils from such patients had defects in the system of activation of the oxidase [26]. Analysis of the defects has been very informative in understanding the complex processes required for activation. A number of proteins necessary for normal function has been identified and fully characterised and their properties are described below. Another fruitful approach to identifying proteins required for oxidase activation has involved the reconstitution of an active oxidase from purified cytosolic proteins or from recombinant cytosolic proteins, together with the membrane components of the oxidase, also purified or recombinant [27, 28]. The key to the *in vitro* reconstitution was the finding that it required not only the protein components but also an anionic amphiphile such as arachidonic acid (or SDS) together with GTP (or GTP-γ-S). The properties of these cytosolic factors and their interactions is described below. Although these are becoming clear, their role in facilitating the electron transfer activity of NADPH oxidase is still somewhat speculative.

p47phox

This was the first of the cytosolic factors to be identified. Neutrophils from patients with an autosomal form of CGD were compared with normal neutrophils after addition of an oxidase stimulus given in the presence of radioactive phosphate. A protein of about Mr 44 kDa was heavily phosphorylated in SDS gels of extracts of control cells but was absent from the CGD cells [29]. This defect has turned out to be the most common failure in the autosomal recessive form of CGD. The protein has been purified and cloned. It is 390 amino acids long and contains multiple serine and threonine phosphorylation sites in the carboxy-terminal region. These become progressively phosphorylated when the neutrophil is activated by the addition of phorbol myristate acetate (PMA), a good activator of the respiratory burst and of the enzyme protein kinase C (PKC). Following activation p47phox translocates to the plasma membrane where it binds tightly. Inhibition of PKC by the addition of staurosporine decreases the activation by PMA, inhibits phosphorylation of p47phox and its translocation to the membrane [30, 31]. Three of the cytosolic factors to be discussed here, including p47[phox], contain Src homology 3 (SH3) domains which are involved in protein-protein interactions by binding to proline-rich regions of proteins. There are two such domains in p47[phox]. These interactions are very important in stabilising cytosolic factors in the resting state and in their association with the membrane in the activated state. Proline-rich regions are found on the cytosolic factors and on the C-terminal [32] region of the cytosolic domain of p22[phox]. A representation of these domains and their interactions [33] is given in Figure 4.

p67[phox]

This cytosolic factor was identified using antibodies raised against partly purified neutrophil cytosol. It was found to be absent from neutrophils of patients with a relatively rare form of autosomal recessive CGD [34]. The p67[phox] cDNA codes for a protein with 526 amino acids with a calculated molecular mass of 60,900 Da, less than the value of 67 kDa derived from SDS-PAGE. It contains two SH3 domains and two possible proline-rich regions [33] (Fig. 4).

p40[phox]

When p67[phox] was purified by gel filtration from neutrophil cytosol it was accompanied by a protein, p40phox, which has high homology [33, 35] with the N-terminal regions of p47[phox]. It contains 339 amino acids and has one SH3 domain. There are no reports of a CGD with defective p40[phox] but its concentration is diminished in the cytosol of neutrophils from CGD patients lacking p67[phox].

p21[rac]

A low molecular weight GTP-binding protein, p21[rac2], is found to be essential for the NADPH oxidase activity of human neutrophils [36, 37]. It was isolated as a tight complex with a guanine-nucleotide exchange factor called *rho*GDI (guanine nucleotide exchange inhibitor) which serves to maintain p21[rac2] in a GDP-bound form [38]. There is a hydrophobic region on *rho*GDI, which binds tightly to an isoprenyl residue [39] on p21[rac]. The dissociation of the *rho*GDI/p21[rac] complex is catalysed by GDS, a GDP dissociation stimulator protein [40]. The released p21[rac] is likely to be converted to the GTP bound form, which is the active form. The dissociation of the *rho*GDI/p21[rac] may follow activation of neutrophil receptors by interaction with target microbes, an event which leads to the release of arachidonate and other active lipids. In human macrophages p21[rac1] is found in place of p21[rac2]. These two species are highly homologous.

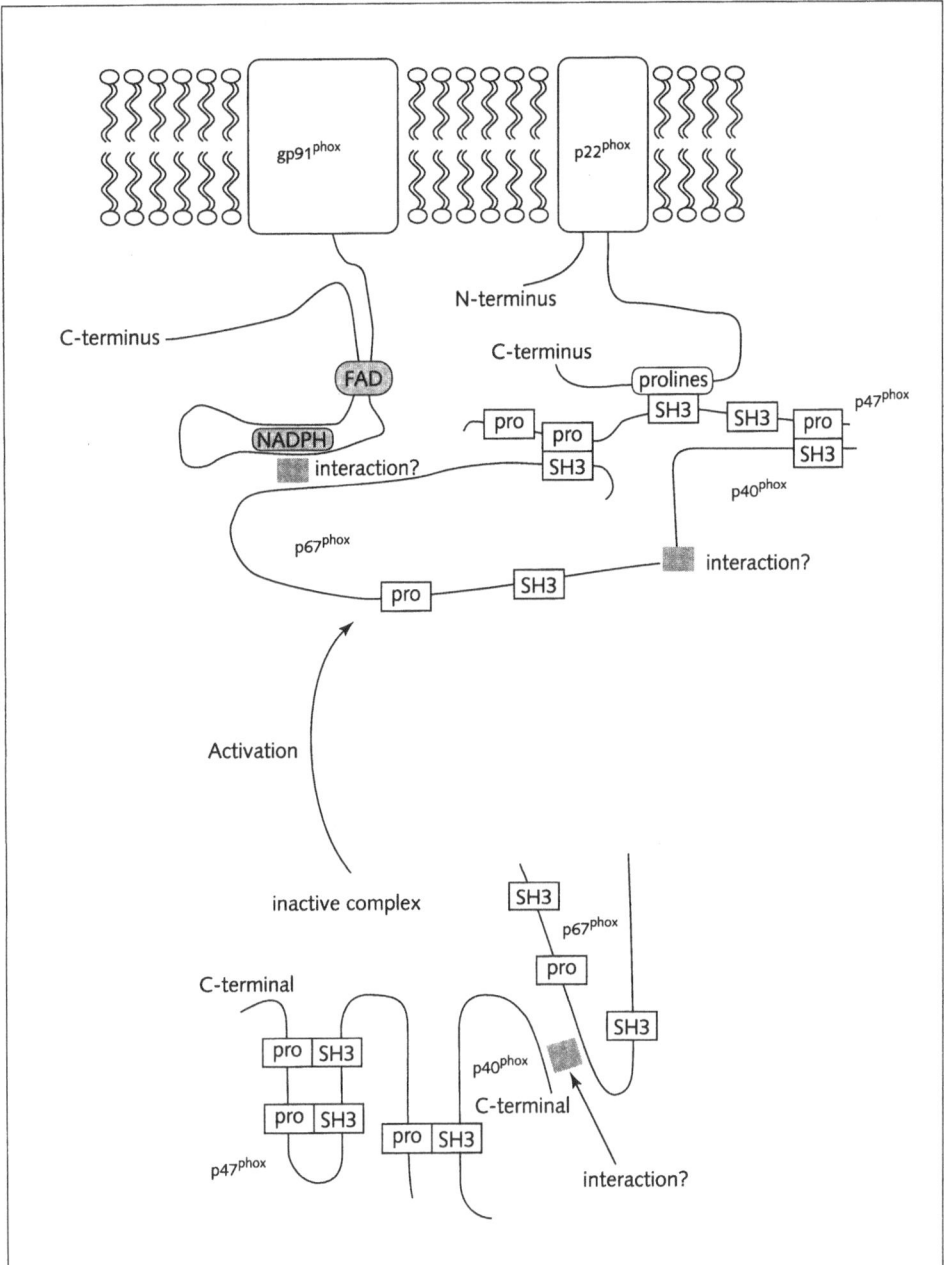

Figure 4
Activation of NADPH oxidase: representation of possible interactions between cytosolic fac-
tors before and after activation. Modified from [33].

Complexes of cytosolic factors

The factors p47^{phox}, p67^{phox}, and p40^{phox} contain SH3 domains, and p47^{phox} and p67^{phox} contain proline-rich regions with a high affinity for SH3 domains. In the unstimulated neutrophil cytosol, these interactions may be involved in stabilising a complex of about 240 kDa which contains these cytosolic factors [41]. The suggested sites of interactions are shown in Figure 4, which summarizes a variety of experimental work. The two SH3 domains of p47^{phox} are internally masked by binding to the two proline-rich regions in its C-terminus, but its third proline-rich region is available to bind to SH3 domains from p40^{phox} or p67^{phox}. Use of the yeast two-hybrid system strongly suggests that p40^{phox} SH3 domain interacts with p47^{phox} proline-rich region residues 360–367 [42]. The association of p40^{phox} with p67^{phox} may not require the intervention of SH3 domains but involve interaction of the charged group at the carboxy terminus of p40^{phox}.

The mechanism of activation of the oxidase complex is not completely defined. The phosphorylation of p47^{phox} by protein kinase could lead to the disruption of the internal bonds between SH3 domains and proline-rich regions of p47^{phox} and the same effect can be produced *in vitro* by arachidonate or SDS [43]. The exposed SH3 domains are now free to bind to proline-rich regions of p22^{phox}. This interaction is obviously crucial because in CGD cells lacking p47^{phox} no binding of p67^{phox} to the plasma membrane occurs on stimulation, whereas in CGD cells lacking p67^{phox}, p47^{phox} is still translocated to the membrane and binds there [44]. The GTP-binding protein p21^{rac} also translocates to the membrane, requires cytochrome b$_{558}$ as a docking site, but is independent [45,46] of the translocation of p47^{phox} and p67^{phox}, although there is evidence for the association of p21^{rac} and the N-terminal regions of p67^{phox} *in vitro* to form a 1:1 complex. Mutation in the 26–45 amino acid sequence region of p21^{rac} diminished the binding of p21^{rac} to p67^{phox}. This region resembles the effector region of *Ras* which is involved in GTP-dependent binding to the *Ras* effector *Raf*1 [47].

The function of p40^{phox} is unclear. In the *in vitro* cell free system of activation its addition does not stimulate activity and there is speculation that it is primarily concerned with the down regulation of the activated oxidase. It can bind to p47^{phox}, and recombinant p40^{phox} inhibits *in vitro* reconstitution activity. Transfection of K562 cells with p40^{phox} lowered the whole cell oxidase activity [48]. Isolated SH3 domains from p40^{phox} were even more effective inhibitors but deletion of its C-terminal region which binds to p67^{phox}, did not relieve the inhibitory effect of p40^{phox} upon oxidase activation, suggesting that the binding of p40^{phox} to p47^{phox}, but not to p67^{phox} is most important in down-regulation of the oxidase.

There are a number of informative CGD patients with single point mutations in the proposed NADPH binding region of the cytosolic C-terminus of gp91^{phox}. In neutrophils from these patients, binding of p67^{phox} to gp91^{phox} is perturbed, and it is possible that binding of p67^{phox} to this protein loop, in close proximity to the NADPH and flavin binding site, could regulate electron transfer activity in the oxidase.

The role of *rap*1A

This small (22 kDa) GTP-binding protein co-purifies with cytochrome b_{558} as a 1:1 complex, although its function is unclear. Like p40^{phox}, it may be concerned with down-regulation of the oxidase. *Rap*1A is not required for the *in vitro* reconstitution of oxidase activity in a cell-free system. Transfection and over-expression of GDP-bound or GTP-bound forms of *rap*1A in B lymphocytes or differentiated (neutrophil-like) HL-60 cells diminished NADPH oxidase activity [50]. GDP bound *rap*1A does not associate with cytochrome b_{558} unlike the GTP-bound form. It is phosphorylated by PKA, leading to loss of interaction with cytochrome b_{558}.

Activation of NADPH oxidase

Human neutrophils respond to a variety of soluble and particulate stimuli by assembling the active oxidase from its cytosolic and membrane components and then generating superoxide by transferring electrons from cytosolic NADPH to dissolved oxygen. Physiological stimuli relate to the function of this microbial oxidase. Such receptor-dependent stimuli include peptides derived from the breakdown of bacterial proteins, which contain N-formyl methionine at the N-terminus, complement fragment C5a, and immune complexes which attach to receptors via their Fc portions. Other receptor-dependent stimuli include cytokines IL-8 and TNFα and leukotriene B4. Non-receptor dependent (and non-physiological) stimuli include phorbol myristate acetate (PMA), an activator of protein kinase C, calcium ionophores, arachidonic acid and other long-chain unsaturated fatty acids. Receptor-independent stimuli tend to persist in their effects for long periods whilst the receptor-dependent stimuli last only 3 or 4 min, as if the receptor is effectively down-regulated. Most of the receptors involved are linked via G proteins to phospholipase C. Phospholipase C attacks phosphatidylinositol bis-phosphate in the membrane with the release of inositol 1,4,5-trisphosphate (IP$_3$) and diacylglycerol (DAG). The concentration of these rises fast in the cytosol of neutrophils stimulated with agonists such as FMLP. IP$_3$ promotes the release of Ca^{2+} from intracellular stores, which acts with DAG to activate protein kinase C (PKC) (Fig. 5). PKC in turn phosphorylates serine residues on p47^{phox} and perhaps other proteins of the oxidase complex. Phosphorylation of p47^{phox} in the region of residues 300 to 380 seems to be a key step in the activation process, with a specific requirement for serine 379 being found in experiments examining the activation of EBV-transformed B lymphocytes (EBVL) by transfection with a mutant gene lacking serine at this posi-

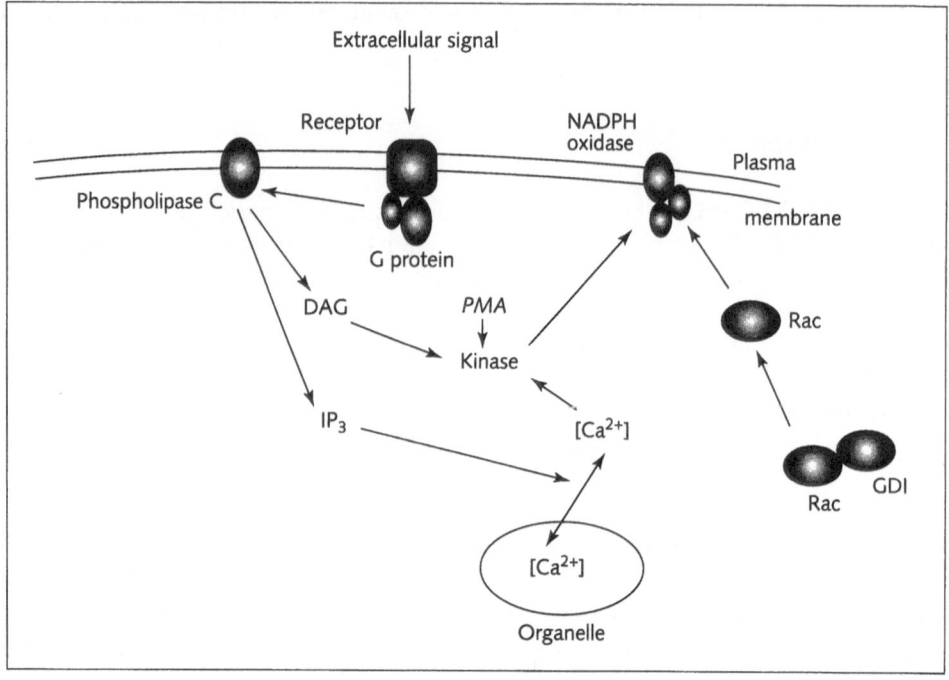

Figure 5

The signalling cascade initiated by the binding of extracellular activators of NADPH oxidase to their specific receptor on the neutrophil plasma membrane.

tion [51] within the p47phox sequence. The NADPH oxidase of such EBVLs could not be activated in reconstitution experiments. *In vitro*, the addition of anionic amphiphiles such as SDS or arachidonate is necessary and it seems likely that these amphiphiles substitute for the phosphorylation of p47phox by inducing a conformational change which mimics that produced by phosphorylation. This conformational change exposes SH3 domains and proline-rich regions which now become available for docking reactions at the cytosolic face of membrane-bound cytochrome b_{558}. The importance of phosphorylation in this process is demonstrated by the stimulatory activity of okadaic acid, an inhibitor of phosphatase activity. This prolongs the respiratory burst response to stimuli suggesting that hydrolysis of phospho-protein bonds is part of the down-regulation process.

The *in vitro* assembly of the active NADPH oxidase by the addition of amphiphiles, such as SDS or arachidonic acid, to a mixture of cytosolic factors and membrane (or recombinant cytochrome b_{558}) has been a much used method of determining the components necessary for activation. It has, however, been found that the amphiphiles can be omitted, and assembly efficiently promoted if the recombinant p47[phox] added was first phosphorylated by protein kinase C (but not by PKA or MAP kinase). Pre-incubation of the mixture in ATP and GTP before adding the phosphorylated p47[phox] was necessary, possibly by phosphorylating some membrane proteins [53].

In neutrophils phospholipase A_2 (PLA_2) is involved in releasing arachidonate from membrane phospholipids. Arachidonate is a potent activator of NADPH oxidase *in vivo* and *in vitro*, possibly by promoting conformational change in p47[phox] to expose SH3 domains. The PLA_2 itself is activated by an increase in intracellular Ca^{2+} and by protein kinase C. The importance of the arachidonate release is clearly shown in experiments where activation of the oxidase by a variety of agonists is blocked by PKC inhibitors, or by inhibitors [52] of PLA_2. The inhibition was overcome by the addition of arachidonate, implicating it in a late role in the activation process. It is possible that PLA_2 is directly activated to release arachidonate by receptors linked to G proteins.

Phospholipase D (PLD) has been implicated in the activation of NADPH oxidase. This enzyme hydrolyses phopholipids (typically phosphatidyl choline) to yield phosphatidic acid. This in turn can be hydrolysed by phosphatidate phosphohydrolase (PAP) to yield diacylglycerol, an activator of PKC. Phosphatidic acid is itself an activator of cytosolic kinase(s) which phosphorylates p47[phox] *in vitro* [53]. The activation of PLD, like PKC, is linked to G protein-coupled receptors [54]. It is regulated by PKC and ADP-ribosylation factor (ARF) in most mammalian cells [55].

Charge compensation during activity of NADPH oxidase

NADPH oxidase is a plasma membrane associated activity. The electron donor, NADPH, is cytosolic and the reduction of O_2 to $O_2^{\cdot-}$ takes place on the outer face of the neutrophil. This is shown with the use of the non-penetrant cytochrome c as an added electron accepting dye which is rapidly reduced by newly formed $O_2^{\cdot-}$ outside the neutrophil. This agonist-induced movement of an electron from inside the cell to the outside is electrogenic, leading to depolarisation of the membrane potential from about -60 mV to around -30 to -40 mV [56]. This depolarisation is stable and is absent from agonist-treated CGD cells. The stabilisation of the lowered membrane potential despite the continuing rapid outward flux of electrons is achieved by the opening of a proton conducting channel. The channel can be blocked by the addition of Cd^{2+} or Zn^{2+} ions leading to greatly increased depolarisation of the activated neutrophil [57]. This H^+ channel also serves to maintain a stable pH in the cytosol, since oxidation of NADPH releases H^+ into the cytosol, and the channel appears to transport approximately 1 H^+ outwards for every 1 e^- moved out. If the NADPH oxidase is blocked by the inhibitor diphenylene iodonium (DPI), the H^+ channel can still be activated by the addition of arachidonate. This channel activity is seen when cells are placed in slightly alkaline conditions. The addition of arachidonate activates the outward flux of H+ down its pH gradient [58]. The channel appears to be associated with the hydrophobic membrane-spanning helices of gp91^{phox}, since its activity can be transfected into non-phagocytic CHO cells [59]. There are reports that this H+ channel is voltage gated and it is possible arachidonate activation and voltage gating act in synergy [60].

It is possible that H+ channel activity is the property of gp91^{phox} itself. However, such activity would require the use of the histidine residues thought to be needed in haem binding (see Fig. 3).

The NADPH oxidase of other cells

Although the NADPH oxidase was originally characterized in neutrophils, reports soon appeared indicating its presence in other cell types. There were early reports of NADPH oxidase activity and components in other phagocytic cells and other white cells, such as macrophages, eosinophils and lymphocytes. However, later reports also indicated that the presence of NADPH oxidase was far more widespread than first envisaged.

Other white blood cells

Macrophages, eosinophils and cultured cells of a similar lineage, such as HL-60 and U937 [61] have been widely studied and the NADPH oxidase found to be almost identical with that of neutrophils and therefore these discussions will concentrate on other cell types.

Other white blood cells which have been investigated extensively include lymphocytes. Superoxide is released albeit at low levels by peripheral blood B lymphocytes and tonsillar lymphocytes [62]. The cytochrome b_{558} was expressed on the surface of such lymphocytes, but was absent from pre-B cells and from terminally differentiated plasma cells [63]. Lymphocytes which have been immortalised by the Epstein-Barr virus (EBV) show respectable rates of superoxide release which continues for almost 1 h [64]. Redox potentiometric analysis of such cells and the use of appropriate antibodies has shown that EBV transformed lymphocytes express cytochrome b_{558} on their plasma membrane [65].Transformed lymphocytes from CGD patients also show defective ROS release, suggesting that their NADPH oxidase is encoded by the same genes. Such cells can be maintained in culture and are used as model systems for the study of correction of genetic defects, perhaps leading to gene therapy for CGD [66]. Similar cell isolation and immortalisation approaches can be used in other diseases in which a neutrophil respiratory burst defect has been identified, such as infantile malignant osteopetrosis [67].

Osteoclasts

Osteoclasts originate through a haemotopoietic lineage common to white blood cells [68] and therefore it is possible that they too express NADPH oxidase. Superoxide is released by these cells and is inhibited by diphenyl iodonium (IDP) and enhanced by the addition of interferon-γ [68], both which suggest the involvement of an NADPH oxidase complex. Using monoclonal antibodies and antisera, expression of both flavocytochrome subunits, i.e. p22^{phox} and gp91^{phox}, along with the expression of the cytosolic p47^{phox} subunit have been detected in osteoclasts [69]. The cytochrome subunits appeared to be localised to the ruffled-border and bone interfaces. By the study of the deposition of formazan by osteoclasts, superoxide production has also been detected in the ruffled-border space and it has been postulated that this release of superoxide is necessary for the bone resorption process [70]. Furthermore, it has been reported that superoxide release by neutrophils is aberrant in patients suffering from the bone thickening disorder, infantile malignant osteopetrosis [67], and it is likely that these patients will have a defect in their osteoclast NADPH oxidase which may contribute to the manifestation of this disease.

Fibroblasts

ROS are also released from fibroblasts and studies here have shown the presence of a cytochrome with a mid-point potential of approximately −243 mV [71]. Further work has established that fibroblasts express mRNA encoding p47^{phox}, p67^{phox} and p22^{phox}, although expression of the gp91^{phox} could not be detected by RT-PCR [72]. Western blot analysis showed the expression of p47^{phox}, while reconstitution experiments, where membranes and cytosol fractions are mixed in the presence of arachidonic acid and GTP-γ-S as stimulators, showed that fibroblast cytosol could initiate low rates of superoxide release when mixed with membranes from either fibroblasts or neutrophils [72].

However, when Meier and her colleagues studied the superoxide release from both fibroblasts and neutrophils from patients suffering from CGD, they found that although the ROS release from the neutrophils was defective, the fibroblasts appeared to be normal. Further analysis by using antibodies suggested that the cytochrome large subunit of the NADPH oxidase complex, that is gp91^{phox}, was different in the two cell types, accounting for this different superoxide release [73]. They therefore hypothesised that the gp91^{phox} subunit existed in at least two isoforms which were both structurally and genetically distinct. Others however, have found the presence of gp91^{phox} in fibroblasts by immunohistochemistry [74]. Using aortic advential fibroblasts, superoxide release was found to be constitutive, but enhanced by the addition of angiotensin.

Using fibroblasts as a model cell type, it has been suggested that the ROS released from the NADPH oxidase are involved in a signalling cascade, rather than in any anti-pathogen role. Here, NADPH oxidase located on the plasma membrane of the cells would be activated by a G-protein downstream from an activated receptor tyrosine kinase, also on the plasma membrane. The superoxide released would either directly, or after dismutation to hydrogen peroxide, lead to the activation of the transcription factor NF-κB, causing an alteration in the expression of the appropriate genes [75, 76] (Fig. 6).

Glomerular mesangial cells

Human glomerular mesangial cells have been shown to contain a cytochrome with a mid-point potential lower than −162 mV [77] which has been reported to be of −250 mV [78, 79]. Further work on these cells showed, by western blotting and RT-PCR, the expression of p22^{phox}, p47^{phox} and p67^{phox}. However, the presence of the large cytochrome subunit, gp91^{phox} was not detected, fitting with the hypothesis [73] that this subunit exists in isoforms in different cells. If these cells were growth-arrested in their cell cycle, it was found that no expression of the NADPH oxidase components could be detected. However, expression of p47^{phox} was seen after 2 h following interleukin-1β (IL-1β) addition, but this expression again declined after 6 h [79]. This suggests that the expression of the NADPH oxidase components in these cells is tightly controlled, although the p22^{phox} mRNA continues to be ubiquitously expressed and does not appear to be controlled by the presence of cytokines.

Chondrocytes

It is well established that oxidative damage occurs in the joints in arthritic disease and it is proposed that the damaging free radicals are produced by invading neutrophils which arrive during the inflammatory response [80]. However, others have shown that chondrocytes resident within the cartilage also have the capacity to produce ROS [81, 82]. Using an immortalised human chondrocyte cell line and isolated porcine articular chondrocytes it has been found that the cytosolic components of NADPH oxidase are expressed both at the mRNA level and at the protein level [83, 84]. Further work by this group has shown that the gp91^{phox} component is expressed at the mRNA level by the immortalised human chondrocyte line and by cells isolated from a patient undergoing joint replacement. Sequence analysis of the gp91^{phox} component from chondrocytes showed that it was different in three places when compared with the published sequence [85] supporting the hypothesis put forward that the NADPH oxidase gp91^{phox} protein exists in isoforms.

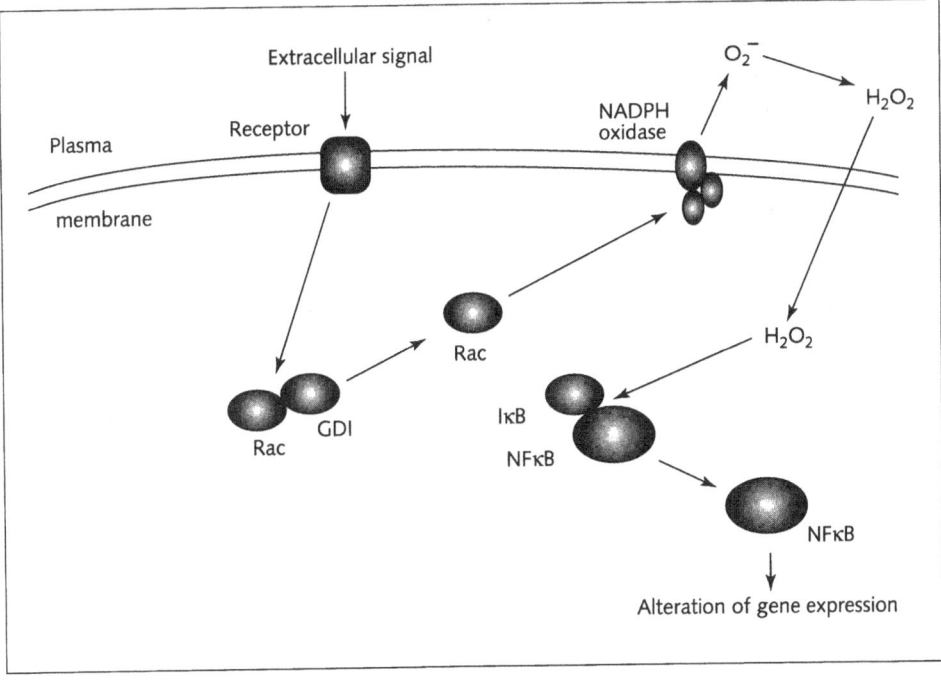

Figure 6
The possible involvement of NADPH oxidase-like systems in controlling gene expression.
Superoxide or hydrogen peroxide causes the activation of the transcription factor NF-κB.

Endothelial cells

Several stimuli have been shown to enhance the ROS release from endothelial cells, and it again has been postulated that NADPH oxidase is responsible for this activity. Diphenyl iodonium inhibits such activity, while RT-PCR has shown the expression of mRNA encoding the NADPH oxidase components gp91^{phox}, p22^{phox}, p67^{phox} and p47^{phox}. Antibodies were used to demonstrate the expression of the cytosolic components at the protein level but haem spectroscopy failed to find the presence of a low potential cytochrome [86], casting doubt on the presence of a functional oxidase system.

Keratinocytes

Keratinocytes release superoxide at a rate of over 8 nmoles/h/10^6 cells and the presence of an NADPH oxidase complex may be suspected. This superoxide release was enhanced by pre-incubation with IL-1β, and was stimulated by the calcium ionophore, ionomycin, supporting the possible involvement of NADPH oxidase. However, the activity was not inhibited by DPI, but was inhibited by lipoxygenase inhibitors [87]. RT-PCR analysis did reveal the expression of mRNA encoding NADPH oxidase cytosolic components although the presence of the polypeptides could not be seen using western blot analysis. It seems probable that there is more than one source of superoxide ions in these cells.

Cells which may use NADPH oxidase as a oxygen sensor

One of the substrates for the NADPH oxidase complex is molecular oxygen and it has been suggested that this enzyme complex may serve as a sensor of the presence of oxygen in, for example, the control of erythropoietin production or in the control of contraction of smooth muscle cells lining the airways of the lung. Therefore the presence of NADPH oxidase components has been sought in such cells.

HepG2 hepatoma cells have been shown to contain a cytochrome with a redox poise lower than -141 mV, the cytochrome b_{558} being the obvious candidate. In such cells the amount of such a cytochrome is a low proportion of the total cytochrome b present, being only approximately 7–8% [88]. Furthermore, this cytochrome has the capacity to bind CO, albeit at low affinity, but suggesting that it also has capacity to bind to molecular oxygen. Reduction of the cytochrome did not follow the addition of cyanide or antimycin, indicating that it is extra-mitochondrial. Both p22^{phox} and p47^{phox} components could be identified by western blotting in these cells, further implicating the role of NADPH oxidase.

Carotid body cells are a second cell type in which the presence of oxygen is monitored. Using spectroscopic analysis a haem containing protein with absorbance maxima at 558, 518 and 425 nm was reported in carotid body type I cells. This cytochrome was found to bind to carbon monoxide, suggesting that oxygen binding was possible [89]. Immunohistochemical studies on type I cells using a bank of eleven antibodies revealed the expression of four of the NADPH oxidase subunits, i.e. p22^{phox}, gp91^{phox}, p47^{phox} and p67^{phox} in cells from humans, guinea pig and rat carotid bodies [90].

Pulmonary neuroepithelial bodies (NEB) are localised widely in the airways of mammalian lungs. These tissues produce hydrogen peroxide which is enhanced by the addition of phorbol esters and inhibited by diphenyl iodonium, suggesting the presence of NADPH oxidase. mRNAs for gp91^{phox} and p22^{phox} have been shown to be present, along with the mRNA for a hydrogen peroxide sensitive potassium channel (KV3.3a). Therefore, a role for NADPH oxidase as a sensor for the presence of oxygen has been suggested, with its action mediated by the formation of hydrogen peroxide acting on this K$^+$ channel [91] (Fig. 7).

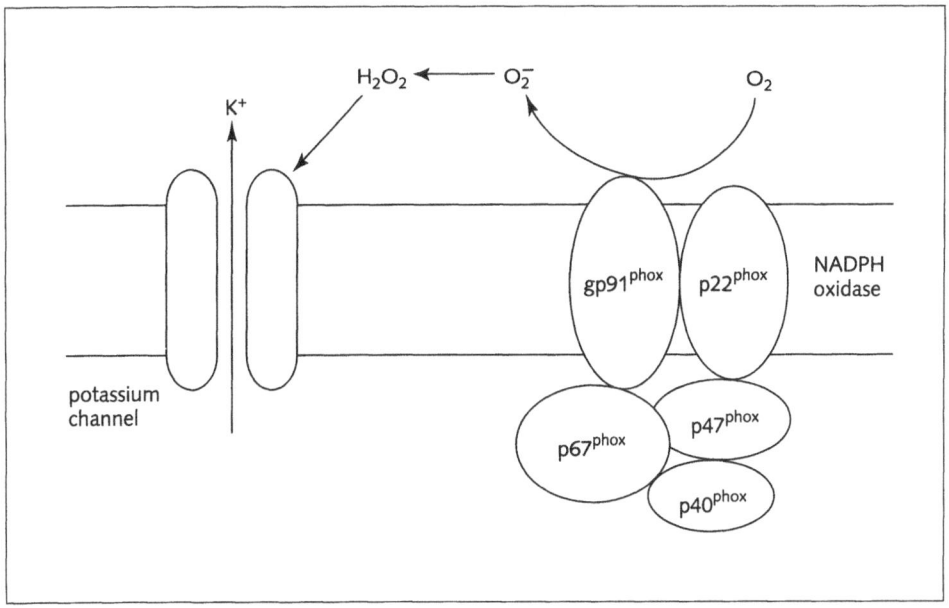

Figure 7
A scheme showing the possible effect of hydrogen peroxide in regulating a K^+ channel.

Angiotensin increases the superoxide release from smooth muscle cells, while inhibition of the superoxide-producing oxidase attenuates vascular hypertrophy [92]. p22phox from rat smooth muscle cells has been cloned, and transfection with antisense p22phox cDNA resulted in both a decrease in cytochrome b content of the cells and an inhibition of the angiotensin stimulated superoxide release [93]. It has therefore been suggested that the NADPH oxidase complex has a central role in the control of vascular hypertrophy.

In further support of this possible role of NADPH oxidase in the vasculature, p22phox, gp91phox, p47phox and p67phox have been identified in aortic advential fibroblasts, using immunohistochemistry, while immunodepletion of p67phox from advential fibroblast particulates caused a loss of NADPH oxidase activity, which was restored by the addition of recombinant p67phox. Constitutive superoxide release by these cells was enhanced by angiotensin [74].

There is a report that vascular smooth muscle cells contain a superoxide generating system which uses NADH rather than NADPH as electron donor. This system is present in membrane fractions, may involve p22phox, and is activated by TNFα [94].

References

1   Baggiolini M, Wymann MP (1990) Turning on the respiratory burst. *TIBS* 15: 69–72

2   Cochrane CG, Gimbrone MA (1992) *Biological oxidants: generation and injurious consequences*. Academic Press, San Diego

3   Baldridge CW, Gerard RW (1993) The extra respiration of phagocytosis. *Am J Physiol* 103: 235–236

4   Zatti M, Rossi F (1965) Early changes of hexose monophosphate pathway activity and of NADPH oxidation in phaogcytosing leucocytes. *Biochem Biophys Acta* 99: 557–561

5   Segal AW, Jones OTG (1979) The subcellular distribution and some properties of the cytochrome component of the microbiocidal oxidase system of human neutrophils. *Biochem J* 182: 181–188

6   Segal AW, Jones OTG (1979) Neutrophil cytochrome b in chronic granulomatous disease. *Lancet* 8124: 1036–1037

7   Cross AR, Jones OTG, Harper AM, Segal AW (1981) Oxidation-reduction properties of the cytochrome b found in the plasma membrane fraction of human neutrophils. *Biochem J* 194: 599–606

8   Cross AR, Heyworth PG, Rae J, Curnutte JT (1995) Cytochrome b-$_{245}$ of the neutrophil superoxide-generating system contains two non-identical heme:. Potentiometric studies of a mutant form of gp91^{phox}. *J Biol Chem* 270: 17075–17077

9   Hurst JK, Loehr TM, Curnutte JT, Rosen H (1991) Resonance Raman and electron paramagnetic resonance structural investigations of neutrophil cytochrome b$_{558}$. *J Biol Chem* 266: 1627–1634

10 Parkos CA, Allen RA, Cochrane CG, Jesaitis AJ (1987) Purified cytochrome b from human granulocyte plasma membrane is comprised of two polypeptides with relative molecular weights of 91,000 and 22,000. *J Clin Invest* 80: 732–742

11 Segal AW (1987) Absence of both cytochromes b$_{245}$ subunits from neutrophils in X-linked chronic granulomatous disease. *Nature* 326: 88–91

12 Wallach TM, Segal AH (1996) Stoichiometry of the subunits of flavocytochrome b$_{558}$ of the NADPH oxidase of phagocytes. *Biochem J* 320: 33–38

13 Dinauer MC, Pierce EA, Bruns GA, Curnutte JT, Orkin SH (1990) Human neutrophil cytochrome b light chain (p22^{phox}). Gene structure, chromosomal location and mutations in cytochrome negative autosomal recessive chronic granulomatous disease. *J Clin Invest* 86: 1729–1737

14 Parkos CA, Dinauer MC, Jesaitis AJ, Orkin SH, Curnutte JT (1989) Absence of both the 91 kD and 22 kD subunits of human neutrophil cytochrome b in two genetic forms of chronic granulomatous disease. *Blood* 73: 1416–1420

15 Quinn MT, Parkes CA, Walker L, Orkin SH, Dinauer MC, Jesaitis AJ (1989) Association of a Ras-related protein with cytochrome b of human neutrophils. *Nature* 342: 198–200

16 Quinn MT, Mullen ML, Jesaitis AJ, Linner JG (1992) Subcellular distribution of the Rap

1A protein in human neutrophils- colocalization and cotranslation with cytochrome b_{559}. *Blood* 79: 1563–73

17   Jesaitis AJ (1995) Structure of human phagocyte cytochrome b and its relationship to microbiocidal superoxide generation. *J Immunol* 155: 3286–3288

18   Hughes EJ (1995) *Studies of the porcine NADPH oxidase*. Ph.D. Thesis, University of Bristol

19   Segal AW, West I, Wientjes F, Nugent JH, Chavan AJ, Haley B, Garcia FC, Rosen H, Scrace G (1992) Cytochrome b_{245} is a flavocytochrome containing FAD and the NADPH-binding site of the microbicidal oxidase of phagocytes. *Biochem J* 284: 781–788

20   Taylor WR, Jones DT, Segal AW (1993) A structural model for the nucleotide-binding domains of the flavocytochrome b_{-245} beta chain. *Protein Sci* 2: 1675–1685

21   Shatwell KP, Dancis A, Cross AR, Klausner RD, Segal AW (1996) The FRE 1 ferric reductase of *Saccharomyces cerevisiae* is a cytochrome b similar to that of NADPH oxidase. *J Biol Chem* 271: 14240–14244

22   Finegold AA, Shatwell KP, Segal AW, Klausner RD, Dancis A (1996) Intramembrane bisheme motif for transmembrane electron transport conserved in a yeast iron reductase and the human NADPH oxidase. *J Biol Chem* 271: 31021–31024

23   Roos D, de Boer M, Kuribayashi F, Meischl C, Weening RS, Segal AW, Ahlin A, Nemet K, Hossle JP, Bernatowska, Matuszklewicz et al (1996) Mutation in the X linked- and autosomal recessive forms of chronic granulomatous disease. *Blood* 87: 1663–1681

24   Dinauer MC, Pierce EA, Bruns GA, Curnutte JT, Orkin SH (1990) Human neutrophil Cytochrome b light chain (p22^{phox}). Gene structure, chromosomal location and mutations in cytochrome negative autsomal recessive chronic granulomatous disease. *J Clin Invest* 86: 1729–1737

25   Thrasher AJ, Keep NH, Wietjes F, Segal AW (1994) Chronic granulomatous disease. *Biochem Biophys Acta* 1227: 1–24

26   Segal AW, Jones OTG (1980) Absence of cytochrome b reduction in stimulated neutrophils from both male and female patients with chronic granulomatous disease. *FEBS Lett* 110: 111–114

27   Bromberg Y, Pick E (1985) Activation of NADPH-dependent superoxide production in a cell-free system by sodium dodecyl sulphate. *J Biol Chem* 260: 13539–13545

28   Rotrosen D, Yeung CL, Katkin JP (1993) Production of recombinant cytochrome b_{558} allows reconstitution of the phagocyte NADPH oxidase solely from recombinant proteins. *J Biol Chem* 268: 14256–14260

29   Segal AW, Heyworth PG, Cockcroft S, Barrowman MM (1985) Stimulated neutrophils from patients with autosomal recessive chronic granulomatous disease fail to phosphorylate a Mr 44000 protein. *Nature* 316: 547–549

30   Heyworth G, Shrimpton CF, Segal AW (1989) Localization of the 47 kDa phosphoprotein involved in the respiratory burst NADPH oxidase of phagocyte cells. *Biochem J* 260: 243–248

31   Rotrosen D, Leto TL (1990) Phosphorylation of neutrophil 47 kDa cytosolic oxidase

factor. Translation to membrane is associated with distinct phosphorylation events. *J Biol Chem* 265: 19910–19915

32 Waite KA, Wallen R,Qualliotine-Mann, Mc Phail L (1997) Phosphatidic acid-mediated phosphorylation of the NADPH oxidase component p47[phox]. *J Biol Chem* 272: 15569–15578

33 Lewsen JHW, Verhoeven AJ, Roos D (1996) Interactions between the components of the human NADPH oxidase family: intrigues in the phox family. *J Lab Clin Med* 128: 461–476

34 Volpp BD, Nauseef WM, Clark RA (1988) Two cytosolic neutrophil oxidase components absent in autosomal chronic granulomatous disease. *Science* 242: 1295–1297

35 Wientjes FB, Hsuan JJ, Totty NF, Segal AW (1993) p40[phox] a third cytosolic component of the activation complex of the NADPH oxidase to contain src homology 3 domains. *Biochem J* 296: 557–561

36 Abo A, Pick E, Hall A, Totty N, Teahan CG, Segal AW (1991) Activation of the NADPH oxidase involves the small GPT-binding protein p21[rac1]. *Nature* 353: 668–670

37 Abo A, Pick E (1991) Purification and characterisation of a third cytosolic component of the superoxide generating NADPH oxidase of macrophages. *J Biol Chem* 266: 23577–23585

38 Abo A, Webb MR, Grogen A, Segal AW (1994) Activation of NADPH oxidase involves the dissociation of p21[rac] from its inhibiting GPD/GTP exchange protein (rho GDI) followed by its translocation to the plasma membrane. *Biochem J* 298: 585–591

39 Chuang TH, Bohl BP, Bokoch GM (1993) Biologically active lipids are regulators of *rac*GDI complexation. *J Biol Chem* 268: 26206–26211

40 Mizuno T, Kaibuchi K, Ando S, Musha T, Hiraoka K,Asada M, Nunoi H, Matsuda I, Takai Y, Takaishi K et al (1992) Regulation of the superoxide-generating NADPH oxidase by a small GTP-binding protein and its stimulatory and inhibitory GDP/GTP exchange proteins. *J Biol Chem* 267: 10215–10218

41 Park JW, El Benn J, Scott KE, Christensen BL, Channock SJ, Babior BM (1994) Isolation of a complex of repiratory burst oxidase components from resting neutrophil cytosol. *Biochemistry* 33: 2907–2911

42 Fuchs A, Dagher MC, Vignais PV (1995) Mapping domains of the interaction of the p40[phox] with both p47[phox] and p67[phox] of the neutrophil oxidase complex using the two hybrid system. *J Biol Chem* 270: 5695–5697

43 Sumimoto H, Kage Y, Nunoi H, Sasaki H, Nose T, Fukumaki Y,Ohno M, Minakami S, Takeshige K (1994) Role of src homology 3 domains in assembly and activation of the phagocyte NADPH oxidase. *Proc Nat Acad Sci* 91: 5345–5349

44 Heyworth PG, Curnutte JT, Nunseef WM, Volpp BD, Pearson DW, Pearson H, Rosen H, Clark RA (1991) Neutrophil nicotinomide adenine dinucleotide phosphate oxidase assembly. Translocation of p47[phox] and p67[phox] requires interaction between p47[phox] and cytochrome b$_{558}$. *J Clin Invest* 87: 352–356

45 Heyworth PG, Bohl BP, Bokoch GM, Curnutte JT (1994) *Rac* translocates indepen-

42

dently of the neutrophil NADPH oxidase components p47^{phox} and p67^{phox}. Evidence for its interaction with flavocytochrome b$_{558}$. *J Biol Chem* 269: 30749–30752

46 Dusi S, Donini M, Rossi F (1996) Mechanism of NADPH oxidase activation: translocation of p40^{phox} Rac1 and Rac2 from the cytosol to the membranes in human neutrophils lacking p47^{phox} or p67^{phox}. *Biochem J* 314: 409–412

47 Nisimoto Y, Freeman JLR, Motalebi SA, Hirschberg M, Lambeth JD (1997) Rac binding to p67 ^{phox}. Structural basis for interactions of Rac1 effector region and insert region with components of the respiratory burst oxidase. *J Biol Chem* 272: 18834–18841

48 Sathyamoorthy M, de Mendez I, Adams AG, Leto TL (1997) p40 ^{phox} down-regulates NADPH oxidase activity through interactions with its SH3 domain. *J Biochem* 272; 9141–9146

49 Leusen JH, de Boer M, Bolscher BG, Hilarius PM,Weening RS,Ochs HD, Roos D, Verhoeven AJ (1994) A point mutation in gp91^{phox} of cytochrome b$_{558}$ of the human NADPH oxidase leading to defective translation of the cytosolic proteins of p47^{phox} and p67^{phox}. *J Clin Invest* 93: 2120–2126

50 Maly FE, Quilham LA, Dorseuil O, Der CJ, Bokoch GM (1994) Activated or dominant inhibitory mutants of Rap 1A decrease the oxidative burst of Epstein-Barr virus-transformed human B lymphocytes. *J Biol Chem* 269: 18743–18746

51 Faust LP, El Benna J, Babior BM, Channock SJ (1995) The phosphorylation targets of p47^{phox}, a subunit of the respiratory burst oxidase. Functions of the individual target series as evaluated by site directed mutagensis. *J Clin Invest* 96: 1499–1505

52 Henderson LM, Chappell JB, Jones OTG (1989) Superoxide generation is inhibited by phospholipase A2 inhibitors. Role for phospholipase A2 in the activation of neutrophils. *Biochem J* 264: 249–255

53 Park JW, Hoyle CR, El Benna J, Babior BM (1997) Kinase-dependent activation of the leucocyte NADPH oxidase in a cell-free system. Phosphorylation of the membranes and p47^{phox} during oxidase activation. *J Biochem* 272: 11035–11043

54 Cockcroft S, (1992) G-protein-regulated phospholipases C, and A2-mediated signalling in neutrophils. *Biochem Biophys Acta* 1113: 135–160

55 Exton JH (1997) New developments in phospholipase D. *J Biochem* 272: 15579–15582

56 Henderson LM, Chappell JB, Jones OTG (1987) The superoxide generating NADPH oxidase of human neutrophils is electrogenic and associated with an H$^+$ channel. *Biochem J* 246: 325–329

57 Henderson LM, Chappell JB, Jones OTG (1988) Internal pH changes associated with the activity of NADPH oxidase of human neutrophils. Further evidence for the presence of an H$^+$ conducting channel. *Biochem J* 251: 563–567

58 Henderson LM, Chappell JB (1992) The NADPH oxidase associated H$^+$ channel is opened by arachidonate. *Biochem J* 283:171–175

59 Henderson LM, Thomas S, Banting G, Chappell JB (1997) The arachidonate-activatable NADPH oxidase-associated H$^+$ channel is contained within the multimembrane-spanning N-terminal region of gp91^{phox}. *Biochem J* 325: 701–705

60 De Coursey TE, Cherry VV (1993) Potential, pH and arachidonate gate hydrogen ion currents in human neutrophils. *Biophys J* 65: 1590–1598

61 Andrew PW, Robertson AK, Lowrie DB, Cross AR, Jones OTG (1987) Induction of synthesis of components of the hydrogen peroxide-generating oxidase during activation of the human monocytic cell line U937 by interferon-γ. *Biochem J* 248: 281–283

62 Maly FE, Jones OTG, Gauchat JF, Urwyler A, Walker C, Dahinden CA, de Weck AL, Nakamura M (1989) Superoxide dependent NBT reduction and expression of cytochrome b_{-245} components by human tonsillar B lymphocytes and B cells. *J Immunol* 142: 1260–1267

63 Kobayashi S, Imajoh-Ohmi S, Nakamura M, Kanegasaki S (1990) Occurrence of cytochrome b_{558} in B cell lineage of human lymphocytes. *Blood* 74: 58–461

64 Jones OTG, Hancock JT, Henderson LM (1991) Oxygen radical production by transformed B lymphocytes. *Mol Aspects Med* 12: 1649–1651

66 Maly FE, Schuerer-Maly CG, Quilliam L et al (1993) Restitution of superoxide generation in autosomal cytochrome negative chronic granulomatomous disease (A22° CGD) derived lymphocyte cell lines by transfection with p22[phox] cDNA. *J Exp Med* 178: 2047–2053

67 Beard CJ, Key L, Newburger PE, Ezekowitz AB, Arceci R, Millar B, Proto P, Ryan T, Anast C, Symons J (1986) Neutrophil defect associated with malignant infantile osteopetrosis. *J Lab Clin Med* 108: 498–505

68 Darden AG, Ries WL, Wolf WC, Rodriguez RM, Key LL,. (1996) Osteoclastic superoxide production and bone-resorption: stimulation and inhibition by modulators of NADPH oxidase. *J Bone Min Res* 11: 671–675

69 Steinbeck MJ, Appel WH, Verhoven AJ, Karnovsky MJ (1994) NADPH-oxidase expression and *in situ* production of superoxide by osteoclasts actively resorbing bone. *J Cell Biol* 126: 765–772

70 Key LL, Wolf WC, Gunberg CM, Ries WL (1994) Superoxide and bone-resorption. *Bone* 15: 431–436

71 Meier B, Cross AR, Hancock JT, Kaup FJ, Jones OTG, (1991) Identification of a superoxide-generating NADPH oxidase system in human fibroblasts. *Biochem J* 275: 241–245

72 Jones OTG, Jones SA, Wood JD, Coffey MJ (1994) The functional expression of p47[phox] and p67[phox] may contribute to the generation of superoxide by NADPH oxidase-like system in human fibroblasts. *FEBS Lett* 355: 178–182

73 Meier B, Jesaitis AJ, Emmendorffer A, Roesler J, Quinn MT (1993) The cytochrome b_{558} molecules involved in the fibroblast and polymorphonuclear leucocyte superoxide-generating NADPH oxidase systems are structurally and genetically distinct. *Biochem J* 289: 481–486

74 Pagano PJ, Clark JK, Cifuentes-Pagano ME, Clark SM, Callis GM, Quinn MT (1977) Localization of a constitutively active phagocyte-like oxidase in a rabbit aortic adventitia: enhancement by angiotensin II. *Proc Natl Acad Sci USA* 94: 1443–1448

75 Irani K, Xia Y, Zweier JL, Sollot SJ, Der CJ, Fearon ER, Sundaresan M, Finkel T, Gold-

schmidt-Clermont PJ (1997) Mitogenic signaling mediated by oxidants in *Ras*-transformed fibroblasts. *Science* 275: 1649–1651

76 Pennisi E (1997) Superoxides relay Ras protein's oncogenic message. *Science* 275: 1567–1568

77 Jones SA, Hancock JT, Topley N, Neubauer A Jones OTG (1995) Expression of NADPH oxidase components in human glomerular mesangial cells. *J Amer Soc Nephrology* 5: 1483–1491

78 Radeke HH, Cross AR, Hancock JT, Jones OTG, Nakamura M Resch K (1991) Functional expression of NADPH – oxidase components α and β subunit of cytochrome b_{558}, 45 kD flavoprotein – by intrinsic human glomerular mesangial cells. *J Biol Chem* 266; 21025–21029

79 Jones OTG, Jones SA, Wood JD (1995) Expression of components of the superoxide-generating NADPH oxidase by human leucocytes and other cells. *Protoplasma* 184: 79–85

80 Eggleton P, Wang L, Penhallow J, Crawford N, Brown KA (1995) Differences in oxidative response of subpopulations of neutrophils from healthy subjects and patients with rheumatoid arthritis. *Ann Rheum Dis* 54: 916–923

81 Tiku ML, Liesch JB, Robertson FM (1990) Production of hydrogen peroxide by rabbit articular chondrocytes: enhancement by cytokines. *J Immunol* 145: 690–696

82 Henrotin Y, Deby-Dupont G, Deby C, De Bruyn M, Lamy M, Franchimont P (1993) Production of active oxygen species by isolated human chondrocytes. *Br J Rheumatol* 32: 562–567

83 Hiran TS, Moulton PJ, Hancock JT (1997) Detection of superoxide and NADPH oxidase in porcine articular chondrocytes. *Free Rad Biol Med* 23: 736–743

84 Moulton PJ, Hiran TS, Goldring MB, Hancock JT (1997) Detection of protein and mRNA of various components of the NADPH oxidase complex in an immortalized human chondrocyte line. *Br J Rheumatol* 36: 522–539

85 Moulton PJ, Hiran TS, Goldring MB, Hancock JT (1998) NADPH oxidase of chondrocytes contains an isoform of the gp91[phox] subunit. *Biochem J* 329: 449–451

86 Jones SA, O'Donnell VB, Wood JD, Broughton JP, Hughes EJ, Jones OTG (1996) Expression of phagocyte NADPH oxidase components in human endothelial cells. *Am J Physiol* 40: H1626–H1634

87 Turner CP, Toye AM, Jones OTG (1998) Keratinocyte superoxide generation. *Free Rad Biol Med* 24: 401–407

88 Gorlach A, Holtermann G, Jelkmann W, Hancock JT, Jones SA, Jones OTG, Acker H, (1993) Photometric characteristics of haem proteins in erythropoietin-producing hepatoma cells (HepG2). *Biochem J* 290: 771–776

89 Cross AR, Henderson LM, Jones OTG, Delpiano MA, Hentschel J, Acker H (1990) Involvement of an NAD(P)H oxidase as a PO_2 sensor protein in the rat carotid body. *Biochem J* 272: 743–747

90 Kummer W, Acker H (1995) Immunohistochemical demonstration of four sub units of

neutrophil NAD(P)H oxidase in type 1 cells of carotid body. *J Appl Physiol* 78: 1904–1909

91   Wang D, Youngson C, Wong V, Yeger H, Dinauer MC, Vega-Saenz De Miera, Rudy B, Cutz E (1996) NADPH-oxidase and a hydrogen peroxide-sensitive K^+ channel may function as an oxygen sensor complex in airway chemoreceptors and small cell lung carcinoma cell lines. *Proc Natl Acad Sci USA* 93: 13182–13187

92   Griendling KK, Minieri CA, Ollerenshaw JD, Alexander RW (1994) Angiotensin-II stimulates NADH and NADPH oxidase activity in cultured vascular. smooth muscle cells. *Circ Res* 74: 1141–1148

93   Ushiofukai M, Zafari AM, Vikui T, Ishizaka N, Griendling KK (1996) p22 [phox] is a critical component of the superoxide generating NADH/NADPH oxidase system and regulates angiotensin II induced hypertrophy in vascular smooth muscle cells. *J Biol Chem* 271: 23317–23321

94   De Keulenaer GW, Alexander RW, Ushio-Fukai M, Ishizaka N, Griendling KK (1998) Tumour necrosis factor α activates a p22[phox]-based NADPH oxidase in vascular smooth muscle. *Biochem J* 329: 653–657

Nitric oxide – a novel antimicrobial agent

Nigel Benjamin

Department of Clinical Pharmacology, St. Bartholomew's and the Royal London School of Medicine and Dentistry, Charterhouse Square, London EC1, UK

Introduction

Nitric oxide is a small molecule with similar chemical and physical characteristics to molecular oxygen. The discovery that this molecule can be manufactured by a variety of vertebrate, invertebrate, plant and bacterial cells has had a profound impact on biological science. The enzymatic synthesis of nitric oxide (NO) from L-arginine, which was only discovered in 1987, seems to be important in a wide variety of bodily systems, affecting a range of biochemical and physiological processes. We now know that NO is synthesised continually in vascular endothelium and the brain, and that many disease processes, particularly those involving infection and inflammation, are associated with enhanced nitric oxide synthesis.

There have been many excellent recent reviews of this system [1–3]. This chapter is intended as an introduction to the subject, stressing the historical development of ideas, and focusing on the evidence that nitric oxide may be an important element in mammalian host defence mechanisms.

Discovery of the arginine-nitric oxide system

The history of this discovery has three main threads which each began about 15 years ago. The first concerns the description of endothelium-derived relaxing factor (EDRF), the second relates to the finding that mammals endogenously synthesise nitrate and the third followed observations on the nature of neurotransmitters in central and peripheral nerves.

EDRF

Before 1980 there was a paradox in vascular pharmacology. When the neurotransmitter acetylcholine (ACh) was infused *in vivo* in experimental animals it was known

Free Radicals and Inflammation, edited by P. G. Winyard, D. R. Blake and C. H. Evans
© 2000 Birkhäuser Verlag Basel/Switzerland

to cause a reduction in blood pressure due to vasorelaxation. Similarly when infused in the brachial artery of the human forearm it causes an increase in flow [4]. However, when segments of blood vessel were removed from animals and tested *in vitro* ACh tended to cause little effect or a vasoconstriction. Robert Furchgott, an already eminent vascular pharmacologist working in New York, was interested in this paradox and was intrigued that in his laboratory there was one researcher who could consistently prepare rabbit aortic vascular rings which dilated in response to ACh whereas others could not. He noted that this particular researcher did not wipe the luminal surface of the vessel clean when setting it up in the organ bath (while others routinely did so). He wondered if the fragile monolayer of endothelial cells was important in conferring the vasodilator effect of ACh. To test this he and his coworker Zawadski [5] prepared rabbit aortic rings in which the luminal surface was untouched or deliberately rubbed with a wooden stick. "Unrubbed" vessels completely dilated when exposed to low doses of ACh whereas rubbed vessels showed no relaxation or even a contraction. Similarly, treatment with collagenase (which is known to selectively remove endothelial cells) also abolished ACh-dependent relaxation. *En face* microscopy confirmed that these treatments had removed the endothelium. They went further and demonstrated that the endothelium was releasing a diffusible factor by showing that a strip of vascular smooth muscle devoid of endothelium would relax to ACh if another strip with intact endothelium was sandwiched next to it. Furchgott called this factor endothelium derived relaxing factor (EDRF).

The nature of EDRF was elusive for several years, mainly because of its evanescent nature. It had a half life of only a few seconds and therefore could not be retrieved from the organ bath. Many assumed it must be an arachidonic acid metabolite like prostacyclin which had recently been described [6]. Therefore many studies were performed to test the effects of drugs which were known to interfere with arachidonic acid metabolism. Although these were generally negative it became clear that a very effective inhibitor of EDRF was haemoglobin [7]. It was then found that the enzyme superoxide dismutase (SOD) enhanced and prolonged the effect of EDRF [8]. Other substances such as bradykinin, substance P and calcium ionophore were found to release EDRF from endothelial cells. It was also found that the second messenger cyclic guanosine monophosphate (cGMP) was elevated in blood vessels exposed to this new dilator substance [9]. Cytosolic cGMP synthesis from the enzyme guanylate cyclase was known to be involved in the vasorelaxant effects of nitrosovasodilators such as glyceryl trinitrate and sodium nitroprusside [10].

This was the situation in 1986 when a large international meeting of vascular pharmacologists took place in Rochester, Minnesota, USA. Here Furchgott related his recent experiments in which he showed (by accident) that inorganic nitrite, when acidified, caused a potent relaxation which was similar in nature to that of EDRF. It was known that nitrite caused relaxation by increasing cGMP and that nitrogen oxides were released when nitrite was acidified. He proposed that EDRF may be an oxide of nitrogen. Most of the audience were very unconvinced, but one who took him quite seriously was Salvador Moncada. He was head of research at the Wellcome Research Institute in Beckenham, UK, and immediately tested the effects of aqueous solutions of nitric oxide on vascular smooth muscle strips. They were identical to that of EDRF. He was in a happy position as he had helped develop the bioassay cascade system which had been important in determining the structure of prostacyclin and also could manufacture large amounts of EDRF by culturing endothelial cells on microscopic beads. It did not take his group long to show that these endothelial cells, when stimulated with bradykinin, released similar amounts of nitric oxide to those required to produce relaxation in the bioassay cascade [11]. These results were a convincing demonstration that vascular endothelium could produce nitric oxide and that it was very likely that EDRF was indeed nitric oxide. Following this there were a spate of publications which suggested that EDRF and NO were not identical [12], but the consensus now seems to be that if EDRF is not NO then it is this substance loosely bound to a carrier molecule.

The identification of EDRF as NO explained the puzzling effects of haemoglobin and superoxide dismutase. NO is known to bind strongly to de-oxygenated haemoglobin to form nitrosohaemoglobin and to oxygenated haemoglobin to form methaemoglobin and nitrate. Superoxide is another biologically important free radical which reacts rapidly with NO to form peroxynitrite (of which more later). Although most reviews of the action of nitric oxide describe this molecule as very reactive, in fact it is relatively unreactive and will combine with few other substances. These tend to be molecules with transition metals (such as iron and copper) and other radicals. It has a physical chemistry very similar to that of molecular oxygen (which is also a free radical as its outer shell electrons are unpaired) and, like oxygen, is soluble in both aqueous and lipid media. This means that passage through biological material is virtually unimpeded.

Endogenous nitrate synthesis

During the late 1970s there was increasing interest in the mammalian metabolism of inorganic nitrate. This ion is absorbed rapidly in the stomach and upper small intestine and then, curiously, concentrated in saliva. When swallowed it is acidified and protonated in the acid conditions of the stomach to form nitrous acid which will react rapidly with secondary amines in the diet to produce N-nitrosamines which are potent carcinogens [13]. Studies of nitrate metabolism in animals and man showed that not all nitrate was derived from the diet, but some was endogenously synthesised [14]. It was first suggested that this may derive from intestinal bacteria but the demonstration that germ-free animals also make nitrate showed it was a mammalian cellular process [15]. By serendipity, long-term nitrate balance studies in man, as well as showing that nitrate is endogenously synthesised in humans, also found that in one volunteer with infective gastroenteritis, nitrate synthesis was greatly enhanced.

This led to experiments in laboratory rats in which nitrate synthesis was very much increased following injection with bacterial lipopolysaccharide. It was considered likely that the source of nitrate was the immune system and subsequent studies by Hibbs et al. [16] showed that isolated mouse peritoneal macrophages synthesise nitrite and nitrate when challenged with lipopolysaccharide. Hibbs' group showed that this nitrite and nitrate derived from the amino acid L-arginine, and that if a methyl group was substituted for a hydrogen on one of the guanidino nitrogen atoms to make L-N^G monomethyl-arginine (L-NMMA), this substance prevented nitrate and nitrite synthesis. Furthermore it was subsequently shown that LNMMA also interferes with the cytotoxic action of murine macrophages against tumour cells and intracellular pathogens such as *Mycobacterium leprae* [17]. It was not realised that the formation of nitrate and nitrite may be due to the oxidation of NO synthesised by these cells until the publication of Moncada's group identifying EDRF as NO.

$$2\,NO + O_2 \longrightarrow 2\,NO_2$$
$$2\,NO_2 + H_2O \longrightarrow 2\,H^+ + NO_2^- + NO_3^-$$

However, it soon became clear that immune cells, as well as a great many other mammalian cells, with appropriate stimulation, could manufacture much larger amounts of nitric oxide than endothelial cells. It was also quickly evident that the source of nitric oxide in both cases was L-arginine which was acted upon by an enzyme which converted L-arginine to citrulline and nitric oxide [18]. The source of oxygen in nitric oxide was not immediately clear, but later shown to be molecular oxygen rather than water [19].

Neuronal nitric oxide synthesis

This element of the nitric oxide story also started about 15 years ago with the investigation of non-adrenergic, non-cholinergic (NANC) autonomic neurotransmission innervating the bovine retractor penis muscle. Gillespie had identified a factor which accumulated in this preparation upon electrical stimulation and caused relaxation of smooth muscle [20]. The factor was labile and inactivated by haemoglobin. Furthermore, it was reactivated by treatment with acid. Again, until EDRF was shown to be NO it was not apparent that the transmitter was NO and that the acid-activatable factor was nitrite [21].

$$NO_2^- + H^+ \longrightarrow HNO_2$$
$$3\,HNO_2 \longrightarrow H_2O + 2\,NO + H^+ + NO_3^-$$

In the central nervous system it was known that guanylate cyclase activation was important in the signal transduction associated with NMDA receptors and it had been shown that L-arginine could increase cGMP production by brain slices [22]. Subsequently, preparations of cerebellar cells [23] were also shown to synthesise NO from L-arginine using an enzyme similar to that shown to be present in endothelium. Studies since then have shown that many central and peripheral nerves use NO as a neurotransmitter.

NO synthase enzymes

The three locations of NO synthesis – the endothelium, neuronal cells and immune cells – are now known to represent three distinct NO synthase (NOS) enzymes which have been cloned and sequenced (reviewed by Sessa [24]). The first to be so characterised, by Bredt and Snyder, was the neuronal NOS from rat cerebellum [25]. They found a high degree of sequence homology between neuronal NOS and cytochrome P450 reductase, itself a cytochrome P450 enzyme. The other two enzymes share considerable sequence homology with the neuronal enzyme. All three enzymes incorporate a haem group, have FMN and FAD and calcium/calmodulin binding sites and require tetrahydrobiopterin as a co-factor.

Endothelial NO synthase

The endothelial enzyme is constitutively expressed and activated by increases in intracellular ionised calcium concentration via the co-factor calmodulin. The main physiological stimulus of endothelial NO synthesis seems to be increase in shear stress at the cell membrane. It may be the pulsatile nature of arterial blood flow which ensures continual NO production from endothelium. The endothelial enzyme is myristylated following synthesis which was originally thought to locate it on the endothelial cell wall [26] where it would be well-placed to respond to shear stress. However, recent work has suggested that the enzyme is tethered to the Golgi apparatus, but the functional significance of this is unknown [27]. The same enzyme is present in platelets [28] and is activated by the same factors which promote platelet aggregation. As NO inhibits platelet aggregation by reducing the rise in calcium consequent to activation, this enzyme can be seen as a negative feedback regulator which limits the process.

Neuronal NO synthase

The neuronal enzyme is also calcium dependent and the main physiological activation in the brain seems to be via NMDA receptors, the normal ligand of which is glutamate. A rise in intracellular calcium will occur in peripheral nitrergic nerves following opening of voltage-dependent calcium channels upon depolarisation. This will activate neuronal NOS in the nerve ending and allow NO to be manufactured and diffuse to the associated smooth muscle cells [29].

Macrophage NO synthase

Unlike the endothelial and neuronal isoforms which are expressed constitutively in healthy cells, the macrophage NO synthase is only expressed following stimulation of cells with lipopolysaccharide or cytokines such as tumour necrosis factor, inter-leukin-1β (IL-1β) and interferon-γ (IFNγ). This isoform of NO synthase can be man-ufactured by most mammalian cells. Rodent cells merely require exposure to lipopolysaccharide to induce iNOS expression whereas human cells need a cocktail of cytokines for maximum induction. Such cocktails work well *in vitro* with hepa-tocytes and mesangial cells [30, 31], but it has been consistently difficult to induce human macrophages to produce appreciable amounts of NO *in vitro* [32]. The mechanism by which these pro-inflammatory cytokines cause induction of inducible NOS (which takes only a matter of a few hours) is not fully understood but may involve the NF-κB pathway [33]. Glucocorticoids such as dexamethasone will effec-tivly suppress but not abolish this [34]. This action may well underlie some of the anti-inflammatory actions of glucocorticoid hormones. The macrophage NOS is distinct from other P450 enzymes in being soluble rather than membrane-bound. This solubility is important in isolating and purifying the protein and is likely to make crystallisation and structural identification possible, which may give impor-tant insights into how P450 enzymes function.

Chemical synthesis of nitric oxide

The mechanism of nitric oxide production for the purpose of microbial killing has been almost universally considered to be via 5 electron oxidation of L-arginine which is accomplished by the inducible (or macrophage) form of nitric oxide syn-thase (NOS) enzyme. In this chapter we also consider another mechanism for the generation of nitric oxide – the enzymatic and chemical reduction of nitrate – and give evidence that this system may be important in protection of humans against pathogenic organisms.

Nitrate (NO_3^-) is ubiquitous in nature, partly as it is a very thermodynamically stable molecule. However it is used by both plants and certain bacteria as a source of nitrogen for incorporation into protein as amine groups (RNH_2). To accomplish this conversion, plants have developed a range of enzymes which accomplish the 8 electron reduction required, using energy derived from photosynthesis. Green, leafy plants such as lettuce often contain large amounts of nitrate, especially if they are grown under low light conditions [35]. Most other food products have a relatively low nitrate and nitrite content.

There has been concern about the amount of nitrate in our diet, as it was found in the mid 1970s that this anion was handled in a peculiar way in the human body [36–38]. When swallowed it is rapidly absorbed and at least 25% is concentrated in the salivary glands by an as yet uncharacterised mechanism, so that the nitrate concentration of saliva is at least 10 times that found in plasma. The nitrate is then rapidly reduced to nitrite (NO_2^-) in the mouth by mechanisms which will be discussed below. Saliva containing large amounts of nitrite will be acidified in the normal stomach to produce nitrous acid which could potentially nitrosate amines to form N-nitrosamines [39] which experimentally are powerful carcinogens [13]. From this theoretical understanding of nitrate metabolism a number of studies have been performed which looked at the relationship between nitrate intake and cancer (particulaly gastric cancer) in humans. In general it was found that there was either no relationship or an inverse relationship, so that those individuals who had a high nitrate intake had a lower rate of cancer [40–42]. Similarly, in animal studies, it has been generally impossible to demonstrate an increased risk of cancer (or any other adverse effect) when nitrate intake is increased [43].

This interest in the metabolism of nitrate stimulated studies in man which confirmed a discovery originally made in 1916 [44] that mammals, including humans, synthesise inorganic nitrate [14, 15, 45, 46]. This means that even on a nitrate-free diet, there are considerable concentrations of nitrate in plasma (around 30 µM) and in the urine (around 800 µmoles/24 h). It was also found that, although it is not protein bound, nitrate has a long half-life of 5–8 h [47], which seems to be because it is about 80% reabsorbed from the renal tubule by an active transport mechanism [48]. It is now thought that endogenous nitrate synthesis derives from constitutive NOS enzymes acting on L-arginine [49]. The NO formed is rapidly oxidised to nitrate when it encounters superoxide or oxidised haemoglobin. It is still not clear whether all endogenous nitrate synthesis derives from this route as following prolonged infusion of ^{15}N-labelled arginine, the enrichment of urinary nitrate with this heavy isotope is only about one-half of the steady state of ^{15}N arginine enrichment [50]. This may mean that nitrate also derives from another source, or that the intracellular enrichment of labelled arginine is less than that in the plasma due to transamination reactions.

This peculiar metabolism of nitrate – renal salvage, salivary concentration and conversion to nitrite in the mouth – made us consider that this may be a purposeful mechanism to provide oxides of nitrogen in the mouth and stomach to provide host defence against swallowed pathogens [51]. The first studies we performed were to investigate the mechanism of nitrate reduction to nitrite in the mouth.

Oral nitrate reduction

Although Tannenbaum and his colleagues had considered that salivary bacteria may be reducing nitrate to nitrite, Sasaki and colleagues [52] showed that in humans this activity is present almost entirely on the surface of the tongue. They contested that the nitrate reductase enzyme was most likely to be a mammalian nitrate reductase. Using a rat tongue preparation, we also found that the dorsal surface of the tongue in this animal had very high nitrate reductase activity, which was confined to the posterior two-thirds [53].

Microscopic analysis of the tongue surface revealed a dense population of gram negative and gram-positive bacteria, 80% of which, *in vitro*, showed marked nitrate reducing activity.

Our suspicion that the nitrate reduction was being accomplished by bacteria was strengthened by the observation that the tongues of rats bred in a germ-free environment, which had no colonisation of bacteria, demonstrated no nitrate reducing activity on the tongue. Furthermore, treatment of healthy volunteers with the broad spectrum antibiotic amoxycillin results in reduced salivary nitrite concentrations [54].

Although we have not been able to characterise the organisms in normal human tongues (this would require a deep biopsy as the majority of the bacteria are at the bottom of the papillary clefts of the tongue surface), the most commonly found nitrite-producing organisms in the rat [55] were *Staphylococcus sciuri*, followed by *Staphylococcus intermedius*, *Pasteurella spp.* and finally *Streptococcus spp.* Both morphometric quantification of bacteria on tongue sections and enumeration of culturable bacteria showed an increase in the density of bacteria towards the posterior tongue.

We now believe that these organisms are true symbionts, and that the mammalian host actively encourages the growth of nitrite-forming organisms on the surface of the tongue. The bacteria are facultative anaerobes which, under hypoxic conditions, use nitrate instead of oxygen as an electron acceptor for oxidation of carbon compounds to derive energy.

For the bacteria, nitrite is an undesirable waste product of this process, but is, we believe, used by the mammalian host for its antimicrobial potential elsewhere.

Acidification of nitrite – production of NO in the mouth and stomach

Nitrite formed on the tongue surface can be acidified in two ways. It can be swallowed into the acidic stomach, or it may encounter the acid environment around the teeth provided by organisms such as *Lactobacillus* or *Streptococcus mutans* which are thought to be important in caries production.

Acidification of nitrite produces nitrous acid (HNO_2) which has an acid dissociation constant of 3.2, so that in the normal fasting stomach (pH 1–2) complete conversion will occur. Nitrous acid is unstable and will spontaneously decompose to NO and nitrogen dioxide (NO_2). Under reducing conditions more NO will be formed than NO_2. Lundberg and his colleagues [56] were the first to show that there was a very high concentration of NO in gas expelled from the stomach in healthy volunteers, which increased when nitrate intake was increased and reduced when stomach acidification was impaired with the proton pump inhibitor omeprazole. We have conducted further studies on the amount of NO produced following ingestion of inorganic nitrate, measured more directly using nasogastric intubation of healthy human volunteers. Following 1 millimole of inorganic nitrate – the amount of nitrate found in a large helping of lettuce – there follows a pronounced increase in stomach headspace gas NO which peaks at about 1 h and continues to be elevated above the control day for at least 6 h [57]. The concentration of NO measured in the headspace gas of the stomach in these experiments would be lethal after about 20 min if breathed continuously.

The concentration of NO in the stomach is much higher than would be expected from the concentration of nitrite in saliva and the measured pH in the gastric lumen. *In vitro* studies suggest that these concentrations of nitrite and acid would generate about one-tenth of the NO that is actually measured (McKnight, Smith and Benjamin, unpublished data). It is likely that a reducing substance such as ascorbic acid [58–60] (which is actively secreted into the stomach) or reduced thiols (which are present in high concentrations in the gastric mucosa) are responsible for the enhanced NO production.

We were surprised to find that NO is also generated in the oral cavity from salivary nitrite [53] as saliva is generally neutral or slightly alkaline.

The most likely mechanism for this production is acidification at the gingival margins as noted above. It will be important to determine if this is the case as the nitric oxide formed in this way may be able to inhibit the growth of organisms which generate acid. Such a mechanism for local NO synthesis from nitrite may in part explain the importance of saliva in protection from caries. As in the stomach, acidification of saliva results in larger amounts of nitric oxide production than would be expected from the concentration of nitrite present.

Nitric oxide synthesis from the skin

Generation of nitric oxide from normal human skin can also readily be detected using a simple apparatus such as a glass jar sealed around the hand, with nitric oxide-free gas passed through it to a chemiluminescence detector [61]. As nitric oxide has the ability to diffuse readily across membranes, we first considered it most likely that we were measuring nitric oxide which had escaped from vascular endothelium to the skin surface, manufactured by constitutive NOS. However, when the NOS antagonist monomethyl arginine was infused into the brachial artery of healthy volunteers in amounts sufficient to maximally reduce forearm blood flow, we found that the release of NO from the hand was not affected. Futhermore, application of inorganic nitrite substantially elevated skin NO synthesis. This coupled with the observations that NO release was enhanced by acidity, and reduced by antibiotic therapy makes it likely that again NO is being formed by nitrite reduction. Normal human sweat contains nitrite at a concentration of about 5 μM, and this concentration is precisely in line with that which we would predict would be necessary to generate the amount of nitric oxide release we observed from the skin. The source of nitrite is not clear, but is likely to be from bacterial reduction of sweat nitrate by skin commensal organisms which are known to elaborate the nitrate reductase enzyme.

This observation has led us to the hypothesis that skin nitric oxide synthesis may also be designed as a host defence mechanism to protect against pathogenic skin infections, especially against fungi. The release of nitric oxide is inevitably increased following licking of the skin (due to the large amount of nitrite in saliva), which may explain why animals and humans have an instinctive urge to lick their wounds [62]. We have also shown that the application of inorganic nitrite and an organic acid is effective in the treatment of patients with tinea [63].

Importance of nitrogen oxides in host defence

Much of the evidence for the importance of the arginine-nitric oxide system in host defence comes from the observation that inhibition of nitric oxide synthesis using arginine analogues impairs the ability of inflammatory cells (such as macrophages) or whole animals to kill invading pathogens [64]. This is particularly the case for intracellular organisms such as *Leishmania major* and *M. tuberculosis* [65–67], where there is particular evidence that the ability of the host to synthesise nitric oxide may be important in containing latent infections. The ability to synthesise adequate amounts of nitric oxide may also be important in reducing the severity of falciparum malaria infections in humans [68].

Mechanisms of nitric oxide-mediated microbial killing

This subject has been extensively reviewed recently by Ferric Fang [69]. It is clear that many organisms are not killed by nitric oxide alone, but require the synthesis of other, more reactive nitrogen oxide species. The reaction of nitric oxide with superoxide anion (which is also produced by activated inflammatory cells) to produce peroxynitrite has received most attention [70].

$$NO + O_2^- \longrightarrow ONOO^-$$

This reaction is very rapid, indeed more rapid than the reaction of superoxide with the enzyme superoxide dismutase. Peroxynitrite is a very reactive species, which can easily be protonated to form peroxynitrous acid (ONOOH) which may then cleave to produce nitrogen dioxide and hydroxyl.

Antimicrobial activity of acidified nitrite

Inorganic nitrates have been used as a food preservative for centuries [71]. It has subsequently become clear that nitrate is generally non-reactive with organic molecules and has to be chemically or enzymatically reduced to nitrite ($NO_2^{\cdot-}$) to be effective as an antimicrobial agent [72], which is much potentiated in an acidic environment. As well as its beneficial effect to limit the growth of serious pathogens such as *Clostridium botulinum* [73], nitrite has also the dubious benefit of rendering muscle tissue a bright pink colour, by the formation of nitrosomyoglobin.

Acidification of nitrite results in a complex mixture of nitrogen oxides as well as nitrous acid. It may also be important to provide the additional stress of acidification to make the organisms more susceptible to these nitrogen oxides. Nitrous acid, dinitrogen trioxide and nitrogen dioxide are all effective nitrosating agents (NO^+ donors) [74]. Nitrosation may occur on the microbial cell surface or due to intermediates such as nitrosothiols, which are also good NO^+ donors. Reduced thiols are in high concentration in gastric mucosa and will inevitably be nitrosated in the presence of nitrite and acid. Thiocyanate is also concentrated in saliva and chloride ions are in high concentration in the stomach. Both of these anions will catalyse nitrosation reactions by the formation of more reactive intermediates and may add to the toxicity of acidified nitrite [74].

Many human pathogens which cause gastrointestinal disease are remarkably resistant to acid alone. Incubation of *Candida albicans* at pH 1 for 1 h has no detectable effect on its future growth. Addition of nitrite to the acid incubation medium at concentrations found in saliva results in nearly complete sterilisation

Similarly, *E. coli* viability is markedly affected by addition of nitrite to an incubation medium buffered to pH 3. As little as 10 μM nitrite will slow the subsequent growth of this organism. The concentration of nitrite in saliva ranges between 100 μM and 1 mM, depending on dietary nitrate intake.

The common enteric pathogens such as *S. typhimurium*, *Y. enterocolitica*, *S. sonnei* and *E. coli 0157* are also similarly sensitive to the combination of acid and nitrite [75]. At pH 3, most of these organisms would not be killed following exposure for 1 h, but would be susceptible to addition of nitrite in the concentration normally found in saliva.

Susceptibilities to the acidified nitrite solutions ranked as follows: *Y. enterocolitica* > *S. enteriditis* > *S. typhymurium* = *Shig. sonnei* (p < 0.05). *E. coli 0157* and *Shig. sonnei* are most resistant to acid; they survive exposure at pH 2.1 for 30 min which kills the other micro-organisms. However, *E. coli 0157* shows inhibition of growth up to pH 4.2 when the other organisms apart from *Y. enterocolitica* manage to maintain growth unless nitrite is present in the solution. It seems that *E. coli 0157* manages to survive a relatively acid environment by slowing down growth activity. Its ability to survive this way is undone by the addition of nitrite to the medium.

Helicobacter pylori clearly must be able to tolerate the nitrosative stress found in the stomach, and indeed, this organism is more resistant than some other organisms to the combination of nitrite and acid [76]. The reason for this is not evident. It may be that it can withstand the effect of nitrogen oxides as it is protected against acid stress by the generation of ammonia from urea via urease enzyme. Alternatively, it may have developed specific biochemical mechanisms for protection. If this is the case, such mechanisms would be an attractive target for eradication of this important pathogen.

Conclusions

The discovery of the L-arginine-nitric oxide system has revealed an important mechanism by which mammalian cells can defend themselves against microbial pathogens. In addition to this classical pathway for nitric oxide synthesis we have described a novel and potentially important mechanism for host defence of epithelial surfaces – the production of reactive nitrogen oxides by the reduction of inorganic nitrate to nitrite and subsequent acidification.

We do not yet completely understand the mechanisms by which nitric oxide and other nitrogen oxides provide selective toxicity towards pathogens, and it is likely that the mechanisms will be different with different organisms.

Whereas it is clear that acidified nitrite is produced on mucosal surfaces, and that this combination is effective in killing a variety of human gut and skin pathogens, we have no definite evidence as yet that this mechanism is truly protective in humans exposed to a contaminated environment.

Further understanding of the complex chemistry of nitrogen oxides may also help develop new antimicrobial therapies based on augmenting what seems to be a simple and effective host defence system.

References

1   Anggard E (1994) Nitric oxide: mediator, murderer, and medicine. *Lancet* 343: 1199–1206

2   Vallance P, Moncada S (1994) Nitric oxide – from mediator to medicines. *J Royal Coll Phys London* 28: 209

3   Moncada S, Higgs A (1993) The L-arginine-nitric oxide pathway. *N Eng J Med* 329: 2002–2012

4   Duff, Greenfield ADM, Shepherd JT, Thomson ID (1953) A quantitative study of the response to acetylcholine and histamine of the blood vessels of the hand and forearm. *J Physiol (Lond)* 120: 160–170

5   Furchgott RF, Zawadzki JV (1980) The obligatory role of endothelial cells in the relaxation of arterial smooth muscle by acetylcholine. *Nature* 288: 373-376

6   Nijkamp FP, Flower RJ, Moncada S, Vane JR (1976) Partial purification of rabbit aorta contracting substance-releasing factor and inhibition of its activity by anti-inflammatory steroids. *Nature* 263 (5577): 479–482

7   Martin W, Villani GM, Jothianandan D, Furchgott RF (1985) Selective blockade of endothelium-dependent and glyceryl trinitrate-induced relaxation by hemoglobin and by methylene blue in the rabbit aorta. *J Pharmacol Exp Ther* 232: 708–716

8   Gryglewski RJ, Palmer RMJ, Moncada S (1986) Superoxide anion is involved in the breakdown of endothelium-derived vascular relaxing factor. *Nature* 320: 454–456

9   Ignarro LJ, Burke TM, Wood KS, Wolin MS, Kadowitz PJ (1984) Association between cyclic GMP accumulation and acetylcholine-elicited relaxation of bovine intrapulmonary artery. *J Pharmacol Exp Ther* 288: 682–690

10   Murad F, Mittal CK, Arnold WP, Katsuki S, Kimura H (1978) Guanylate cyclase: activation by azide, nitro compounds, nitric oxide, and hydroxyl radical and inhibition by hemoglobin and myoglobin. *Adv Cyclic Nucleo Res* 9: 145–158

11   Palmer RMJ, Ferrige AG and Moncada S (1987) Nitric oxide release accounts for the biological activity of endothelium-derived relaxing factor. *Nature* 327: 524–526

12   Myers PR, Minor RL Jr, Guerra R Jr, Bates JN, Harrison DG (1990) Vasorelaxant properties of the endothelium-derived relaxing factor more closely resemble S-nitrosocysteine than nitric oxide. *Nature* 345 (6271): 161–163

13   Crampton RF (1980) Carcinogenic dose-related response to nitrosamines. *Oncology* 37: 251

14   Green LC, Ruiz de Luzuriaga K, Wagner DA, Rand W Istfan N, Young VR, Tannenbaum SR (1981) Nitrate biosynthesis in man. *Proc Natl Acad Sci USA* 78: 7764–7768

15   Green LC, Tannenbaum SR, Goldman P (1981) Nitrate synthesis in the germfree and conventional rat. *Science* 212: 56–58

16   Hibbs JBJr, Taintor RR, Vavrin Z (1987) Macrophage cytotoxicity: role for L-arginine deiminase and imino nitrogen oxidation to nitrite. *Science* 235: 473–476

17   Adams LB, Franzblau SG, Vavrin Z, Hibbs JB Jr (1991) L-arginine-dependent macrophage effector functions inhibit metabolic activity of *Mycobacterium leprae*. *J Immunol* 147: 1642–1646

18   Palmer RMJ, Ashton DS, Moncada S (1988) Vascular endothelial cells synthesize nitric oxide from L-arginine. *Nature* 333: 664–666

19   Leone AM, Palmer RM, Knowles RG, Francis PL, Ashton DS, Moncada S (1991) Constitutive and inducible nitric oxide synthases incorporate molecular oxygen into both nitric oxide and citrulline. *J Biol Chem* 266: 23790–23795

20 Gillespie JS, Martin W (1980) A smooth muscle inhibitory material from the bovine retractor penis and rat anococcygeus muscles. *J Physiol* 309: 55–64

21 Furchgott RF (1988) Studies on the relaxation of rabbit aorta by sodium nitrite: the basis for the proposal that the acid-activatable factor from retractor penis is inorganic nitrite and the endothelium-derived relaxing factor is nitric oxide. In: PM Vanhoutte (ed): *Vasodilatation: Vascular smooth muscle, peptides, autonomic nerves and endothelium*. Raven Press, New York, 401–414

22 Deguchi T, Yoshioka M (1982) L-arginine identified as an endogenous activator for soluble guanylate cyclase from neuroblastoma cells. *J Biol Chem* 257: 10147–10152

23 Garthwaite J, Charles SL, Chess-Williams R (1988) Endothelium-derived relaxing factor release on activation of NMDA receptors suggests role as intercellular messenger in the brain. *Nature* 336: 385–388

24 Sessa WC (1994) The nitric oxide synthase family of proteins. *J Vas Res* 31: 131–143

25 Bredt DS, Hwang PM, Glatt CE, Lowenstein C, Reed RR, Snyder SH (1991) Cloned and expressed nitric oxide synthase structurally resembles cytochrome P-450 reductase. *Nature* 351: 714–178

26 Pollock JS, Klinghofer V, Förstermann U, Murad F (1992) Endothelial nitric oxide synthase is myristylated. *FEBS Lett* 309: 402–404

27 Sessa WC, Garcia-Cardenas G, Liu J, Keh A, Pollock JS, Bradley J, Thiru S, Braverman IM, Desai KM (1995) The Golgi association of endothelial nitric oxide synthase is necessary for the efficient synthesis of nitric oxide. *J Biol Chem* 270: 17641–17644

28 Radomski MW, Palmer RMJ, Moncada S (1990) Characterization of the L-arginine: nitric oxide pathway in human platelets. *Br J Pharmacol* 101: 325–328

29 Garthwaite J, Boulton CL (1995) Nitric oxide signaling in the central nervous system. *Physiol Rev* 57: 683–706

30 Curran RD, Billiar TR, Stuehr DJ, Ochoa JB, Harbrecht BG, Flint SG, Simmons RL (1990) Multiple cytokines are required to induce hepatocyte nitric oxide production and inhibit total protein synthesis. *Ann Surg* 212: 462–469

31 Nicolson AG, Haites NE, McKay NG, Wilson HM, MacLeod AM, Benjamin N (1993) Induction of nitric oxide synthase in human mesangial cells. *Biochem Biophys Res Comm* 193(3): 1269–1274

32 Hibbs JB Jr, Westenfelder C, Taintor R, Vavrin Z, Kablitz C, Baranowski RL, Ward JH, Menlove RL, McMurry MP, Kushner JP et al (1992) Evidence for cytokine-inducible nitric oxide synthesis from L-arginine in patients receiving interleukin-2 therapy. *J Clin Invest* 89: 867–877

33 Xie QW, Kashiwabara Y, Nathan C (1994) Role of transcription factor NF-kappa B/Rel in induction of nitric oxide. *J Biol Chem* 269 (7): 4705–4708

34 Rees DD, Cellek S, Palmer RMJ, Moncada S (1990) Dexamethasone prevents the induction by endotoxin of a nitric oxide synthase and the associated effects on vascular tone: an insight into endotoxin shock. *Biochem Biophys Res Commun* 173: 541–547

35 Cantliffe DJ (1972) Nitrate accumulation in vegetable crops as affected by photoperiod and light duration. *J Amer Soc Hort Sci* 97: 414–418

36 Committee on Nitrite and Alternative Curing Agents in Food (1981) The health effects of nitrate, nitrite, and N-nitroso compounds, Part 1. National Academy Press, Washington DC, 5.41–5.52

37 Hadara M, Ishiwata H, Nakamura Y, Tanimura A, Ishidate M (1975) Studies on the *in vivo* formation of nitroso compounds 1. Changes of nitrite and nitrate concentration in human saliva after ingestion of salted Chinese cabbage. *J Food Hyg Soc* 16: 11

38 Spiegelhalder B, Eisenbrand G, Preussman R (1976) Influence of dietary nitrate on nitrite content of human saliva: possible relevance to *in vivo* formation of N-nitroso compounds. *Foods Cosmet Toxicol* 14: 545–548

39 Tannenbaum SR, Weisman M, Fett D (1976) The effect of nitrate intake on nitrite formation in human saliva. *Food Cosmet Toxicol* 14: 549–552

40 Forman D, Al-Dabbagh S, Doll R (1985) Nitrate, nitrites and gastric cancer in Great Britain. *Nature* 313: 620–625

41 Knight TM, Forman D, Pirastu R, Comba P, Iannarilli R, Cocco PL, Angotzi G, Ninu E, Schierano S (1990) Nitrate and nitrite exposure in Italian populations with different gastric cancer rates. *Int J Epidemiol* 19: 510–515

42 Al-Dabbagh S, Forman D, Bryson D, Stratton I, Doll R,(1986) Mortality of nitrate fertiliser workers. *Brit J Indus Med* 43: 507–515

43 Vittozzi L (1992) Toxicology of nitrates and nitrites. *Food Additives & Contaminants* 9: 579–585

44 Mitchell HH, Shonle HA, Grindley HS (1916) The origin of the nitrates in the urine. *J Biol Chem* 24: 461–490

45 Tannenbaum SR (1979) Nitrate and nitrite: origin in humans. I, B (4413): 1332, 1334–1337

46 Tannenbaum SR, Fett D, Young VR, Land PD, Bruce WR. Nitrite and nitrate are formed by endogenous synthesis in the human intestine. I, 200: 1487–1489

47 Wagner DA, Schultz DS, Deen WM, Young VR, Tannenbaum SR (1983) Metabolic fate of an oral dose of ^{15}N-labeled nitrate in humans: effect of diet supplementation with ascorbic acid. *Cancer Res* 43: 1921–1925

48 Kahn T, Bosch J, Levitt MF, Goldstein MH (1975) Effect of sodium nitrate loading on electrolyte transport by the renal tubule. *Am J Physiol* 229: 746–753

49 Hibbs JB Jr, Westenfelder C, Taintor R, Vavrin Z, Kablitz C, Baranowski RL, Ward JH, Menlove RL, McMurry MP, Kushner JP et al (1992) Evidence for cytokine-inducible nitric oxide synthesis from L-arginine in patients receiving interleukin-2 therapy. *J Clin Invest* 89: 867–877 (published erratum appears in *J Clin Invest* 90: 295)

50 Macallan DC, Smith LM, Ferber J, Milne E, Griffin GE, Benjamin N, McNurlan MA (1997) Measurement of NO synthesis in humans by L-[15N2]arginine: application to the response to vaccination. *Am J Physiol* 272: R1888–R1896

51 Benjamin N, O'Driscoll F, Dougall H, Duncan C, Smith L, Golden M, McKenzie H (1994) Stomach NO synthesis. *Nature* 368: 6471–6502

52 Sasaki T, Matano K (1979) Formation of nitrite from nitrate at the dorsum linguae. *J Food Hyg Soc* 20: 363–369

53 Duncan C, Dougall H, Johnston P, Green S, Brogan R, Leifert C, Smith L, Golden M, Benjamin N (1995) Chemical generation of nitric oxide in the mouth from the enterosalivary circulation of dietary nitrate. *Nature Med* 1: 546–551

54 Dougall HT, Smith L, Duncan C, Benjamin N (1995) The effect of amoxycillin on salivary nitrite concentrations: an important mechanism of adverse reactions? *Br J Clin Pharm* 39: 460–462

55 Li H, Duncan C, Townend J, Killham K, Smith LM, Johnston P, Dykhuizen R, Kelly D, Golden M, Benjamin N, Leifert C (1997) Nitrate-reducing bacteria on rat tongues. *Appl Environ Microbiol* 63: 924–930

56 Lundberg JON, Weitzberg E, Lundberg JM, Alving K (1994) Intragastric nitric oxide production in humans: measurements in expelled air. *Gut* 35: 1543–1546

57 McKnight GM, Smith LM, Drummond RS, Duncan CW, Golden M, Benjamin N (1997) Chemical synthesis of nitric oxide in the stomach from dietary nitrate in humans. *Gut* 40: 211–214

58 Schorah CJ, Sobala GM, Sanderson M, Collis N, Primrose JM (1991) Gastric juice ascorbic acid: effects of disease and implications for gastric carcinogenesis. *Am J Clin Nutr* 53: 287S–293S

59 Sobala GM, Pignatelli B, Schorah CJ, Bartsch H, Sanderson M, Dixon MF, King RFG, Axon ATR (1991) Levels of nitrite, nitrate, N-nitroso compounds, ascorbic acid and total bile acids in gastric juice of patients with and without precancerous conditions of the stomach. *Carcinogenesis* 12: 193–198

60 Sobala GM, Schorah CJ, Sanderson M, Dixon MF, Tompkins DS, Godwin P, Axon ATR (1989) Ascorbic acid in the human stomach. *Gastroenterology* 97: 357–363

61 Weller R, Pattullo S, Smith L, Golden M, Ormerod A, Benjamin N (1996) Nitric oxide is generated on the skin surface by reduction of sweat nitrate. *J Invest Dermatol* 107: 327–331

62 Benjamin N, Pattullo S, Weller R, Smith L, Ormerod A (1997) Wound licking and nitric oxide. *Lancet* 349: 1776

63 Weller R, Ormerod AD, Hobson R, Benjamin N (1998) A randomised trial of acidified nitrite cream in treatment of tinea pedis. *J Am Acad Dermatol* 38: 559–563

64 DeGroote MA, Fang FC (1995) NO inhibitions: antimicrobial properties of nitric oxide. *Clin Infect Dis* 21: S162–S165

65 Stenger S, Donhauser N, Thuring H, Rollinghoff M, Bogdan C (1996) Reactivation of latent leishmaniasis by inhibition of inducible nitric oxide synthase. *J Exp Med* 183: 1501–1514

66 MacMicking JD, North RJ, LaCourse R, Mudgett JS, Shah SK, Nathan CF (1997) Identification of NOS2 as a protective locus against tuberculosis. *Proc Natl Acad Sci USA* 94: 5243–5248

67 Mannick JB, Asano K, Izumi K, Kieff E, Stamler JS (1994) Nitric oxide produced by human B lymphocytes inhibits apoptosis and Epstein-Barr virus reactivation. *Cell* 79: 1137–1146

68 Anstey NM, Weinberg JB, Hassanali MY, Mwaikambo ED, Manyenga D, Misukonis

MA, Arnelle DR, Hollis D, McDonald MI, Granger DL (1996) Nitric oxide in Tanzanian children with malaria. Inverse relationship between malaria severity and nitric oxide production/nitric oxide synthase type 2 expression. *J Exp Med* 184: 557–567

69 Fang FC (1997) Perspectives series: host/pathogen interactions. Mechanisms of nitric oxide-related antimicrobial activity. *J Clin Invest* 99: 2818–2825

70 Beckman JS, Koppenol WH (1996) Nitric oxide, superoxide, and peroxynitrite: the good, the bad, and ugly. *Am J Physiol* 271: C1424–C1437

71 Binkert EF, Kolari OE (1975) The history and use of nitrate and nitrite in the curing of meat. *Food Cosmet Toxicol* 13: 655–661

72 Brooks J, Haines RB, Moran T, Pace J (1940) *The function of nitrate, nitrite and bacteria in curing bacon and hams.* Department of Scientific and Industrial Research, Food Investigation Board Special Report No 49. His Majesty's Stationery, London, UK

73 Reddy D, Lancaster JR, Cornforth DP (1983) Nitrite inhibition of *Clostridium botulinum*: electron spin resonance detection of iron-nitric oxide complexes. *Science* 221: 769–770

74 Williams DHL (1988) *Nitrosation.* Cambridge University Press, Cambridge

75 Dykhuizen RS, Frazer R, Duncan C, Smith CC, Golden M, Benjamin N, Leifert C (1996) Antimicrobial effect of acidified nitrite on gut pathogens: importance of dietary nitrate in host defense. *Antimicrob Agents Chemo* 40: 1422–1425

76 Dykhuizen RS, Fraser A, McKenzie H, Golden M, Leifert C, Benjamin N (1978) *Helicobacter pylori* is killed by nitrite under acidic conditions. *Gut* 42: 334–337

Xanthine oxidoreductase

Roger Harrison

Department of Biology and Biochemistry, University of Bath, Bath BA2 7AY, UK

Xanthine oxidoreductase (XOR) and ischaemia-reperfusion injury

Xanthine oxidoreductase (XOR) is a widely-distributed molybdenum-containing flavoenzyme, being particularly rich in mammary epithelial cells and in capillary endothelium in a range of tissues [1, 2]. While its conventionally accepted role is in purine catabolism, catalysing the oxidation of hypoxanthine to xanthine and xanthine to uric acid, such a general housekeeping function is somewhat at odds with its specialised cellular distribution. In fact, the enzyme has a broad specificity for reducing substrates, accepting electrons from many purines, other heterocyclic compounds and even simple aldehydes [3]. It also has a choice of oxidising substrate. XOR exists in two interconvertible forms, xanthine dehydrogenase (XDH, EC 1.1.1.204) and xanthine oxidase (XO, EC 1.1.3.22). XDH, which is believed to predominate *in vivo*, preferentially reduces NAD^+, whereas XO does not reduce NAD^+, preferring molecular oxygen. Reduction of oxygen yields superoxide anion, $O_2^{\cdot-}$, and hydrogen peroxide and it is the ability to generate these reactive oxygen species (ROS) that has led to a great deal of interest in XOR as a pathogenic factor in many instances of ischaemia-reperfusion injury [4].

Attention was directed towards XOR by Granger et al. who identified the enzyme as the source of destructive oxygen radicals in ischaemia-reperfusion injury of the feline small intestine [5]. On the basis of their results, Granger and colleagues [6] proposed a mechanism of ROS generation. According to this scheme (Fig. 1), during the ischaemic period ATP is catabolised to hypoxanthine, which accumulates in the tissues. As a result of the low energy state there is an influx of Ca^{2+} into the cells. The intracellular Ca^{2+} then triggers the conversion of XDH to XO via a calmodulin-regulated protease. On reperfusion, molecular oxygen is reintroduced into the tissues and interacts with XO and hypoxanthine to generate a burst of superoxide anion and hydrogen peroxide, which, in their turn, interact to produce the more reactive hydroxyl radical The mechanism outlined in Figure 1 has served as a stimulus and a working hypothesis for many hundreds of subsequent studies in a range of species and tissues. While the conclusions of such studies have been var-

Free Radicals and Inflammation, edited by P. G. Winyard, D. R. Blake and C. H. Evans
© 2000 Birkhäuser Verlag Basel/Switzerland

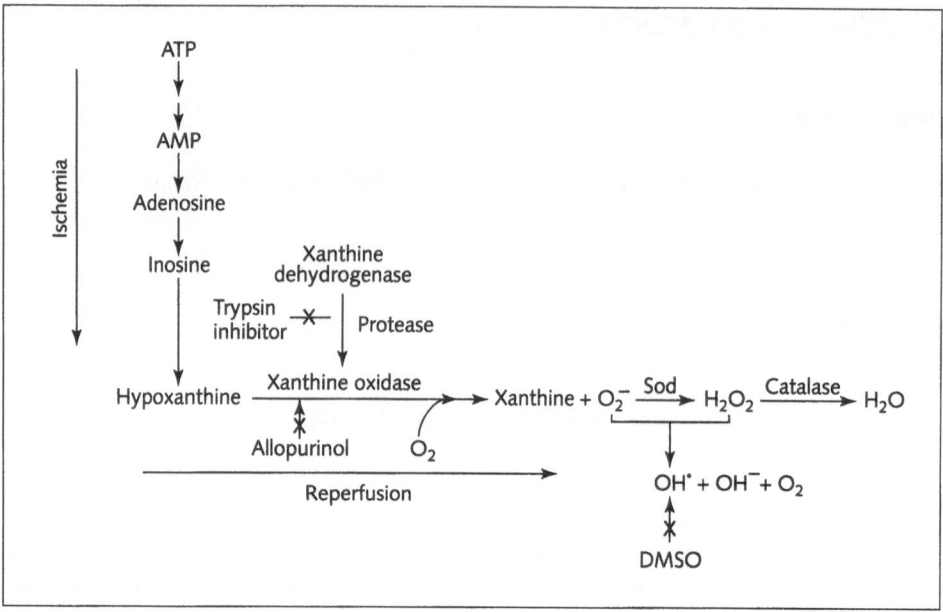

Figure 1
Mechanism of generation of ROS in ischaemia-reperfusion proposed by Granger et al. [6].
Reproduced, with permission, from [6].

ied in their support for the details of the basic hypothesis, particularly the extent and time scale of XDH to XO conversion [7–11], many positive clinical advances have accrued, including the now routine use of antioxidants and XOR inhibitors in organ preservation [12, 13].

XOR and inflammation

One of the consequences of the above research activity has been to focus attention on the physiological role of XOR in microvascular endothelial cells. Clearly, the primary function of endothelial XOR is unlikely to be as an autodestructive agent in ischaemia-reperfusion, the relevance of which in a natural environment is, in any case, questionable. Work in a number of laboratories has combined to suggest complementary roles for endothelial XOR and neutrophils in the inflammatory response. One scenario envisioned by Ward and colleagues [14] is illustrated in Figure 2. In increasingly well understood processes, inflammatory stimuli lead to upregulation of adhesion molecules on the surfaces of both endothelial cells and

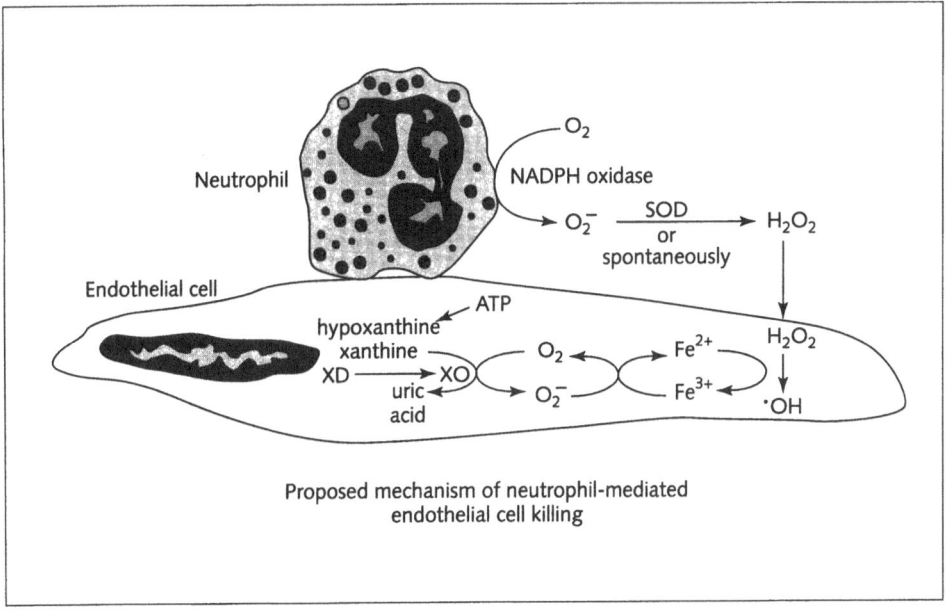

Proposed mechanism of neutrophil-mediated
endothelial cell killing

Figure 2
*Mechanism of neutrophil-mediated endothelial cell killing proposed by Varani and Ward
[14]. Reproduced, with permission, from [14].*

neutrophils, and consequently to the "rolling", tethering and eventual diapedesis of the latter. It is proposed that, once in contact with the endothelial cell, the neutrophil is stimulated to generate a "respiratory burst" via its membrane-bound NADPH oxidase system (see Blake et al., this volume). The resulting superoxide anion is rapidly dismutated, either by superoxide dismutase or spontaneously to generate hydrogen peroxide, which can readily cross the endothelial cell membrane. The endothelial cell then actively participates in its own destruction by providing Fe^{2+}, which, in a Fenton reaction, reduces hydrogen peroxide to the highly reactive hydroxyl ion:

$$Fe^{2+} + H_2O_2 = Fe^{3+} + {}^{\cdot}OH + OH^-$$

Because most intracellular iron is stored in the form of its Fe^{3+}-ferritin complex, a reducing agent is required to reduce and release free Fe^{2+}. Superoxide anion is proposed as this agent and endothelial cell XOR as its source. As in the case of ischaemia-reperfusion injury, XDH to XO conversion is an integral part of this scheme and evidence has been presented that the conversion is a consequence of the exposure of endothelial cell to activated neutrophils [15]. Tumour necrosis factor α (TNFα), a macrophage-derived inflammatory cytokine, has also been shown to effect XDH to XO conversion [16].

A related scheme involving cooperation of endothelial XOR and neutrophils in the inflammatory process has been proposed by Bulkley [12, 13]. His proposed mechanism (Fig. 3) differs from that of Figure 2 in that endothelial XOR is seen as directly involved in the recruitment of neutrophils to the endothelial cell surface. Thus, XOR-derived oxidants are envisaged as participating in the upregulation of adhesion molecules on endothelial cells and also in activating circulating neutrophils. The latter function would be facilitated if at least some of the endothelial cell XOR were exposed on the outer cell surface; evidence for which Bulkley and his colleagues have briefly reported [17]. The mechanism of Figure 3 depends critically on cytokine-induced conversion of XDH to XO in the endothelial cell, described in the case of TNFα by Ward and coworkers [16], and also on cytokine-driven , XOR-dependent neutrophil adhesion, again reported in the particular case of TNFα [13].

The inflammatory mechanism outlined in Figure 3 proposes a role for ROS in signal transduction rather than as purely destructive agents. Such a concept is not new and indeed is receiving rapidly-increasing attention [18–20], particularly in view of the explosion of research activity concerning nitric oxide [21]. An especially well-documented case of signal transduction involving ROS, that is relevant to inflammation, concerns the transcription factor, NF-κB. Targets for NF-κB include a growing list of genes intrinsically linked to a coordinated inflammatory response, including those encoding TNFα, interleukins (IL)-1, -6 and -8 and inducible nitric oxide synthase [22]. The DNA-binding form of NF-κB is a protein heterodimer comprising p65 and p50 subunits. In non-stimulated cells, NF-κB is cytosolic and inactive, bound to the inhibitory protein, IκB. Activators of NF-κB, which, among many others, include TNFα and IL-1, induce the dissociation of IκB and translocation of the remaining p65–p50 dimer to the nucleus, where it controls expression of the relevant genes. The role of ROS in this process has been elucidated by Baeuerle and his colleagues [23], who showed that activation of NF-κB could be induced by hydrogen peroxide in a human T cell line and inhibited by a range of antioxidants. Dissociation of IκB involves its phosphorylation and proteolytic degradation [24] and it is the phosphorylation step that is promoted by ROS [25].

In few of the increasing number of cases involving ROS in signal transduction is their origin known with certainty. Xanthine oxidase is commonly a plausible candidate and a number of inflammatory cytokines, including TNFα, certain interleukins and interferon upregulate XOR activity in a range of experimental systems [26–29]. One particularly well-characterised example is the involvement of XOR in the propagation of synovial inflammation [30]. Other sources of ROS are, in many cases, also possible, including NADPH oxidase, arachidonate metabolism, and leakage from the mitochodrial electron transport chain [31]. In the following part of this

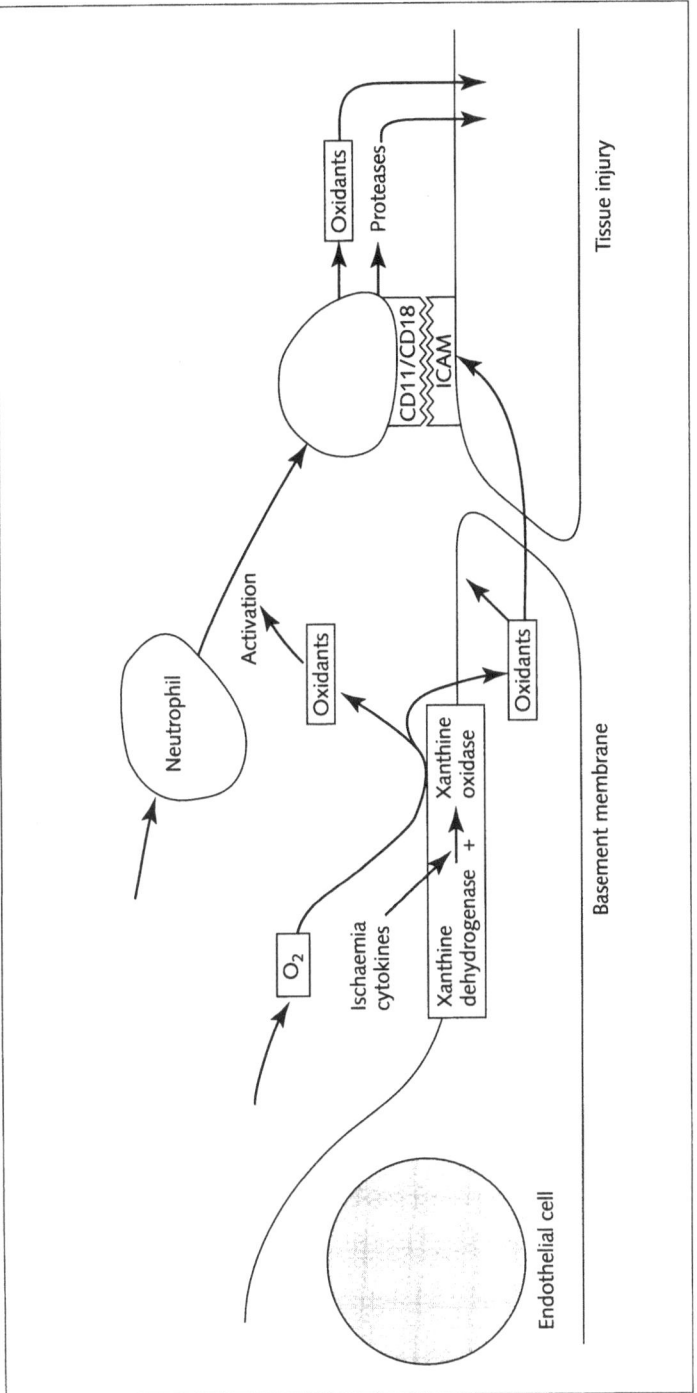

Figure 3
Mechanism of reticuloendothelial activation proposed by Bulkley [12]. Reproduced, with permission, from [12].

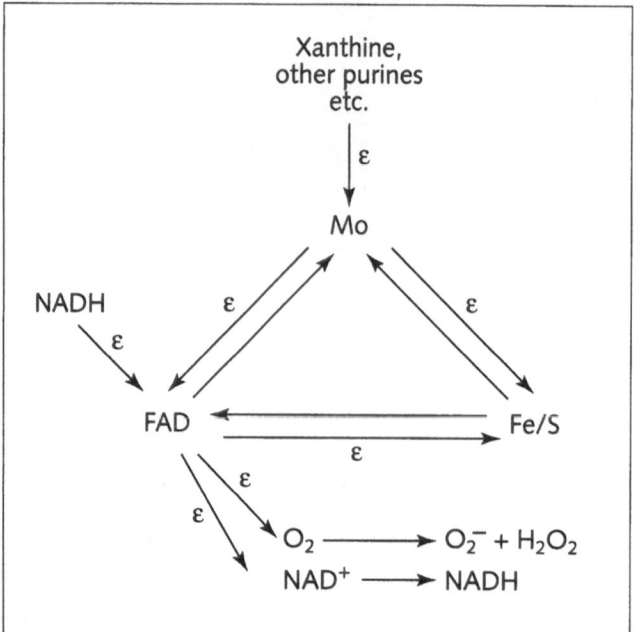

Figure 4
Schematic representation of electron transfers catalysed by XOR.

chapter, I shall attempt to examine the suitability of XOR as a source of ROS in signal transduction generally and in inflammation in particular.

Bovine milk XOR

XOR is a major protein component of the membrane surrounding fat droplets in whole milk; the membrane itself being derived from the mammary epithelial cell in the exocytotic secretion process. Consequently, cow's milk is a rich and convenient source of the enzyme, which has been known for at least 95 years and studied in its essentially pure form for nearly 60 years [32]. The bovine milk enzyme is complex, existing as a homodimer, each 150 000 Da subunit of which contains one molybdenum atom, one FAD and two iron-sulphur redox centres [1, 33]. As already mentioned, XOR has a wide specificity for reducing substrates and, depending on its form (XDII or XO) preferentially reduces NAD$^+$ or molecular oxygen. As shown schematically in Figure 4, most reducing substrates donate electrons to the molybdenum site. Following rapid equilibration between the three redox centres (the two iron-sulphur groupings are shown here as a single centre) electrons are passed on, at the FAD centre, either to NAD^+ or to molecular oxygen. XOR can also act as an NADH oxidase, and NADH is unique among reducing substrates in donating its electrons directly to the FAD site.

As much as 60% of purified bovine milk XOR is inactive towards conventional reducing substrates like hypoxanthine or xanthine. Such "inactive" enzyme comprises two forms. "Demolybdo" XOR lacks molybdenum and commonly makes up 30–40% of the total. Of the remaining 60–70% molybdenum-containing enzyme, about one-third is "desulpho" form, in which an $Mo = S$ grouping, essential for activity, is replaced by $Mo = O$. The origin and function of these "inactive" forms of XOR are unknown and will be discussed below in the context of the human enzyme.

XOR from other non-human vertebrates

XOR has also been characterised from rat [34], chicken [35] and turkey [36] livers. Although much less information is available than for the bovine milk enzyme, their properties are generally very similar to those of the latter. There is, however, one noteworthy difference between bovine and rat enzymes on the one hand and chicken and turkey enzymes on the other. Rat XOR, like the bovine enzyme, can exist as a dehydrogenase (XDH) or an oxidase (XO) form. These forms can be interconverted reversibly by means of sulphide reagents or irreversibly (XDH to XO) by proteolysis [37, 38]. The avian enzymes, in contrast, occur only in the XDH forms.

Human XOR

Most discussions of the pathophysiological role of XOR are based on the properties of the bovine milk or rat liver enzymes and although results obtained in experimental animal systems are commonly extrapolated, at least implicitly, to humans, relatively little is known about the human enzyme. We have purified human XOR from breast milk and found it to have surprising properties [39]. Starting from 1500 ml frozen breast milk, it is possible to routinely obtain 20–25 mg of high purity enzyme [40], yields comparable with those obtainable from fresh bovine milk. The human milk enzyme, while very similar in its physicochemical properties to the well-characterized bovine milk enzyme, shows striking differences in its catalytic activity towards 'conventional' reducing substrates. Thus, activity to xanthine is only 1–2% that of purified bovine milk XOR; an observation that can be largely explained in terms of an exceptionally low molybdenum content of the human enzyme. Purified human milk XOR appears to contain at least 95% "demolybdo" enzyme, as opposed to 30–40% for the bovine milk enzyme [41].

Clearly, the question arises as to the nature of XOR in other human tissues. Levels of XOR enzymic activity are very low in most human tissues [42–44], suggesting the possibility that like breast milk, they may contain XOR of low specific activity. Indeed, immunoaffinity purification of XOR from human heart yielded a protein with specific activity towards xanthine similar to that of purified human milk XOR [45, 46]. Liver and intestine, on the other hand, may differ from most other human tissues in that they show relatively high xanthine oxidase activity [42, 44] and enzyme purified from human liver showed specific activity very similar to those of the bovine milk and rat liver enzymes [47]. It appears possible, accordingly, that human XOR might be tissue-specific, with "high activity" enzyme in a limited number of tissues (e.g. liver and intestine) and "low activity" enzyme, similar to that in breast milk, in the rest.

If, in anticipation of further information, we accept the idea that many human tissues contain low activity breast milk-like XOR, we are left with the question, why? In the context of XOR as a generator of ROS in signal transduction, the concept of a low activity enzyme that is potentially subject to post-translational activation is attractive. We have, in fact, obtained evidence of such activation *in vivo*, although its physiological relevance is presently obscure. XOR enzymic activity was measured in serial samples of breast milk, obtained from 14 mothers during the first few weeks after giving birth [48]. In all cases, a peak of enzymic activity, lasting 6–10 days, was observed during the first few weeks following parturition. Thereafter, activity fell to basal levels which were largely maintained. Throughout these events, the levels of XOR protein remained essentially unchanged with the consequence that specific activity varied by as much as 50-fold between peak and basal levels. These findings raise many questions, particularly as the role of XOR in milk is by no means clear. It appears that in response to some, presumably hormonal stimulus, XOR is subjected to post-translational activation-deactivation cycles. Concerning the mechanism of such activation-deactivation, it is intriguing to speculate on the possible role of molybdenum content. This content is very low in purified breast milk XOR; a fact which largely determines the low specific activity of this enzyme to xanthine and related reducing substrates [41]. It is conceivable that the peaks of activation described above could result from controlled incorporation of molybdenum into enzyme of low basal activity. There is, to my knowledge, no precedent for such a means of regulation, which would probably require incorporation also of the molybdopterin cofactor [41, 49], in what might appear to be a cumbersome process. Although not directly relevant to this discussion, it is worth noting that the well known mouse L929 fibroblastic cell line has been shown to contain inactive XOR protein which can be activated by addition of molybdenum salts to the culture medium [50].

There is another potential mechanism for post-translational activation of XOR, about which rather more is known. "Desulpho" XOR commonly makes up at least one-third of the molybdenum-containing enzyme from most sources (see above) and can be converted to the active "sulpho" form *in vitro* by incubation of the reduced enzyme with sulphide ion [51]. Moreover, "desulpho"-"sulpho" conversion *in vivo* has been suggested as the basis of activation of XOR in response to increased protein diet in chickens [52] and rats [53]. Apparent post-translational activation of similar (two to five-fold) magnitude has been reported in response to hypoxia in bovine aortic endothelial cells [54] and in 3T3 cells [55] and we, ourselves, have demonstrated two to three-fold post-translational activation of XOR in the human mammary epithelial cell line, HB4a, in response to interferon-γ (IFNγ) [28]. Activation of these magnitudes would be consistent with the content of "desulpho" XOR from most sources and, indeed, "desulpho"-"sulpho" activation has been proposed as a general mechanism of regulation of relevant enzymes [56–58].

The low activity of human XOR, in breast milk and in at least some other tissues, to "conventional" reducing substrates prompted us to investigate the relevance of other catalytic activities of the enzyme *in vivo*. NADH oxidase activity is possessed by XORs generally but has been relatively little studied [59–61]. NADH differs from other reducing substrates in donating its electrons directly to the FAD site [1], rather than to the molybdenum (Fig. 4) and so might be expected to be unaffected by variations in the latter site. Indeed, the NADH oxidase activity of purified human milk XOR was found to be very similar to that of the bovine milk enzyme. Both human and bovine enzymes, particularly in their dehydrogenase (XDH) forms, are capable of oxidising NADH to generate superoxide anion in the presence of molecular oxygen. For either enzyme, the maximal rate of superoxide production is approximately 0.2 μmol/min/mg [40]. In the case of the human enzyme, this rate is some four times faster than that shown by the oxidase form in the presence of xanthine [40]; the activity with respect to which XOR would normally be assessed as a source of ROS. Accordingly, it seems entirely possible that XOR, particularly the human enzyme, may play a physiological role as an NADH oxidase. In this context, it is worth noting that the naturally predominant dehydrogenase form of the enzyme is actually more effective than the oxidase form, conversion to which need not be a prerequisite for activity [62]. The involvement of XOR as a source of ROS in experimental or clinical situations is commonly assessed on the basis of the effects of inhibitors such as allopurinol or oxypurinol [63], although other inhibitors, such as amflutizole [64] or BOF 4272 [65] have also been used. All of these inhibitors interact specifically with the molybdenum centre of XOR and have no effect on NADH oxidation [40]. Similar considerations apply to studies based on incorporation of tungsten [66], which takes the place of molybdenum and renders XOR inactive in those reactions that depend upon the latter atom. In so far, therefore, as XOR acts as a source of ROS by virtue of its NADH oxidase activity, this is unlikely to have been detected in most systems hitherto studied and may be more widespread than generally supposed. There is currently no specific inhibitor of XOR-derived NADH oxidase activity. It is strongly blocked by diphenyleneiodonium [40], which is, however, a relatively non-specific inhibitor of flavoenzymes, including NADPH oxidase and nitric oxide synthase [67, 68].

In summary, XOR, especially human XOR has the capacity to generate ROS in the presence of molecular oxygen from a range of reducing substrates, including NADH, and also has the potential for activation by at least one mechanism at the post-translational level. As such, the enzyme is an attractive candidate as a source of ROS in signal transduction, including inflammatory processes.

Subcellular location of XOR

XOR is generally understood to be cytosolic although there have actually been very few published investigations of its subcellular location. Jarasch et al. [2] used both light and electron microscopic immunohistochemical procedures to show that the enzyme is located throughout the cytoplasm of bovine capillary endothelial cells. This was found to be the case in the activity-based ultrastructural studies of rat liver endothelial cells by Angermuller et al. [69], who also reported localisation of the enzyme in the peroxisomes of hepatocytes: a finding confirmed by Dikov and coworkers [70], using the same tissue and similar techniques. A peroxisomal location of XOR in rat liver hepatocytes was, however, subsequently refuted in the immunoelectron microscopic studies of Ichikawa et al. [71], who concluded the enzyme to be exclusively cytosolic with no significant association with intracellular organelles, including endoplasmic reticulum, Golgi apparatus, lysosomes or peroxisomes. In 1991, Bulkley and coworkers reported, in the form of conference abstracts [17], immunolocalisation of XOR on the outer surface of cultured bovine aorta endothelial cells; a localisation that is crucial to their proposed role of XOR as a trigger in the inflammatory response (Fig. 3). Following these reports, Adachi and colleagues [72] proposed that XOR binds to sulphated glycosylaminoglycans on the endothelial cell surface and went on to identify a heparin-binding site on the surface of the human enzyme [73]. The kinetics of ROS production by heparin-bound XOR were subsequently studied by Radi et al. [74].

We (M. Rouquette et al., unpublished data) have recently made use of both monoclonal and polyclonal anti-(human XOR) antibodies in confocal microscopy to confirm the presence of XOR on the outer surface of human endothelial and epithelial cells in culture. The enzyme was also seen in the cytoplasm of all cell types examined, with a clearly higher intensity of staining in the perinuclear region. The latter localisation in particularly intriguing in the context of XOR as a cytoplasmic source of ROS involved in signal tranduction and activation of nuclear transcription factors (see above).

Circulating anti-XOR antibodies

The occurrence of anti-XOR antibodies in human serum has been recognised for many years [75–78] and we have recently reexamined this phenomenon [79]. Levels of IgM anti-XOR antibodies in healthy adults were found to be high, representing approximately 3% of total IgM. ELISAs using both bovine milk and human XOR as antigen indicated that such antibodies are generated in response to endogenous XOR rather than to XOR from ingested milk. Levels of these autoantibodies depend on age and sex and are significantly elevated in patients with coronary heart disease [77]. It is suggested that they constitute a natural defence against excess levels of serum XOR, clearing them from the circulation in the form of immune complexes [79]. The presence of circulating anti-XOR autoantibodies adds an extra factor in considerations of XOR on the surface of vascular endothelial cells. It might be expected that heparin and the autoantibodies will compete for binding to the enzyme, in which context it should be noted that activity is largely retained in either complex [74, 79].

XOR as a source of nitric oxide

A further dimension to discussions of pathophysiological roles of XOR has recently been added by observations that the enzyme can generate nitric oxide. While not generally known, the ability of XOR to reduce inorganic nitrate to nitrite, under conditions of low oxygen tension, was reported many years ago [80–82]. It has now been demonstrated that, in the presence of xanthine or NADH as reducing substrate, XOR can reduce either nitrate or nitrite to nitric oxide [30, 83, 84]. Nitric oxide generation is inhibited in the presence of molecular oxygen, presumably because oxygen competes for electrons, yielding superoxide anion and hydrogen peroxide.

Nitric oxide is an important component of the inflammatory response (see Evans and Stefanovic-Racic, this volume) and is generally understood to be produced by the nitric oxide synthases in the presence of arginine, NADPH and molecular oxygen. In contrast to nitric oxide synthase, XOR will only generate nitric oxide in the absence of oxygen and so can be seen as complementary to the former enzyme, metabolising endogenous nitrate and/or nitrite to nitric oxide under hypoxic conditions. The situation is further complicated by the possibility that, at low oxygen tension, both nitric oxide and superoxide might be produced concurrently, leading to the generation of peroxynitrite, yet another ROS of metabolic significance [85]. While potentially of the greatest importance, these findings are still essentially preliminary and require detailed investigation before their full significance is known.

Summary

XOR, known for almost 100 years, became a focus of intense research activity in the early 1980s because of its hypothesised involvement as a source of ROS in ischaemia-reperfusion injury. More recently, the enzyme has been also seen as a generator of ROS in inflammation and signal transduction generally, as the importance of ROS in these contexts is increasingly recognised. Most discussions of the pathophysiological involvement of XOR are based on the properties of the well-characterised bovine milk or rat liver enzymes, although extrapolation to the human system is usually implicit. In fact, human XOR, in at least some tissues, is surprisingly different in showing only very low activity to conventional reducing substrates, such as xanthine. Such low "conventional" activity of human XOR prompts consideration of its possible activation, for which there are two potential mechanisms. It is conceivable that, in response to specific stimuli, XOR could be activated by "desulpho"-"sulpho" interconversion or even by incorporation of molybdenum. While very largely speculative, the concept of post-translational control of an enzyme that is capable of producing ROS for signal transduction is attractive. Alternatively, XOR could have a cellular role as an NADH oxidase; an activity which is no less in the human enzyme than in XOR from other species.

The subcellular location is clearly relevant to its function and evidence for its occurrence both on the cell surface and in the cytoplasmic perinuclear region is in accord with its suggested roles in signal transduction. The presence of high levels of circulating anti-XOR autoantibodies should be borne in mind in any discussions of the role of XOR on the endothelial cell surface.

Finally, recent evidence that XOR is capable of reducing nitrate to nitric oxide adds a new dimension to the potential role of the enzyme in the inflammatory process.

Acknowledgements
Work at Bath described here was supported by the Medical Research Council in a project grant to the author together with Dr. R. Eisenthal and Dr. A. Wolstenholme (Bath University) and Professor R.C. Bray (Sussex University). Further support has been obtained from the BBSRC, The Wellcome Trust and the Arthritis and Rheumatism Research Council. The latter funding was held jointly with Professor D. Blake and Dr. C. Stevens (Bath University).

References

1   Bray RC (1975) Molybdenum iron-sulfur flavin hydroxylases and related enzymes. In: PD Boyer (ed): *The enzymes*. Academic Press, New York, 299–419

2   Jarasch E-D, Grund,C, Bruder G, Heid HW, Keenan TW, Franke WW (1981) Localization of xanthine oxidase in mammary gland epithelium and capillary endothelium. *Cell* 25: 67–82

3   Krenistsky TA, Nei SM, Elion GB, Hitchings GH (1972) A comparison of the specificities of xanthine oxidase and aldehyde oxidase. *Arch Biochem Biophys* 150: 585–599

4   McCord JM Oxygen-derived free radicals in postischemic tissue injury. *New Engl J Med* 312: 159–163

5   Granger DN, Rutili G, McCord JM (1981) Superoxide radicals in feline intestine. *Gastroenterology* 81: 22–29

6   Granger DN, Hollwarth ME, Parks DA (1986) Ischemia-reperfusion injury: role of oxygen-derived free radicals. *Acta Physiol Scand Suppl* 548: 47–63

7   Lindsay S, Liu T-H, Xu J, Marshall PA, Thompson JK, Parks DA, Freeman BA, Hsu CY, Beckman JS (1991) Role of xanthine dehydrogenase and oxidase in local cerebral ischaemic injury to rat. *Am J Physiol* 261: H2051–2057

8   Marubayashi S, Dohi K, Yamada K, Kawasaki T Role of conversion of xanthine dehydrogenase to oxidase in ischemic rat liver cell injury. *Surgery* 110: 537–543

9   Partridge CA, Blumenstock FA, Malik AB Pulmonary microvascular endothelial cells constitutively release xanthine oxidase. *Arch Biochem Biophys* 294: 184–187

10   Kooij A, Schiller HJ, Schijns M, Van Noorden CJF, Frederiks WM (1994) Conversion of xanthine dehydrogenase into xanthine oxidase in rat liver and plasma at the onset of reperfusion after ischemia. *Hepatology* 19: 1488–1495

11   Frederiks WM, Bosch KS (1996) The proportion of xanthine oxidase activity of total xanthine oxidoreductase activity *in situ* remains constant in rat liver under various (patho) physiological conditions. *Hepatology* 24: 1179–118

12   Bulkley GB (1994) Reactive oxygen metabolites and reperfusion injury: aberrant triggering of reticuloendothelial function. *Lancet* 344: 934–936

13   Bulkley GB (1997) Physiology of reactive oxidant-mediated signal transduction: an overview. *Biochem Soc Trans* 25: 804–81

14   Varani J, Ward PA (1994) Mechanisms of endothelial cell injury in acute inflammation. *Shock* 2: 311–319

15   Phan SH, Gannon DE, Varani J, Ryan US, Ward PA (1989) Xanthine oxidase activity in rat pulmonary artery endothelial cells and its alteration by activated neutrophils. *Am J Pathol* 134: 1201–1209

16   Friedl HP, Till GO, Ryan US, Ward PA (1989) Mediator-induced activation of xanthine oxidase in endothelial cells. *FASEB J* 3: 2512–2516

17   Schiller H, Vickers S, Hildreth J, Mather I, Kuhajda F, Bulkley G (1991) Immunoaffinity localization of xanthine oxidase on the outside surface of the endothelial cell plasma membrane. *Circ Shock* 34: A435

18   Saran M, Bors W (1989) Oxygen radicals acting as chemical messengers: a hypothesis. *Free Rad Res Commun* 7: 213–220

19   Suzuki YJ, Forman HJ, Sevanian A (1997) Oxidants as stimulators of signal transduction. *Free Rad Biol Med* 22: 269–285

20   Hancock JT (1997) Superoxide, hydrogen peroxide and nitric oxide as signalling molecules: their production and role in disease. *Br J Biomed Sci* 54:38–46

21   Stamler JS, Singel DJ, Loscalzo J (1994) Biochemistry of nitric oxide and its redox-activated forms. *Science* 258: 1898–1902

22   Baeuerle PA, Henkel T (1994) Function and activation of NF-κB in the immune system. *Ann Rev Immunol* 12:141–171

23   Schreck R, Albermann K, Baeuerle PA (1992) Nuclear factor κB: An oxidative stress-responsive transcription factor of eukaryotic cells (a review). *Free Rad Res Commun* 17: 221–237

24   Brown K, Gerstberger S, Carlson L, Franzoso G, Siebenlist U (1995) Control of IκB-α proteolysis by site-specific signal-induced phosphorylation. *Science* 267: 1485–1488

25   Traencker E B-M, Wilk S, Baeuerle PA (1994) A proteasome inhibitor prevents activation of NF-κB and stabilises a newly phophorylated form of IκB. *EMBO J* 13: 5433–5441

26   Dupont GP, Huecksteadt TP, Marshall BC, Ryan US, Michael JR, Hoidal JR (1992) Regulation of xanthine dehydrogenase and xanthine oxidase activity and gene expression in cultured rat pulmonary endothelial cells. *J Clin Invest* 89: 197–202

27   Pfeffer KD, Huecksteadt TP, Hoidal JR (1994) Xanthine dehydrogenase and xanthine oxidase activity and gene expression in renal epithelial cells. *J Immunol* 153: 1789–1797

28   Page S, Benboubetra M, Blake D, Powell D, Selase F, Stevens C, Wolstenholme A, Harrison R (1997) Cytokine-induced activation of xanthine oxidase in human mammary epithelial cells. *Biochem Soc Trans* 25: 95S

29   Terao M, Kurosaki M, Zanotta S, Garattini E (1997) The xanthine oxidoreductase gene: structure and regulation. *Biochem Soc Trans* 25: 791–796

30   Blake DR, Stevens CR, Sahinoglu T, Ellis G, Gaffney K, Edmonds S, Benboubetra M, Harrison R, Jawed S, Kanczler J, Millar TM, Winyard PG, Zhang Z (1997) Xanthine oxidase: four roles for the enzyme in rheumatoid pathology. *Biochem Soc Trans* 25: 812–816

31   Winyard PG, Blake DR (1997) Antioxidants, redox-regulated transcription factors and inflammation. *Adv Pharmacol* 38: 403–421

32   Massey V, Harris CM (1997) Milk xanthine dehydrogenase: the first one hundred years. *Biochem Soc Trans* 25: 750–755

33   Hille R (1996) The mononuclear molybdenum enzymes. *Chem Rev* 96: 2757–2816

34   Saito T, Nishino T (1989) Differences in redox and kinetic properties between NAD-dependent and O_2 dependent types of rat liver xanthine dehydrogenase. *J Biol Chem* 264: 10013–10022

35   Nishino T, Nishino T, Scopfer LM, Massey V (1989) The reactivity of chicken liver xanthine dehydrogenase with molecular oxygen. *J Biol Chem* 264: 2518–2527

36   Cleere WF, Coughlan MP (1975) Avian xanthine dehydrogenases I. Isolation and characterisation of the turkey liver enzyme. *Comp Biochem Physiol* 508: 311–322

37   Batelli MG, Lorenzoni E, Stirpe F (1973) Milk xanthine oxidase type D (dehydrogenase) and typeO (oxidase). *Biochem J* 131: 191–198

38   Batelli MG (1980) Enxymic conversion of rat liver xanthine oxidase from dehydroge-
     nase (D form) to oxidase (O form). *FEBS Lett* 113: 47–51
39   Abadeh S, Killacky J, Benboubetra M, Harrison R (1992) Purification and partial char-
     acterization of xanthine oxidase from human milk. *Biochim Biophys Acta* 1117: 25–32
40   Sanders SA, Eisenthal R, Harrison R (1997) NADH oxidase activity of human xanthine
     oxidoreductase. Generation of superoxide anion. *Eur J Biochem* 245: 541–548
41   Godber B, Sanders S, Harrison R, Eisenthal R, Bray RC (1997) > 95% of xanthine oxi-
     dase in human milk is present as the demolybdo form, lacking molybdopterin. *Biochem
     Soc Trans* 25: 519S
42   Parks DA, Granger DN (1986) Xanthine oxidase: biochemisty, distribution and physi-
     ology. *Acta Physiol Scand Suppl* 548: 87–99
43   De Jong JW, Van der Meer P, Nieukoop AS, Huizer T, Stroeve RJ, Bos E (1990) Xan-
     thine oxidoreductase activity in perfused hearts of varous species, including humans.
     Circ Res 67: 770–773
44   Sarnesto A, Linder N, Raivio KO (1996) Organ distribution and molecular forms of
     human xanthine dehydrogenase, xanthine oxidase protein. *Lab Invest* 74: 48–56
45   Abadeh S, Case PC, Harrison R (1992) Demonstration of xanthine oxidase in human
     heart. *Biochem Soc Trans* 20: 346S
46   Abadeh S, Case PC, Harrison R (1993) Purification of xanthine oxidase from human
     heart. Biochem Soc Trans 21: 99S
47   Krenitsky TA, Spector T, Hall WW (1986) Xanthine oxidase from human liver: purifi-
     cation and characterisation. *Arch Biochem Biophys* 247: 108–119
48   Brown A-M, Benboubetra M, Ellison M, Powell D, Reckless JD, Harrison R (1995)
     Molecular activation-deactivation of xanthine oxidase in human milk. *Biochim Biophys
     Acta* 1245: 248–254
49   Rajagopalan KV (1997) Biosynthesis and processing of the molybdenum cofactors.
     Biochem Soc Trans 25:757–761
50   Falciani F, Terao M, Goldwurm S, Ronchi A, Gotti A, Minoia C, Li Calzi M, Salmon
     M, Cazzaniga G, Garattini E (1994) Molybdenum (VI) salts convert the xanthine oxi-
     doreductase apoprotein into the active enzyme in mouse L929 fibroblast cells. *Biochem
     J* 298: 69–77
51   Massey V, Edmondson D (1970) On the mechanism of inactivation of xanthine oxidase
     by cyanide. *J Biol Chem* 245: 6595–6598
52   Itoh R, Nishino T, Usami C, Tsushima K (1972) An immunochemical study of the
     changes in chicken liver xanthine dehydrogenase activity during dietary adaptation. *J
     Biochem* 84: 19–26
53   Furth-Walker D, Amy NK (1987) Regulation of xanthine oxidase activity and immuno-
     logically detectable protein in rat in response to dietary protein and iron. *J Nutrition*
     117: 1697–1703
54   Poss WB, Huecksteadt TP, Panus PC, Freeman BA, Hoidal JR (1996) Regulation of xan-
     thine deydrogenase and xanthine oxidase activity by hypoxia. *Am J Physiol* 270:
     L941–L946

55 Terada LS, Piermattei D, Shibao GN, McManaman JL, Wright RM (1997) Hypoxia regulates xanthine dehydrogenase activity at pre- and posttranslational levels. *Arch Biochem Biophys* 348: 163–168

56 Nishino T, Usami C, Tsushima K (1983) Reversible interconversion between sulfo and desulfo xanthine oxidase in a system containing rhodanese, thiosulfate and sulfhydryl reagent. *Proc Natl Acad Sci USA* 80: 1826–1829

57 Nishino T (1986) Reversible interconversion between sulfo and desulfo xanthine oxidase. In: WL Nyham, LF Thompson, RWE Watts (eds): *Purine and pyrimidine metabolism in man.* Plenum Press, New York, 259–262

58 Coughlan MP (1981) Is protein function regulated by the reversible incorporation of sulphur? *Biochem Soc Trans* 9: 307–308

59 Fhaolain IN, Coughlan MP (1976) Turkey liver xanthine dehydrogenase. Relation between nicotinamide adenine dinucleotide oxidoreductase activity and the content of functional enzyme. *Biochem J* 157: 283–285

60 Nishino T, Nishino T, Schopfer LM, Massey V (1989) The reactivity of chicken liver xanthine dehydrogenase with molecular oxygen. *J Biol Chem* 264: 2518–2527

61 Nakamura M (1991) Allopurinol insensitive oxygen radical formation by milk xanthine oxidase systems. *J Biochem* 110: 450–456

62 Harrison R (1997) Human xanthine oxidase: in search of a function. *Biochem Soc Trans* 25: 786–791

63 Moorhouse PC, Grootveld M, Halliwell B, Quinlan JG, Gutteridge MCJ (1987) Allopurinol and oxypurinol are hydroxyl radical scavengers. *FEBS Lett* 213: 23–28

64 Werns SW, Grum CM, Ventura A, Hahn RA, Ho PPK, Towner RD, Fantone JC, Schork MA, Lucchesi BR (1991) Xanthine oxidase inhibition does not limit canine infarct size. *Circulation* 83: 995–1005

65 Okamoto K, Nishino T (1995) Mechanism of inhibition of xanthine oxidase with a new tight binding inhibitor. *J Biol Chem* 270: 7816–7821

66 Terada LS, Willingham IR, Guidot DM, Shibao GN, Kindt GW, Repine JE (1992) Tungsten treatment prevents tumour necrosis factor-induced injury of brain endothelial cells. *Inflammation* 16: 13–19

67 Stuehr DJ, Fasehum OA, Kwon NS, Gross SS, Gonzalez JA, Levi R, Nathan CF (1991) Inhibition of macrophage and endothelial cell nitric oxide synthase by diphenyleneiodonium and its analogs. *FASEB J* 5: 98–103

68 O'Donnell VB, Smith GCM, Jones OTG (1994) Involvement of phenyl radicals in iodonium inhibition of flavoenzymes. *Mol Pharmacol* 46: 778–785

69 Angermuller S, Bruder G, Volkl A, Wesch H, Fahimi HD (1987) Localization of xanthine oxidase in crystalline cores of peroxisomes. A cytochemical and biochemical study. *Eur J Cell Biol* 45: 137–144

70 Dikov VA, Alexandrov I, Roussinova A, Boyajieva-Michailova A (1988) Ultracytochemischer Nachweis von Enzymen durch Reduktion von Kalium hexacyanoferrat (III). I Eine Methode zum Nachweis der Xanthinoxidase. *Acta Histochem* 83: 107–115

71 Ichikawa M, Nishino T, Nishino T, Ichikawa A (1992) Subcellular localization of xan-

thine oxidase in rat hepatocytes. High resolution immunoelectron microscopic study combined with biochemical analysis. *J Histochem Cytochem* 40: 1097–1103

72   Adachi T, Fukushima T, Usami Y, Hirano K (1993) Binding of human xanthine oxidase to sulphated glycosaminoglycans on the endothelial cell surface. *Biochem J* 289: 523–527

73   Fukushima T, Adachi T, Hirano K (1995) The heparin-binding site of human xanthine oxidase. *Biol Pharm Bull* 18: 156–158

74   Radi R, Rubbo H, Bush K, Freeman BA (1997) Xanthine oxidase binding to glycosaminoglycans: kinetics and superoxide dismutase interactions of immobilized xanthine oxidase-heparin complexes. *Arch Biochem Biophys* 339: 125–135

75   Oster KA, Oster JB, Ross DJ (1974) Immune response to bovine xanthine oxidase in atherosclerotic patients. *Am Lab* 6: 41–47

76   Bruder G, Jarasch E-D, Heid HW (1984) High concentrations of antibodies to xanthine oxidase in human and animal sera. *J Clin Invest* 74: 783–794

77   Harrison R, Benboubetra M, Bryson S, Thomas RD, Elwood PC (1990) Antibodies to xanthine oxidase: elevated levels in patients with acute myocardial infarction. *Cardioscience* 1: 183–189

78   Lewis WHP, Ng YLE (1991) Human xanthine oxidase antibody levels: variation between males and females in Chinese and Europeans. *Med Lab Sci* 48: 84–88

79   Benboubetra M, Gleeson A, Harris CPD, Khan J, Arrar L, Brennand D, Reid J, Reckless JD, Harrison R (1997) Circulating anti-(xanthine oxidoreductase) antibodies in healthy human adults. *Eur J Clin Invest* 27: 611–619

80   Fridovich I, Handler P (1962) Differential inhibition of the reduction of various electron acceptors. *J Biol Chem* 237: 916–921

81   Hackenthal E, Hackenthal R (1966) Competitive inhibitors of nitrate reduction by xanthine oxidase. *Naturwissenschaften* 53: 81

82   Sergeev NS, Ananiadi LI, L'vov NP, Kretovich WL (1985) The nitrate reductase activity of milk xanthine oxidase. *J Appl Biochem* 7: 86–92

83   Zhang Z, Naughton DP, Blake DR, Benjamin N, Stevens CR, Winyard PG, Symons CR, Harrison R (1997) Human xanthine oxidase converts nitrite ions into nitric oxide. *Biochem Soc Trans* 25: 524S

84   Millar TM, Stevens CR, Blake DR (1997) Xanthine oxidase can generate nitric oxide from nitrate in ischaemia. *Biochem Soc Trans* 25: 528

85   Beckman JS, Koppenol WH (1996) Nitric oxide, superoxide and peroxynitrite: the good, the bad and the ugly. *Am J Physiol* 271: C1424–C1437

Inflammatory mediators, free radicals and gene transcription

Vanessa Gilston[1], David R. Blake[2] and Paul G. Winyard[1]

[1]Bone and Joint Research Unit, St. Bartholomew's and the Royal London School of Medicine and Dentistry, Queen Mary and Westfield College, University of London, 25–29 Ashfield Street, London E1 2AD, UK; [2]School of Postgraduate Medicine, University of Bath, Claverton Down, Bath BA2 7AY, UK

Introduction

A key feature of inflammatory diseases such as rheumatoid arthritis (RA) is the increased expression of certain genes which encode "inflammatory" proteins. These include a variety of adhesion molecules, as well as cytokines such as tumour necrosis factor α (TNFα) and interleukin-1 (IL-1). The proteinases involved in inflammatory tissue destruction include the metalloproteinases; collagenases, gelatinases and stromelysins. An important characteristic of gene expression is the control of gene transcription by specific proteins, transcription factors, which bind to short DNA sequence elements located adjacent to the promoter or in enhancer regions of genes. Once bound to DNA, transcription factors interact with each other and with the proteins of the transcriptional apparatus itself (e.g. RNA polymerase) to regulate gene expression. Recently, there has been considerable interest in the idea that transcription factors may be useful targets for novel therapeutic strategies in the treatment of human diseases, including inflammatory diseases [1].

Amongst the array of transcription factors which regulate inflammatory gene transcription, a number appear to be redox regulated. In particular, two transcription factors, activator protein-1 (AP-1) and NF-κB, can both be regulated by intracellular reactive oxygen intermediates (ROI) which contribute to the redox state of the cell [2, 3]. They have been implicated in the transcriptional regulation of a wide range of genes involved in cellular inflammatory responses and tissue destruction. Inappropriate activation, such as the overexpression of pro-inflammatory genes, may be involved in the progression of inflammatory diseases, such as RA. The activation of both AP-1 and NF-κB within the cell may be relevant to the dual proliferative/inflammatory response characteristic of rheumatoid synovitis, which has sometimes been referred to as "tumour-like proliferation" [4].

Certain "heat shock", or stress protein, transcription factors also appear to be influenced by ROI. In this case, ROI activity plays a critical role in regulating the

Free Radicals and Inflammation, edited by P. G. Winyard, D. R. Blake and C. H. Evans
© 2000 Birkhäuser Verlag Basel/Switzerland

transcription of genes that encode proteins able to act in a protective fashion, such as heat shock protein (hsp) 32, also known as haem oxygenase [5]. In addition, the expression of genes that modulate the activity of transcription factors may, in turn, be induced by oxidative stress. An example is gadd153 (a gene induced by growth arrest and DNA damage [6]) the murine product of which has been shown to bind to NF-IL6 (also known as C/EBPβ) and form a heterodimer that cannot bind to DNA [7].

The overproduction of ROI may, in part, be counteracted through the use of antioxidants. Nevertheless, it should be remembered that these processes, when properly controlled, are physiological. Therefore, both ROI and reactive nitrogen intermediates (RNI) can no longer be regarded solely as damaging species, whose complete elimination by antioxidant therapy is bound to have beneficial effects on human health. Thus far there is still no convincing evidence from the clinical studies conducted that supplementation with antioxidant nutrients can influence the process of on-going joint inflammation [8], although a small analgesic effect of vitamin E has been noted in RA patients [9]. As a result, recent studies have focused on specifically targeting transcription factors that may represent important targets for both existing and new antioxidant drugs and selective inhibitors of ROI-generating enzymes.

The redox regulation of NF-κB

As mentioned at the start of this review, the co-ordinated inflammatory response is linked to the increased transcription of a defined set of genes. Many of these "inflammatory genes" are target genes for NF-κB. Examples include genes encoding tumour necrosis factor α (TNFα), IL-1, IL-6, IL-8, the IL-2 receptor β chain, inducible nitric oxide synthase (iNOS), MHC class I antigens, E-selectin, vascular cell adhesion molecule-1, serum amyloid A precursor, c-Myc [10] and the H-chain of ferritin [11]. The DNA binding, nuclear form of NF-κB is a protein heterodimer made up of one Rel-A (p65) subunit and one p50 subunit. In non-stimulated cells, NF-κB exists in an inactive, cytosolic form bound to its inhibitor, IκB. Activators of NF-κB (such as TNFα, IL-1, phorbol esters, viruses, lipopolysaccharide, calcium ionophores, cycloheximide and ionising radiation) induce the dissociation of IκB from the NF-κB-IκB complex and positively charged nuclear location sequences (NLS) in Rel-A and p50 are unmasked. NF-κB is then translocated to the nucleus, where it controls gene expression. The events of NF-κB activation are summarised in Figure 1. The importance of ROI in the expression of the genes coding for these proteins has been highlighted by Baeuerle and colleagues [12]. They showed that NF-κB activity was induced by hydrogen peroxide in an human T cell line. This effect was blocked by the antioxidant N-acetylcysteine. Other more recently reported activators include oxidised LDL [13] and nitric oxide (endothelial-derived relaxing factor) [14] although the latter effect is disputed [15].

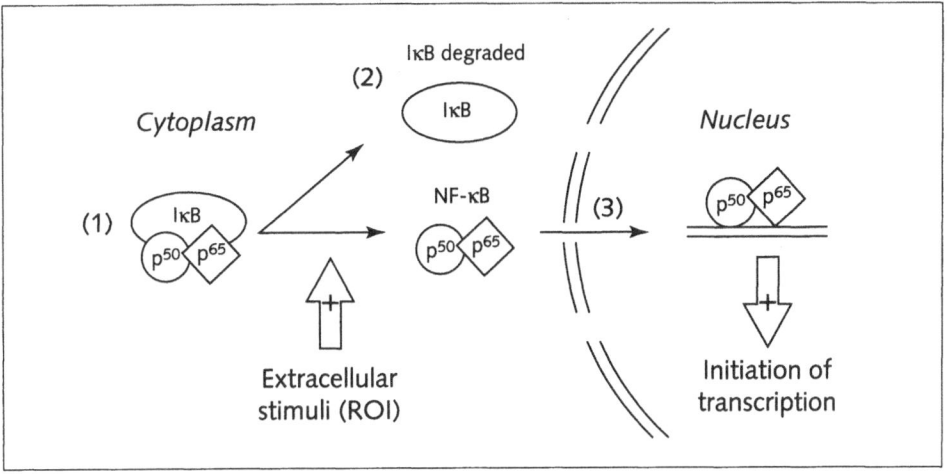

Figure 1
The activation of NF-κB
(1) Within the cell NF-κB exists in an inactive form bound to its inhibitory subunit, IκB.
(2) When the cell is challenged by extracellular stimuli (e.g. ROI) IκB is released and prote-
olytically degraded.
(3) The release of IκB "unmasks" the nuclear location sequence of NF-κB enabling it to
translocate to the nucleus and initiate transcription.

Not only N-acetylcysteine, but also other antioxidants such as pyrrolidine dithiocarbamate (PDTC), diethyl dithiocarbamate, 2-mercaptoethanol, ortho-phenanthroline and desferrioxamine inhibited the activation of NF-κB by the recognised stimuli of this transcription factor mentioned above. In addition, α-tocopherol was recently reported to suppress NF-κB activation [15]. However, some of the effects of α-tocopherol on cellular signalling may not be due solely, or at all, to an antioxidant effect, since α-tocopherol has been shown to inhibit protein kinase C activity via a mechanism that does not involve the antioxidant action of α-toco-pherol [16].

A further important control step in the activation of both AP-1 and NF-κB, appears to be the signal responsible for the DNA binding of these two transcription factors to their responsive element. In both cases it appears that the reduction of specific cysteine residues within the DNA recognition sites of AP-1 and NF-κB is an important regulatory signal for the induction of DNA binding [17–19]. One particular enzyme involved in this reduction is thioredoxin which is discussed by Okamoto and Tetsuka, this volume.

ROI and IκB kinases

In vivo, phosphorylation of IκB occurs when it is complexed with NF-κB, but dissociation and proteolytic degradation cannot occur without ubiquitination of the complex [20]. ROI appear to control IκB phosphorylation which may explain why NF-κB activation is blocked by a host of antioxidants. The precise mechanism by which ROI control the phosphorylation of IκB remains unclear. Experiments using specific inhibitors of different protease classes indicated that the intracellular proteinase activity responsible for the degradation of the phosphorylated form of the NF-κB-IκB complex was the 26S proteosome [10, 16, 21].

Chen and co-workers [22] were the first to report the identification of a kinase complex that specifically phosphorylated IκBα at the serine residues, S36 and S32. They showed that ubiquitination was required for the activation of the IκB kinase. More recently, several groups have purified a cytokine-activated protein kinase complex that also phosphorylates at these cysteine residues but has a slightly different molecular weight [23, 24]. ROI's may effect NF-κB activation by activating either an IκB kinase or an "NF-κB kinase" that phosphorylates the subunits of NF-κB directly and dissociates it from IκB [25]. ROI may also indirectly effect NF-κB activation by triggering a stress response within the cell. However, the precise location and mechanism of action remains unclear. Future studies should examine the intricate signalling pathways triggered by receptor-stimulus interaction to determine the role of ROI in the cascades preceding IκB kinase activation.

NF-κB activation by the enzymic generation of ROI/RNI

There are many potential sources of ROI/RNI which may be involved in inflammatory cell signalling. These include NADPH oxidase, cytochrome P450, nitric oxide synthases, cyclo-oxygenases and lipoxygenases, the mitochondrial respiratory chain and xanthine oxidase. Some of these systems have been discussed in earlier chapters, in the context of their radical-generating properties. It appears that the relative importance of different sources of ROI, and therefore the potential source of ROI involved in activating NF-κB, may be dependent on the type of cell and possibly the nature of the stimulus.

As discussed by Jones and Hancock, this volume, the plasma membrane bound NADPH oxidase of polymorphonuclear leucocytes (PMN's) contains cytochrome b_{245} and catalyses the univalent reduction of molecular oxygen to generate the superoxide anion radical, $O_2^{\cdot-}$ [26, 27]. In addition to phagocytic cells, other cell types such as lymphocytes [28] and glomerular mesangial cells [29] also possess a plasma membrane NADPH oxidase. For example, in glomerular mesangial cells, the NADPH oxidase inhibitor, 4'-hydroxy-3'-methoxy-acetophenone (apocynin) inhibited the activation of NF-κB in response to TNFα or aggregated IgG [29].

In contrast, aspirin (acetylsalicylic acid), a potent cyclooxygenase inhibitor, has been shown to block the activation of NF-κB in the human Jurkat T cell line, albeit at high concentrations [30] and also in TNFα stimulated human endothelial cells [31, 32]. However, certain other nonsteroidal anti-inflammatory drugs (NSAID) that exert their effects by inhibiting the cyclooxygenase activity of prostaglandin H synthase-1 (PGHS1) (e.g. indomethacin), did not block NF-κB activation [30, 33]. It has been demonstrated that a NSAID-insensitive peroxidase activity of PGHS1 exists that mediates NF-κB activation through an intracellular ROI signalling pathway, separable from its role in prostaglandin synthesis [33]. This may explain why certain non-selective cyclooxygenase inhibitors do not entirely suppress NF-κB activation.

Nitric oxide may also play a role, as Lander et al. [34] showed that NO˙ generating compounds such as S-nitroso-N-acetylpenicillamine (SNAP) induced the activation of NF-κB binding *in vitro* in human peripheral blood mononuclear cells. Furthermore, the transcription of the iNOS gene is itself induced by NF-κB [2, 35].

Recently, Los et al. [36] studied the activation of the CD28-responsive complex, which has been shown to consist of protein subunits of the NF-κB family, as a consequence of the triggering of the CD28 surface receptor of isolated human peripheral blood T lymphocytes. It was shown that the intracellular formation of ROI was a required step in this process. To identify the source of the ROI, the effects of inhibitors of the ROI-generating enzymes discussed above were tested. No significant effects were seen with the NADPH oxidase inhibitor, diphenylene iodonium, the respiratory chain inhibitor, rotenone, or the xanthine oxidase inhibitor, allopurinol. However, specific inhibitors of either 5-lipoxygenase (such as ICI 230487) or phospholipase A_2 (such as *p*-bromophenacyl bromide) prevented the activation of the NF-κB/CD28-responsive complex. These results are of particular interest, because the experiments were carried out in primary human cells. Many experiments which have been carried out in relation to the role of ROI/RNI as cellular messengers that induce gene expression, have been done in cell lines. In such cells, some signalling pathways may be redundant.

In contrast to the study by Los et al [36] experiments in the TNFα-sensitive, L929 fibrosarcoma cell line [37] showed that the activation of NF-κB by TNFα was blocked by rotenone, a specific inhibitor of the electron flow within the mitochondrial electron transport chain, which inhibits ROI generation. L929 subclones which lacked a functional respiratory chain were resistant to NF-κB activation by TNFα. These subclones were likewise resistant to the cytotoxicity of TNFα, which also appears to involve ROI production. In addition, whilst rotenone reduced TNFα cytotoxicity, inhibitors of two of the other potential ROI sources (xanthine oxidase and NADPH oxidase) had no effect [38].

A recent study has shown inhibition of ceramide mediated NF-κB activation as well as apoptosis by rotenone in U937 cells, implicating mitochondrial derived ROI's as early mediators of these events [39]. Likewise, mitochondrial respiratory chain uncoupling in isolated rat hepatocytes was associated with NF-κB activation [40]. Further studies are required in order to determine the importance of cell type, and stimulus, in determining the origin of ROI/RNI involved in NF-κB activation.

Inhibition of NF-κB by anti-inflammatory drugs

The anti-inflammatory action of several well-known drugs, including sodium salicylate [30, 31, 32] and gold(I) thiolate compounds such as aurothioglucose [41] (see Okamoto and Tetsuka, this volume), has been suggested to be due to the inhibition of NF-κB activation. The DNA-binding activity of NF-κB is thought to be Zn^{2+}-dependent. Yang et al. [41] suggested that cysteine residues may be involved in the binding of Zn^{2+}. Thus, in the case of aurothioglucose, it was proposed that Au(I) oxidises the Zn^{2+}-associated thiolate anions to disulphides, thereby preventing the binding of NF-κB to DNA.

It has also recently been suggested that glucocorticoids exert their immunosuppressive activity by inducing the synthesis of IκB [42, 43], which blocks the NF-κB-mediated expression of the genes described above. Another mechanism which may contribute to immunosuppression is the direct interaction of the glucocorticoid-receptor complex with NF-κB, thereby preventing its association with DNA (see [42, 43]). For example, Kleinert et al. [44] have recently shown that glucocorticoids can inhibit the induction of inducible nitric oxide synthase (iNOS) in the human epithelial cell line A549/8 cells by down-regulating cytokine-induced activity of NF-κB. This suggested that the activated glucocorticoid receptor prevents the binding of NF-κB to the iNOS promoter thereby inhibiting the induction of iNOS transcription. Glucocorticoids may, therefore, exert their anti-inflammatory effects by blocking the increased NO production associated with inflammatory conditions such as RA [45].

NF-κB has also been shown to interact with the oestrogen receptor [46]. This receptor physically interacts with NF-κB and another transcription factor, C/EBPß (NF-IL6). Both NF-κB and C/EBPβ regulate IL-6 gene expression in human osteoblasts. Their interaction with the oestrogen receptor results in inhibition of the IL-6 promoter. This oestrogen effect may be involved in the bone resorption associated with osteoporosis (the most common form is postmenopausal in women) and, possibly, in the marked preponderance of RA in females.

The redox regulation of AP-1

Activator protein-1 (AP-1) is a protein dimer composed of the proto-oncogene products, Fos and Jun. mRNA levels for c-*fos* and c-*jun* are strongly induced in response to hydrogen peroxide and other oxidative stresses such as ultraviolet light and ionising radiation, in both fibroblasts and T cells [47]. In contrast, AP-1 binding activity is only weakly induced by hydrogen peroxide [48]. Treatment with antioxidants such as pyrrolidine dithiocarbamate activates AP-1 and it has been suggested that the AP-1 DNA binding site is an antioxidant response element [48].

The matrix metalloproteinases (MMP's), collagenase and stromelysin, are thought to play a key part in cartilage destruction and inactivation of proteinase inhibitors in inflammatory joint disease [49, 50] and possibly in atherosclerosis [51]. The AP-1 site, also referred to as the tetradeconyl phorbol acetate responsive element (TRE) is found in various genes, including those encoding human collagenase, stromelysin, transforming growth factors (TGFs) α and β, IL-2 and tissue inhibitor of metalloproteinases-1 (TIMP-1) [52]. In fact, the AP-1 site is a necessary, but not sufficient, element for the transcription of MMPs [53]. Several other elements are also required for maximal transcription rates, such as the recognition motif for the transcription factor, PEA-3, and the sequence 5'-TTCA-3' [54]. TGFβ induces the expression of collagen type I and III genes, down-regulates collagenase production and induces TIMP-1 – an inhibitor of stromelysin and collagenase [55].

Transcription factor activation in rheumatoid arthritis and osteoarthritis

The inflamed rheumatoid joint serves as a good example of chronic inflammation. Typically cells of the synovial tissue within the inflamed knee-joint proliferate (for example, fibroblast-like cells also known as "type B synoviocytes"), and the tissue is infiltrated by other cells (such as lymphocytes) which are characteristic of a chronic inflammatory response. Osteoarthritis (OA) is considered to be a "non-inflammatory" joint disease, although some degree of inflammation is often present.

An immunohistochemical and *in situ* hybridisation study of synovial tissue from RA patients showed numerous cells expressing *jun*-B and c-*fos* (the genes encoding AP-1 subunits) [56]. These positive cells were within the lining layer and diffuse infiltrates of the synovial membrane. They were identified as fibroblast-like, using cell-specific markers. Expression of *jun*-B/c-*fos* was not detected in lymphocytes or macrophage-like cells, whilst the number of cells which were positive was considerably smaller in osteoarthritis and healthy control synovia. The spontaneous expression of c-*fos* and other proto-oncogenes in rheumatoid synovial cells has been reviewed [57]. The cellular distribution of Jun/Fos within the rheumatoid synovium contrasts with that seen for the p50 and p65 subunits of NF-κB in a recent immunohistochemical study by Handel et al. [58]. These authors found that p50/p65 was present in the nuclei of macrophage-like cells of the synovial lining and sublining areas, as well as in endothelial cells. There was little staining in normal control synovium. The contrast in subunit distribution highlights the importance of cell type specific signalling and gene expression.

We have used antibodies specific for the DNA binding, nuclear form of NF-κB to perform immunohistochemical studies in the synovium of RA and OA patients [59]. The basis of such "activity specific" antibodies is that they were raised against the NLS of Rel-A. Binding of IκB to the p50-Rel-A heterodimer sterically masks the NLS ([60], see also above). In agreement with Handel et al. [58] we found that in the synovium of RA patients, both vascular endothelial cells and macrophage-like cells showed the presence of the activated form of NF-κB. Again, staining was nuclear – as would be expected – and synovial tissue from controls exhibited either no staining or only weak staining. We also found that the relative amounts of staining in these two cell types was dependent on the chronicity of the disease. Interestingly, we recently observed positive staining for NF-κB in patients with "early synovitis" (joint inflammation of < 6 months) [61]. Staining was predominantly located within the microvasculature with only relatively weak staining observed in the lining layer.

Staining for activated NF-κB in the synovium of RA patients was not associated with lymphocyte aggregates. This result is consistent with previous observations of an apparent lack of recent activation of T lymphocytes within the rheumatoid synovium. Thus, whilst synovial T cells have been implicated in the pathology of RA, T cell derived cytokines and other markers of recent T cell activation such as the IL-2 receptor have only been demonstrated at low levels in the rheumatoid joint [62].

Recently, Crofford and co-workers [63] have shown NF-κB to be involved in the regulation of COX-2 expression in rheumatoid synoviocytes induced by IL-1β. Early passage rheumatoid synoviocytes were treated with IL-1β and DNA binding of NF-κB to the COX-2 promoter/enhancer was examined by electrophoretic mobility shift assay (EMSA). Supershift assays using antibodies raised against specific subunits of the NF-κB family members, revealed the activation of the p50-p65 heterodimer. Pretreatment of rheumatoid synoviocytes with NF-κB p65 antisense oligonucleotides resulted in decreased binding to the COX-2 promoter and decreased COX-2 protein expression as analysed by western blotting [63]. This data demonstrated that signalling via the NF-κB pathway is involved in the regulation of COX-2 expression induced by IL-1β in RA synoviocytes.

Tsao et al. [64] have recently investigated the activation of NF-κB in the rat adjuvant arthritis model in a 28-day time-course experiment using immunohistochemistry. Using an antibody raised against the NLS of the Rel-A (p65) subunit of NF-κB, staining was detected in the synovial lining layer and around blood vessels in the inflamed synovium as early as day 3 post adjuvant injection. The cells that expressed p65 in the synovial lining were thought to be macrophage-like synoviocytes. Dexamethasone treatment at 1 mg/kg (days 0–20) suppressed both the hindpaw oedema and the increase in p65 expression [64]. This is consistent with the fact that that the anti-inflammatory action of dexamethasone may be through inhibition of NF-κB activation [65].

Anderson et al. [66] have shown an increased expression of COX-2 mRNA in rat adjuvant arthritis, and TNFα and IL-1 levels were also increased. Since Tsao's group [64] observed an increased activation of NF-κB in this animal model, it would be interesting to speculate that NF-κB may be mediating COX-2 expression in this model of inflammation as is shown to be the case in the human synovium [63], an hypothesis that is yet to be explored.

It has also recently been shown that there is an increase in the expression of COX-2 as well as inducible nitric oxide synthase (iNOS) in rats injected with lipopolysaccharide (LPS) [67]. When these LPS-treated animals were then treated with calpain inhibitor-1, an inhibitor of the proteolysis of IκB, iNOS and COX-2 expression was attenuated. As both iNOS and COX-2 lead to the production of NO˙ and prostaglandins synthesis respectively, the prevention of the activation of NF-κB *in vivo* may be useful in the therapy of disorders associated with local or systemic inflammation.

Recently, we have screened a panel of bone resorptive stimuli for their ability to activate NF-κB in human osteoblastic cells [68]. Using the electrophoretic mobility shift assay (EMSA), we demonstrated dose- and time-related increases in NF-κB-DNA binding in cells treated with the structurally unrelated bone resorptive agents, TNFα, IL-1β and parathyroid hormone. In contrast, 1,25-dihydroxyvitamin D_3 produced no effect on NF-κB activation at any dose or time period studied. This is consistent with the previously reported lack of effect of steroid hormones, including 1,25-dihydroxyvitamin D_3, on the human osteoblast cell line, Saos-2. Based on these results we suggested that activation of NF-κB in osteoblastic cells may constitute an important pathway in the progression of pathological bone loss.

NF-κB has also been shown to play a role in upregulating NO˙, in human OA-affected cartilage [69]. In *ex vivo* experiments, spontaneous NO˙ accumulation by OA cartilage was observed, which could be inhibited by > 90% by the NF-κB inhibitor PDTC (see above). This indicated that NF-κB may, in part, regulate NOS activity where NO˙ synthesis contributes to chondrocyte dysfunction and damage to cartilage integrity [69].

Apoptosis, nitric oxide and NF-κB

A theme of this chapter, and indeed this book, is the increasing recognition of the cellular control aspects of free radical action. Endothelium-derived relaxing factor (EDRF) has been identified as NO˙ (reviewed in [70]). Moreover, ROI can activate apoptosis, a programmed form of cell death, at least in some circumstances [71]. Many studies have now begun to focus on the importance of NF-κB in the apoptotic pathway.

NF-κB has been reported not only to mediate apoptosis [72], but also to block apoptotic cell death in response to a variety of stimuli, including exposure to TNFα

[73, 74]. Goodman and Mattson [75] have extended this NF-κB protection paradigm, showing that a TNFα ceramide pathway (which suppresses ROI) protects neurones from excitotoxic damage. The explanation for these conflicting findings may be that the different subunit components comprising NF-κB family members control the delicate balance between apoptosis and cell survival, or it may be possible that the same dimers have opposing effects in disparate cell types or with different stimuli [10]. At present the precise role for NF-κB in the paradox of "anti-apoptotic" versus "pro-apoptotic" remains unclear.

Interestingly, NO˙ has been shown to inhibit Fas-induced apoptosis in human leucocytes [76] suggesting that Fas activity is regulated by the NO˙ signalling pathway. This, in turn, suggests a new role for NO˙ in the human immune response. One could speculate that the inhibition of Fas-mediated apoptosis by NO˙ may be regulated by the activation of NF-κB. Since certain forms of NOS have been shown to contain the NF-κB binding site within their promoter region (see above), NO˙ production may be facilitated by way of NF-κB-DNA binding in some cell types. This hypothesis would then be consistent with a protective role of NF-κB in the apoptotic pathway. The role of nitric oxide in the apoptotic pathway is further examined in the chapter by Bombeck et al., this volume.

Conclusion

The cellular signalling events leading to NF-κB activation may be initiated by a wide variety of receptor-stimulus interactions. The environment associated with a particular cell type may also influence the nature of the signalling cascades that precede NF-κB activation, where the ultimate event is IκB phosphorylation. Certain cytokines, such as TNFα and IL-1β, have been shown to stimulate ROI production in the signalling events that lead to NF-κB activation [37], so even if the initial cellular stimulus for NF-κB activation is not a ROI, the apparent merging of all the pathways of signal transduction involving NF-κB on a ROI-dependent step suggests a possible therapeutic target.

The reducing systems that exist within the cell are presumably as important in redox-regulated transcriptional events as those contributing to oxidative stress. NF-κB is reduced by the cellular reducing catalyst, thioredoxin which is important for the binding of NF-κB to DNA [77]. Therefore, the redox balance within the cell plays a key role in events which both precede and follow, the dissociation of IκB from NF-κB. Okamoto and Tetsuka discuss further the roles of thioredoxin in inflammatory diseases later in this volume.

The redox state of the cell also needs to be delicately balanced so as not to perturb the physiological function of the transcription factor AP-1. The expression of c-jun/c-fos genes, whose protein products form the AP-1 heterodimer, is also required for the transcription of matrix metalloproteinases (MMPs) [53], that may lead to cartilage destruction and the inactivation of proteinase inhibitors in inflammatory diseases [54]. The induction of MMPs in the chondrocytes of cartilage is examined by Lo et al., this volume.

This chapter has introduced new and exciting areas of study that examine the signalling cascades and consequent responses in inflammatory disease. The following chapters review these events in more detail, revealing insights into potential new drug targets.

References

1   Lee JI, Burckart GJ (1998) Nuclear factor kappa B: Important transcription factor and therapeutic target. *J Clin Pharmacol* 38: 981–993

2   Baeuerle PA, Henkel T (1994) Function and activation of NFκB in the immune system. *Annu Rev Immunol* 12: 141–179

3   Blake DR, Winyard PG, Marok R (1994) The contribution of hypoxia-reperfusion injury to inflammatory synovitis: the influence of reactive oxygen intermediates on the transcriptional control of inflammation. *NY Acad Sci* 723: 308–317

4   Fassbender HG (1984) Current understanding of rheumatoid arthritis. *Inflammation* 8: (Suppl), S27–S42

5   Keyse SM, Tyrrell RM (1990) Induction of the heme oxygenase gene in human skin fibroblasts by hydrogen peroxide and UVA (365nm) radiation: Evidence for the involvement of the hydroxyl radical. *Carcinogenesis* 11: 787–791

6   Fornace AJ, Nerbert DW, Hollander MC, Luethy JD, Papathanasiou M, Fargnoli J, Holbrook NJ (1989) Mammalian genes coordinately regulated by growth arrest signals and DNA-damaging agents. *Mol Cell Biol* 9: 4196–4203

7   Ron D, Habner JF (1992) CHOP, a novel developmentally regulated nuclear protein that dimerises with transcription factors C/EBP and LAP and functions as a dominant-negative inhibitor of gene transcription. *Genes Dev* 6: 439–453

8   Kus ML, Fairburn K, Blake DR, Winyard PG (1995) A vascular basis for free radical involvement in inflammatory joint disease. In: DR Blake, PG Winyard (eds): *Immunopharmacology of free radical species*. Academic Press, London, 97–112

9   Edmonds SE, Winyard PG, Guo R, Kidd B, Merry P, Langrish-Smith A, Hansen C, Ramm S, Blake DR (1997) Putative analgesic activity of repeated oral doses of vitamin E in the treatment of rheumatoid arthritis. Results of a prospective placebo controlled double blind trial. *Ann Rheum Dis* 56: 649–655

10   Baeuerle PA, Baichwal VR (1998) NF-κB as a frequent target for immunosuppressive and anti-inflammatory molecules. *Adv Immunol* 65: 111–137

11   Kwak EL, Larochelles DA, Beaumont C, Torti SV, Torti FM (1995) Role for NF-κB in the regulation of ferritin H by tumour necrosis factor-α. *J Biol Chem* 270: 15285–15293

12   Schreck R, Rieber P, Baeuerle PA (1991) Reactive oxygen intermediates as apparently

widely used messengers in the activation of the NF-κB transcription factor and HIV-1. *EMBO J* 10: 2247–2258

13 Liao F, Andalibi A, deBeer FC, Fogelman AM, Lusis AJ (1993) Genetic control of inflammatory gene induction and NF-κB like transcription factor activation in response to an atherogenic diet in mice. *J Clin Invest* 91: 2572–2579

14 Lander HM, Sehajpal P, Levine DM, Novogrodsky A (1993) Activation of human peripheral blood mononuclear cells by nitric oxide-generating compounds. *J Immunol* 150: 1509–1516

15 Schreck R, Albermann K, Baeuerle PA (1992) Nuclear factor κB: an oxidative stress-responsive transcription factor of eukaryotic cells (a review). *Free Rad Res Comm* 17: 221–237

16 Traenckner EB-M, Wilk S, Baeuerle PA (1994) A proteosome inhibitor prevents activation of NF-κB and stabilises a newly phosphorylated form of IκB that is still bound to NF-κB. *EMBO J* 13: 5433–5441

17 Gilston V, Blake DR, Winyard PG (1997) The rheumatoid joint: Redox paradox? In: L Montagnier, R Olivier, C Pasquier (eds): *Oxidative stress in cancer, aids, and neurodegenerative diseases*. Marcel Dekker Inc., New York, 49: 517–535

18 Xanthoudakis S, Miao G, Wang F, Yu ching E. Pan, Curran T (1992) Redox activation of Fos and Jun DNA binding activity is mediated by a DNA repair enzyme. *EMBO J* 11: 3323–3335

19 Matthews JR, Waksasugi N, Virelizier JL, Yodoi J, Hay RT (1992) Thioredoxin regulates the DNA binding activity of NF-κB by a reduction of a disulphide bond involving cysteine 62. *Nucleic Acids Res* 20: 3821–3830

20 Mercurio F, Manning AM (1999) Multiple signals converging on NF-κB. *Curr Op Cell Biol* 11: 226–232

21 Brown K, Gerstberger S, Carlson L, Franzoso G, Siebenlist U (1995) Control of IκB-α proteolysis by site-specific, signal-induced phosphorylation. *Science* 267: 1485–1488

22 Chen JZ, Parent L, Maniatis T (1996) Site-specific phosphorylation of IκB-α by a novel ubiquitination-dependent protein kinase activity. *Cell* 84: 853–862

23 DiDonato JA, Hayakawa M, Rothwarf DM, Zandi E, Karin M (1997) A cytokine-responsive IκB kinase that activates the transcription factor NF-κB. *Nature* 388: 548–554

24 Mercurio F, Zhu H, Murray BW, Shevchenko A, Bennett B, Li J, Young DB, Barbosa M, Mann M, Manning A, Rao A (1997) IKK-1 and IKK-2: cytokine activated IkappaB kinases essential for NF-kappaB activation. *Science* 281: 860–866

25 Hayashi T, Ueno Y, Okamoto T (1993) Oxidoreductive regulation of nuclear factor κB: involvement of a cellular reducing catalyst thioredoxin. *J Biol Chem* 268: 11380–11388

26 Forman HJ, Thomas MJ (1986) Oxidant production and bactericidal activity of phagocytes. *Annu Rev Physiol* 48: 669–680

27 Segal AW (1991) Components of the microbicidal oxidase of phagocytes. *Biochem Soc Trans* 49: 49–50

28 Hancock JT, Maly FE, Jones OTG (1989) Properties of the superoxide-generating oxi-

dase of B-lymphocyte cell lines. Determination of Michaelis parameters. *Biochem J* 262: 373–375

29   Satriano J, Schlondorff D (1994) Activation and attenuation of transcription factor NF-κB in mouse glomerular mesangial cells in response to tumor-necrosis-factor-alpha, immunoglobulin G, and adenosine 3'/5'-cyclic monophosphate – evidence for involvement of reactive oxygen species. *J Clin Invest* 94: 1629–1636

30   Kopp E, Ghosh S (1994). Inhibition of NF-κB by sodium salicylate and aspirin. *Science* 265: 956–959

31   Weber C, Erl W, Pietsch A, Weber PC (1995) Aspirin inhibits nuclear factor-kappa B mobilisation and monocyte adhesion in stimulated human endothelial cells. *Circulation* 91: 1914–1917

32   Pierce JW, Read MA, Ding H, Luscinskas FW, Collins T (1996) Salicylates inhibit IκB phosphorylation, endothelial-leukocyte adhesion molecule expression, and neutrophil transmigration. *J Immunol* 156: 3961–3969

33   Munroe DG, Wang EY, MacIntyre JP, Tam SC, Lee DHS, Taylor GR, Zhou L, Plante RK, Kazmi SMI, Baeuerle PA, Lau CY (1995) Novel intracellular signalling function of prostaglandin H synthase-1 in NF-κB activation. *J Inflammation* 45: 260–268

34   Lander HM, Sehajpal P, Levine DM, Novogrodsky A (1993) Activation of human peripheral blood mononuclear cells by nitric oxide generating compounds. *J Immunol* 150: 1509–1516

35   Barnes PJ (1995) Anti-inflammatory mechanisms of glucocorticoids. *Biochem Soc Trans* 23: 940–945

36   Los M, Schenk H, Hexel K, Baeuerle PA, Droge W, Schulze-Osthoff, K (1995) IL-2 gene expression and NF-κB activation through CD28 requires reactive oxygen production by 5-lipoxygenase. *EMBO J* 14: 3731–3740

37   Schulze-Osthoff K, Beyaert R, Vandevoorde V, Haegeman G, Fiers W (1993) Depletion of the mitochondrial electron transport abrogates the cytotoxic and gene-inductive effects of TNF. *EMBO J* 12: 3095–3104

38   Schulze-Osthoff K, Akker AC, Vanhaesebroeck B, Beyaert R, Jacob WA, Fiers W (1992) Cytotoxic activity of tumor necrosis factor is mediated by early damage of mitochondrial functions. Evidence for the involvement of mitochondrial radical generation. *J Biol Chem* 267: 5317–5323

39   Quillet-Mary A, Jaffrezou JP, Mansat V, Bordier C, Naval J, Laurent G (1997) Implication of mitochondrial hydrogen peroxide generation in ceramide-induced apoptosis. *J Biol Chem* 272: 21388–21395

40   Garciaruiz C, Colell A, Morales A, Kaplowitz N (1993) Role of oxidative stress generated from the mitochondrial electron-transport chain and mitochondrial glutathione status in loss of mitochondrial-function and activation of transcription factor nuclear factor-kappa-B – studies with isolated mitochondria and rat hepatocytes. *Mol Pharmacol* 48: 825–834

41   Yang JP, Merin JP, Nakano T, Kato T, Kitade Y, Okamoto T (1995) Inhibition of the DNA-binding activity of NF-κB by gold compounds *in vitro*. *FEBS Lett* 361: 89–96

42   Scheinman RI, Cogswell PC, Lofquist AK, Baldwin AS (1995) Role of transcriptional activation of IκB-α in mediation of immunosuppression by glucocorticoids. *Science* 270: 283–286

43   Auphan N, DiDonato JA, Rosette C, Helmberg A, Karin M (1995) Immunosuppression by glucocorticoids: inhibition of NF-κB activity through induction of IκB synthesis. *Science* 270: 286–29

44   Kleinert H, Euchenhofer C, Ihrig-Biedert I, Forstermann U (1996) Glucocorticoids inhibit the induction of nitric oxide synthase II by down-regulating cytokine induced activity of transcription factor nuclear factor-kappa B. *Mol Pharmacol* 49: 15–21

45   Farrell AJ, Blake DR, Palmer RM, Moncada S (1992) Increased concentrations of nitrite in synovial fluid and serum samples suggest increased nitric oxide synthesis in rheumatic diseases. *Ann Rheum Dis* 51: 1219–1222

46   Stein B, Yang MX (1995) Repression of the interleukin-6 promoter by estrogen receptor is mediated by NF-κB and C/EBPβ. *Mol Cell Biol* 15: 4971–4979

47   Amstad PA, Krupitza G, Cerutti PA (1992) Mechanism of c-fos induction by active oxygen. *Cancer Res* 52: 3952–3960

48   Meyer MR, Schreck R, Baeuerle PA (1993) Hydrogen peroxide and antioxidants have opposite effects on activation of NF-κB and AP-1 in intact cells: AP-1 as secondary antioxidant-responsive factor. *EMBO J* 12: 2005–2015

49   Gravallese EM, Darling JM, Ladd AL, Katz JN, Glimcher LH (1991) *In situ* hybridization studies of stromelysin and collagenase messenger RNA expression in rheumatoid synovium. *Arthritis Rheum* 34: 1076–1084

50   Winyard PG, Zhang Z, Chidwick K, Blake DR, Carrell RW, Murphy G (1991) Proteolytic inactivation of human α₁ antitrypsin by human stromelysin. *FEBS Lett* 279: 91–94

51   Henney AM, Wakeley PR, Davies MJ, Foster K, Hembry R, Murphy G, Humphries S (1991) Localization of stromelysin gene expression in atherosclerotic plaques by *in situ* hybridization. *Proc Natl Acad Sci USA* 88: 8154–8158

52   Karin M (1991) The AP-1 complex and its role in transcriptional control by protein kinase C. In: P Cohen P, JG Foulkes (eds): *Molecular aspects of cellular regulation. Vol 6: The hormonal control of gene transcription*. Elsevier, Amsterdam 235–253

53   Matrisian LM (1990) Metalloproteinases and their inhibitors in matrix remodelling. *Trends in Genet* 6: 121–125

54   Auble DT, Brinckerhoff CE (1991) The AP-1 sequence is necessary but not sufficient for phorbol induction of collagenase in fibroblasts. *Biochemistry* 30: 4629–4635

55   Edwards DR, Murphy G, Reynolds JJ, Whitlam SE, Docherty AJP, Angel P, Heath JK (1987) Transforming growth factor beta modulates the expression of collagenase and metalloproteinase inhibitor. *EMBO J* 6: 1899–1904

56   Kinne RW, Boehm S, Iftner T, Aigner T, Vornehm S, Weseloh G, Bravo R, Emmrich F, Kroczek RA (1995) Synovial fibroblast-like cells strongly express *jun*-B and c-*fos* protooncogenes in rheumatoid- and osteoarthritis. *Scand J Rheumatol* 24 (Suppl 101): 121–125

57   Gay S, Gay RE, Koopman WJ (1993) Molecular and cellular mechanisms of joint destruction in rheumatoid arthritis: two cellular mechanisms explain joint destruction? *Ann Rheum Dis* 52: S39–S47

58   Handel ML, McMorrow LB, Gravallese EM (1995) Nuclear factor-κB in rheumatoid synovium. Localisation of p50 and p65. *Arthritis Rheum* 38: 1762–1770

59   Marok R, Winyard PG, Coumbe A, Kus ML, Gaffney K, Mapp PI, Blades S, Morris CJ, Blake DR, Kaltschmidt C, Baeuerle PA (1996) Activation of the transcription factor NF-κB in the inflamed human synovium. *Arthritis Rheum* 39: 583–591

60   Kaltschmidt C, Kaltschmidt B, Henkel T, Stockinger H, Baeuerle PA (1995) Selective recognition of the activated form of transcription factor NF-κB by a monoclonal antibody. *Biol Chem Hoppe-Seyler* 376: 9–16

61   Gilston V, Jones HW, Soo CC, Coumbe, Blades S, Kaltschmidt C, Baeuerle PA, Morris CJ, Blake DR, Winyard PG (1997) NF-kappa B activation in human knee-joint synovial tissue during the early stage of joint inflammation. *Biochem Soc Trans* 25: 518S

62   Salmon M, Gaston JSH (1995) The role of T-lymphocytes in rheumatoid arthritis. *Br Med Bull* 51: 332–345

63   Crofford LJ, McCarthy IB, Hla T (1997) Involvement of nuclear factor κB in the regulation of cyclooxygenase-2 expression by IL-1 in rheumatoid synoviocytes. *Arthritis Rheum* 40: 226–236

64   Tsao PW, Suzuki T, Totsuka R, Murata T, Takagi T, Ohmachi Y, Fujimura H, Takata I (1997) The effect of dexamethasone on the expression of activated NF-κB in adjuvant arthritis. *Clin Immunol Immunopathol* 83: 173–178

65   Ray A, Prefontaine KE (1994) Physical association and functional antagonism between the p65 subunit of transcription factor NF-kappa B and the glucocorticoid receptor. *Proc Natl Acad Sci USA* 91: 752–756

66   Anderson GD, Hauser SD, McGarity KL, Bremer ME, Isakson PC, Gregory SA (1996) Selective inhibition of cyclooxygenase (COX)-2 reverses inflammation and expression of COX-2 and interleukin 6 in rat adjuvant arthritis. *J Clin Invest* 97: 2672–2679

67   Reutten H, Thiemermann C (1997) Effect of calpain inhibitor I, an inhibitor of the proteolysis of I kappa B, on the circulatory failure and multiple organ dysfunction caused by endotoxin in the rat. *Br J Pharmacol* 121: 695–704

68   Gilston V (1999) NF-κB activation, antioxidants and inflammation. PhD Thesis, University of London

69   Amin AR, Di Cesare PE, Vyas P, Attur M, Tzeng E, Billiar R, Stuchin SA, Abramson SB (1995) The expression and regulation of nitric oxide synthase in human osteoarthritis-affected chondrocytes: Evidence for up-regulated neuronal nitric oxide synthase. *J Exp Med* 182: 2097–2102

70   Synder SH (1995) No endothelial NO. *Nature* 377: 196–197

71   Jacobson MD (1996) Reactive oxygen species and programmed cell death. *TIBS* 21: 83–86

72   Grilli M, Pizzi M, Memo M, Spano P (1996) Neuroprotection by aspirin and sodium salicylate through blockade of NF-κB activation. *Science* 274: 1383–1385

73 Beg AA, Baltimore D (1996) An essential role for NF-κB in preventing TNF-α-induced cell death. *Science* 274: 782–784

74 Wang C-Y, Mayo MW, Baldwin AS (1996) TNF-α and cancer therapy-induced apoptosis potentiation by inhibition of NF-κB. *Science* 274: 784–787

75 Goodman Y, Mattson MP (1996) Ceramide protects hippocampal neurones against excitotoxic and oxidative insults, and amyloid β-peptide toxicity. *J Neurochem* 66: 869–872

76 Mannick JB, Miao XQ, Stamler JS (1997) Nitric oxide inhibits Fas-induced apoptosis. *J Biol Chem* 272: 24125–24128

77 Okamoto T, Ogiwara H, Hayashi T, Mitsui A, Kawabe T, Yodoi J (1992) Human thioredoxin/adult T cell leukemia-derived factor activates the enhancer binding protein of human immunodeficiency virus type 1 by thiol redox control mechanism. *Int Immunol* 4: 811–819

Reactive metabolites of oxygen and nitrogen, adhesion molecule expression and chronic joint inflammation

Matthew B. Grisham[1] and Robert E. Wolf[2]

Departments of [1]Molecular and Cellular Physiology and [2]Medicine, Louisiana State University Medical Center, 1501 Kings Highway, P.O. Box 33932, Shreveport, LA 71130-3932, USA

Introduction

One of the hallmark features of rheumatoid arthritis (RA) is the infiltration of large numbers of mononuclear leukocytes (monocytes, lymphocytes) into the inflamed synovium. In addition, extensive polymorphonuclear leukocyte (neutrophil) infiltration is observed in synovial fluid. This inflammatory infiltrate is accompanied by extensive articular damage including cartilage and bone erosion, edema and enhanced vascular permeability suggesting an important role for these leukocytes in the pathophysiology of RA. Recent studies have demonstrated that the enhanced leukocyte infiltrate and some of the pathophysiology observed in different models of synovitis and in human RA may be mediated by the interaction between leukocytes and specific endothelial cell adhesion molecules (ECAMs) [1–6]. These observations have prompted us to propose that the synovial microvasculature regulates chronic joint inflammation by virtue of its ability to modulate the infiltration of immune-modulating and/or potentially injurious leukocytes into the synovial interstitium. Indeed, one of the earliest histopathological events observed in the development of RA is activation and/or injury to the endothelial cell lining of the synovial microvasculature [7–9]. This discussion will review the data implicating ECAMs as important determinants in the pathogenesis of RA and discuss the molecular mechanisms that regulate ECAM expression in the chronically inflamed joint, and indicate the roles of oxygen- and nitrogen-derived free radicals in these processes.

Role of cytokines in the pathogenesis of RA

The etiology of RA remains undefined, however, it is thought that the initiation and pathogenesis of this disease is multi-factorial, involving interactions among genetic, immune and possibly infectious agents [9–11]. Indeed, there is a growing body of experimental and clinical evidence to suggest an immune-mediated pathogenesis of RA.

The first step in the immune response to antigen is the uptake and processing of the antigen by macrophages and/or other antigen presenting cells. Antigen recognition by T lymphocytes activates these cells to synthesize and release interleukin-2 (IL-2) and interferon γ (IFNγ). IL-2 promotes the clonal expansion of cytotoxic T cells and enhances the function of helper T cells and B cells, whereas IFNγ activates macrophages and enhances ECAM expression on endothelial cells. Activated macrophages produce large amounts of tumor necrosis factor α (TNFα), IL-1, IL-6 and IL-8, all of which are thought to be important in initiating and/or promoting the inflammatory response via activation of PMNs and macrophages as well as enhancing ECAM expression. Indeed, RA is associated with the local overproduction of many of the proinflammatory cytokines [12, 13]. The importance of cytokines as mediators of chronic joint inflammation can be seen in clinical studies where investigators have demonstrated that administration of IL-1 receptor antagonist or antibodies specific for T helper cell 1 (Th1)- and macrophage-derived cytokines such as TNF attenuate the chronic joint inflammation observed in different animal models of synovitis as well as human RA (14,15). It is well known that one mechanism by which certain cytokines initiate and/or perpetuate inflammation is via their ability to upregulate surface expression of certain ECAMs.

Leukocyte/endothelial cell interactions

Leukocyte adhesion to microvascular endothelium involves a complex sequence of interactions between circulating leukocytes and vascular endothelial cells (Fig. 1). The initial event is believed to be a weak adhesive interaction which results in leukocytes "rolling" along the endothelium. Subsequently, there is a strengthening of these adhesive forces, such that the leukocytes become firmly attached to the endothelium and remain stationary. Finally, the leukocytes begin to change shape, send pseudopodia between endothelial cells, and extravasate into the interstitium. These adhesive interactions are regulated in an orderly fashion by sequential activation of different families of membrane adherence receptors on leukocytes and endothelial cells. Although much of our current understanding of leukocyte-endothelial cell interactions has come from studies describing PMN/endothelial cell interactions, more recent data suggest a very similar, multi-step process for monocyte- or lymphocyte-endothelial cell interactions both of which involve the sequential rolling, activation, firm adhesion and diapedesis of the leukocyte (Fig. 1) [16]. The following overview briefly outlines the general concepts involved in leukocyte-endothelial cell interactions.

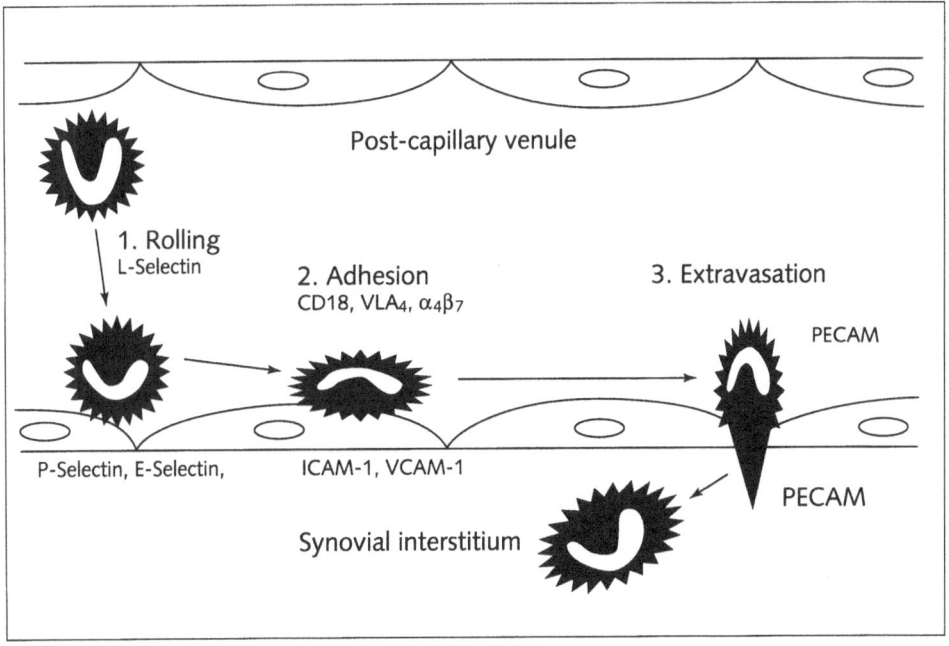

Figure 1

Leukocyte-endothelial cell interactions involving rolling, adhesion and extravasation of leukocytes from post-capillary venules into the synovial interstitium.

Rolling

In vivo the initial adhesive interaction of leukocytes with vascular endothelium involves the movement of leukocytes from the central stream of circulating blood cells toward the vessel wall and subsequent rolling along the endothelium [17, 18]. The movement of leukocytes toward the venular wall may be due to a hydrodynamic interaction between red blood cells and leukocytes as they pass from the smaller diameter capillaries to the larger diameter postcapillary venules, i.e., the faster moving red blood cells displace the leukocytes from the axial stream toward the venular endothelium [18]. The rolling of leukocytes along the endothelium is considered to be a result of weak adhesive interactions which are insufficient to overcome the effects of the shear stress along the vessel wall.

The selectins, L-selectin of leukocytes and the P- and E-selectins of endothelial cells have been implicated as the major ECAMs involved in rolling of leukocytes along the endothelium (Tab. 1) [19]. L-selectin is constitutively expressed on quiescent PMNs and lymphocytes, whereas, P- and E- selectins appear only on the surface of activated endothelium (Tab. 1) [20, 21]. E-selectin mobilization to the surface of the endothelial cell is stimulated by certain Th1-derived cytokines (e.g. IFNγ, TNFα) and maximum surface levels are achieved several hours after activation with a return to basal levels within 12–24 h. P-selectin, on the other hand, is rapidly mobilized to the endothelial cell surface, reaching peak levels within 10–30 min. The expression of P-selectin is very transient, decreasing to negligible levels within minutes due to internalization of the selectin via endocytosis. Interestingly, some stimuli (e.g. reactive oxygen species) can activate endothelial cells in such a manner that P-selectin expression is prolonged for up to 3 h [22].

The ligands for the selectins have not been firmly established, but are thought to be Sialyl-Lewis x and other fucosylated carbohydrates (Tab. 1) [23]. A direct interaction between the selectins is also possible, i.e. PMN or lymphocyte L-selectin with the P- or E-selectin on endothelium [24]. L-selectin has been shown to be important for PMN or lymphocyte-endothelial rolling [16]. Although there are some differences in the mechanisms by which PMNs, monocytes or lymphocytes are initially "tethered" to the endothelium to initiate rolling, by and large, the ligands and their counter receptors are very similar.

Adhesion

It is believed that the rolling of leukocytes along the venular endothelium keeps these cells in close apposition to the endothelium, thereby facilitating their activation by inflammatory mediators generated by the endothelium or resident interstitial cells (e.g. mast cells) [17]. For example, activated PMNs (or monocytes), and to a lesser extent lymphocytes, adhere to venular endothelium (despite the shear stress of flowing blood) by virtue of the strong adhesive interactions between β_2 integrins (CD11/CD18) on these leukocytes and ICAM-1 on endothelial cells (Tab. 1). *In vivo* studies indicate that neutralization of L-selectin function or removal of L-selectin from the PMNs prevents firm adhesion to venules exposed to inflammatory mediators [25]. These latter observations support the contention that selectin mediated rolling is a prerequisite for CD11/CD18-ICAM-1 mediated adhesion.

Upon activation, PMNs shed their L-selectin and upregulate and/or activate their integrins [25, 26]. The β_2 integrins on PMNs are heterodimers consisting of a common subunit (CD18) noncovalently linked to one of three immunologically distinct subunits designated CD11a, CD11b, and CD11c (Tab. 1). CD11a/CD18 is basally expressed on the surface of PMNs and lymphocytes and interacts with ICAM-1 and ICAM-2 on endothelial cells to promote adhesive interactions [27]. Addition of unstimulated PMNs to naive or cytokine stimulated endothelial cell monolayers *in vitro* results in PMN adherence to the endothelial cells which is inhibitable by monoclonal antibodies (mAbs) directed against CD11a/CD18 or ICAM-1 [28]. A vari-

Table 1 - Leukocyte-endothelial cell interactions: Role of adhesion glycoproteins.

Adhesion molecule	Alternative designation	Localization	Ligand
Selectin family			
L-selectin	LAM-1	All leukocytes	P-selectin
	LECAM-1		E-selectin
	MEL-14 Ag		GlyCAM
	CD62L		CD14
			MAdCAM
P-selectin	PAGDEM	Endothelial	L-selectin
	GMP-140	cells	PSGL-1
	CD62P	platelets	120 kDa PSL
E-selectin	ELAM-1	Endothelial	L-selectin
	CD62L	cells	CLA
			SSEA-1
			250 kDa ESL
Immunoglobulin supergene family			
ICAM-1	CD54a	Endothelium	LFA-1
		Monocytes	Mac-1
			CD43
ICAM-2	CD102	Endothelium	LFA-1
VCAM-1	CD106	Endothelium	VLA-4 ($\alpha_4\beta_1$)
PECAM-1	CD31	Endothelium	PECAM-1
MAd-CAM-1	–	Endothelium	VLA-4 ($\alpha_4\beta_1$)
		(intestine)	L-selectin
			CD49d/β_7
Integrin family			
CD11a/CD18	LFA-1	All leukocytes	ICAM-1
	$\alpha_L\beta_2$		ICAM-2
CD11b/CD18	Mac-1, MO1	Granulocytes	ICAM-1
	CR3, $\alpha_M\beta_2$		
CD11c/CD18	p150,95	Granulocytes	Fb; iC3b?
	$\alpha_x\beta_2$		
CD49d/CD29	VLA-4 ($\alpha_4\beta_1$)	Monocytes	VCAM-1
		Lymphocytes	MAdCAM-1
		PMNs (?)	

103

ety of inflammatory mediators or cytokines are unable to increase the expression of CD11a/CD18 on the surface of PMNs. By contrast, most of the CD11b/CD18 and CD11c/CD18 adherence glycoproteins are stored in PMN granules and can be rapidly (within minutes) mobilized to the surface of PMNs by fusion of granule membranes with the cell membrane upon stimulation [29, 30]. Stimulation of PMNs with inflammatory mediators or cytokines results in a 3–10-fold increase in the expression of CD11b/CD18 and CD11c/CD18 on the PMN surface. Both anti-CD11a and anti-CD11b MAb can inhibit the adherence of activated PMNs to cytokine stimulated endothelial cell monolayers.

ICAM-1 and ICAM-2 are endothelial cell adhesion molecules which are members of the immunoglobulin supergene family (Tab. 1) [29, 31, 32]. ICAM-1 contains 5 Ig-like extracellular domains of which the first NH_2-terminal Ig-like domain recognizes CD11a/CD18 and the third lg-like domain recognizes CD11b/CD18 [33]. ICAM-1 is basally expressed on endothelial cells and its expression is increased in response to activation of endothelial cells with certain Th1-derived cytokines or bacterial products (Tab. 1). Maximal expression of ICAM-1 is achieved within 4–8 h after activating the endothelial cells and is associated with maximal levels of PMN adherence. The mechanism by which ICAM-1 is increased on the cell surface is unclear, but the process appears to require activation of certain transcription factors (see below). ICAM-2 is a truncated form of ICAM-1, containing only two Ig-like extracellular domains [34]. Like ICAM-1, ICAM-2 is also basally expressed on endothelial cells, but its level of expression is higher (10-fold) than that of ICAM-1 [35]. In contrast to ICAM-1, ICAM-2 expression is not increased on cytokine activated endothelial cells.

PMN and monocyte adhesion and extravasation can be markedly inhibited by the use of monoclonal antibodies directed against the CD11/CD18 complex or ICAM-1, however, these same antibodies are only weakly effective at inhibiting adhesion of lymphocytes to cytokine-activated endothelium. Indeed, it is now known that lymphocytes, monocytes, and eosinophils possess a β_1 integrin called very-late activation antigen-4 (VLA-4; $\alpha_4\beta_1$) which binds to the inducible vascular cell adhesion molecule-1 (VCAM-1) and mucosal addressin cell adhesion molecule-1 (MAdCAM-1) expressed on the surface of cytokine-activated endothelial cells (Tab. 1). The kinetics of VCAM-1 expression on vascular endothelial cells closely resembles that seen with ICAM-1.

More recent studies have identified an additional ligand/counter receptor pair in lymphocytes which is thought to be important in cell-cell adhesion, signaling, trafficking and regulation of the immune responses in mucosal tissues, especially in the gastrointestinal tract [16, 36]. MAdCAM-1 is a member of the Ig supergene family that is expressed on gastrointestinal mucosal endothelial cells and high endothelial cells in lymph nodes and Peyer's patches and is involved in the selective homing of lymphocytes to mucosal tissue [16, 36]. Surface expression of MAdCAM-1 is induced by certain cytokines and bacterial products and may last for several days.

Its lymphocyte-associated counter-receptor, $\alpha_4\beta_7$, is found primarily on a subpopulation of memory lymphocytes involved in mucosal immunity. The role of MAdCAM-1 in RA is not known.

Transendothelial migration

Following adhesion of leukocytes to the endothelium they send pseudopodia between endothelial cells, and migrate into the interstitium. Based on studies using blocking antibodies, PMN transmigration across endothelial cell monolayers appears to require CD18-ICAM-1 interactions. Recently, an adhesion molecule, PECAM-1, has been identified which appears to be intimately involved in PMN transmigration [37]. PECAM-1 is preferentially distributed between endothelial cells (intercellular junctions) and the transmigration process appears to involve homotypic adhesive interactions between PECAM-1 on PMNs and endothelial cells. MAb directed to PECAM-1 blocks PMN transmigration without preventing adhesion [37]. Taken together, these studies suggest that some ECAMs may be very important in promoting and/or sustaining joint inflammation.

A number of different studies have demonstrated that ECAM expression is enhanced in synovial tissue obtained from patients with active RA [38–44]. Indeed, these observations have prompted clinical studies using neutralizing antibodies to certain ECAMs as a potential therapy to treat RA [1–3].

Regulation of adhesion molecule expression in chronic joint inflammation

Nuclear transcription factor κ B (NF-κB) and reactive oxygen metabolism

It is becoming increasingly apparent that the chronic joint inflammation observed in rheumatoid arthritis (RA) is associated with increased production of reactive oxygen metabolites of oxygen and nitrogen [45–59]. Historically, it has been thought that these oxidants and free radicals promote synovitis as well as bone and cartilage damage directly via their ability to degrade important cellular constituents and biopolymers such as hyaluronic acid proteoglycans and collagen (Tabs. 2 and 3) [47]. More recent data suggest that reduced oxygen species may also initiate and/or perpetuate chronic joint inflammation by activating the transcription of a variety of different genes known to be important in the inflammation response. For example, certain reactive oxygen species are known to activate specific transcription factors such as nuclear transcription factor κ B (NF-κB). It is well appreciated that Th1-derived cytokines such as TNFα, TNFβ (lymphotoxin-α) and IFNγ either alone or in combination promote leukocyte adhesion *in vitro* and *in vivo* [60]. The mechanisms by which this diverse group of pro-inflammatory agents promote leukocyte

Table 2 - Evidence suggesting enhanced oxidant production in RA*

- Decreased ascorbate levels in synovial fluid and serum
- Decreased α-tocopherol content in synovial fluid
- Increased levels of lipid peroxidation products in synovial fluid, serum or expired air
- Hydroxylated derivatives of salicylate
- Decreased α_1-antiproteinase activity
- Degradation of hyaluronic acid
- Increased levels of protein carbonyls and fluorescent products
- Increased concentrations of uric acid oxidation products
- Increased levels of 8-OH-DG

*Compiled from Odeh [13] and Halliwell [47]

Table 3 - Oxidant-dependent reactions thought to contribute to the pathophysiology of RA

- Hyaluronic acid degradation
- Inactivation of α_1-antiprotease activity
- Activation of metalloproteinase activity (e.g. collagenase, gelatinase)
- Fragmentation of collagen
- Degradation of proteoglycans
- Activation of osteoclastic activity
- Inhibition of proteoglycan synthesis
- Oxidation of immunoglobulin G
- Lipid oxidation

adhesion *in vivo* is not clear, however, recent *in vitro* data suggest that cytokine-receptor interaction may activate NF-κB. This heterodimer protein is a ubiquitous transcription factor and pleiotropic regulator of numerous inflammatory and immune responses. Once activated, NF-κB translocates to the nucleus of the cell where it binds to its consensus sequence on the promoter-enhancer region of different genes thereby activating the transcription of genes known to be important in the immune and inflammatory responses [60]. For example, NF-κB appears to regulate the transcription of a variety of different cytokines (e.g., IL-1, IL-2, TNF, IL-6, IL-8) as well as certain ECAMs such as ICAM-1, VCAM-1, E-selectin and MAdCAM-1 [60–63]and the inducible form of nitric oxide synthase (iNOS). Thus, NF-κB may regulate ECAM expression directly or indirectly via its ability to activate transcription of inflammatory cytokines. NF-κB belongs to the Rel family of transcription factors [60] where members share a region of about 300 amino acids known as the Rel homology domain. The heterodimeric NF-κB is composed of p50 and p65 subunits and is normally sequestered in the cytoplasm associated with its inhibitor IκB [64]. A large number of different bacterial and viral products, cytokines and lipid mediators activate NF-κB [60]. It is unlikely that each of these stimuli activates the cytoplasmic NF-κB-IκB complex via completely different pathways. Indeed, there is a growing body of experimental data to suggest that many, if not all, of these stimuli activate multiple signaling pathways which converge to enhance reactive oxygen metabolism within the cell (Fig. 2) [65–69]. This has been shown for the NF-κB activators TNF, IL-1, lipopolysaccharide, phorbol esters, UV light, γ radiation, anti-IgM, okadaic acid and anti-CD28. Further supporting this concept is the recognition that certain lipophilic, membrane-permeable oxidants, such as H_2O_2 and oxidant producing xenobiotics (e.g. menendione) active NF-κB as well [69]. The identity of the specific intracellular source(s) for this enhanced oxidative metabolism has (have) not been identified, however prostaglandin synthase, xanthine oxidase, mitochondria, NADPH oxidase and cytochrome P-450 are likely candidates [70–73]. Sources of exogenous oxidants *in vivo* that could activate NF-kB include activated phagocytic leukocytes (e.g. PMNs, monocytes, macrophages, eosinophils). Furthermore, NF-κB activation has been shown to be inhibited *in vitro* by a wide variety of structurally diverse enzymatic or non-enzymatic antioxidants or free radical scavengers such as SOD, catalase, GSH peroxidase, N-acetylcysteine, vitamin E derivatives, a-lipoic acid and certain dithiocarbamates (reviewed in [65–69]). Furthermore, two recent studies have demonstrated that certain antioxidants inhibit NF-κB *in vivo* and protect the lung from inflammatory tissue injury [74, 75]. Indeed, it is intriguing to speculate that the observed protective effects of antioxidants in various models of RA may be due more to inhibition of NF-κB activation than inhibition of oxidant-induced toxicity. Recent data demonstrate activation and nuclear translocation of NF-κB in synovial tissue obtained from patients with RA [76]; see also preceding chapter and references cited therein.

The mechanisms by which oxidants activate NF-κB have not been defined. This intracellular oxidative stress is thought to then activate via several intermediate reactions, one or more redox-sensitive kinases which specifically phosphorylate IκB [77, 78] (Fig. 2). Once phosphorylated, IκB is selectively ubiquinated and then degraded via the non-lysosomal, ATP-dependent 26S proteolytic complex [79, 80]. Thus, the 26S proteasome represents an important step in the activation of NF-κB (Fig. 2). Because the proteolytic degradation of the post-translationally modified IκB is known to be mediated by the 26S proteasome complex we recently assessed the therapeutic anti-inflammatory activity of a selective proteasome inhibitor in a model of chronic polyarthritis [81]. Chronic polyarthritis with granulomatous liver inflammation was induced in female Lewis rats via the intraperitoneal injection of peptidoglycan polysaccharide (PG/PS). Twenty-one rats were randomized into three groups consisting of a saline-injected control group, a PG/PS arthritic group given vehicle (methylcellulose) p.o. daily beginning 7 days following the induction of arthritis, and a PG/PS arthritic group given 0.3 mg/kg^{-1}/day^{-1} PS-341 (proteasome

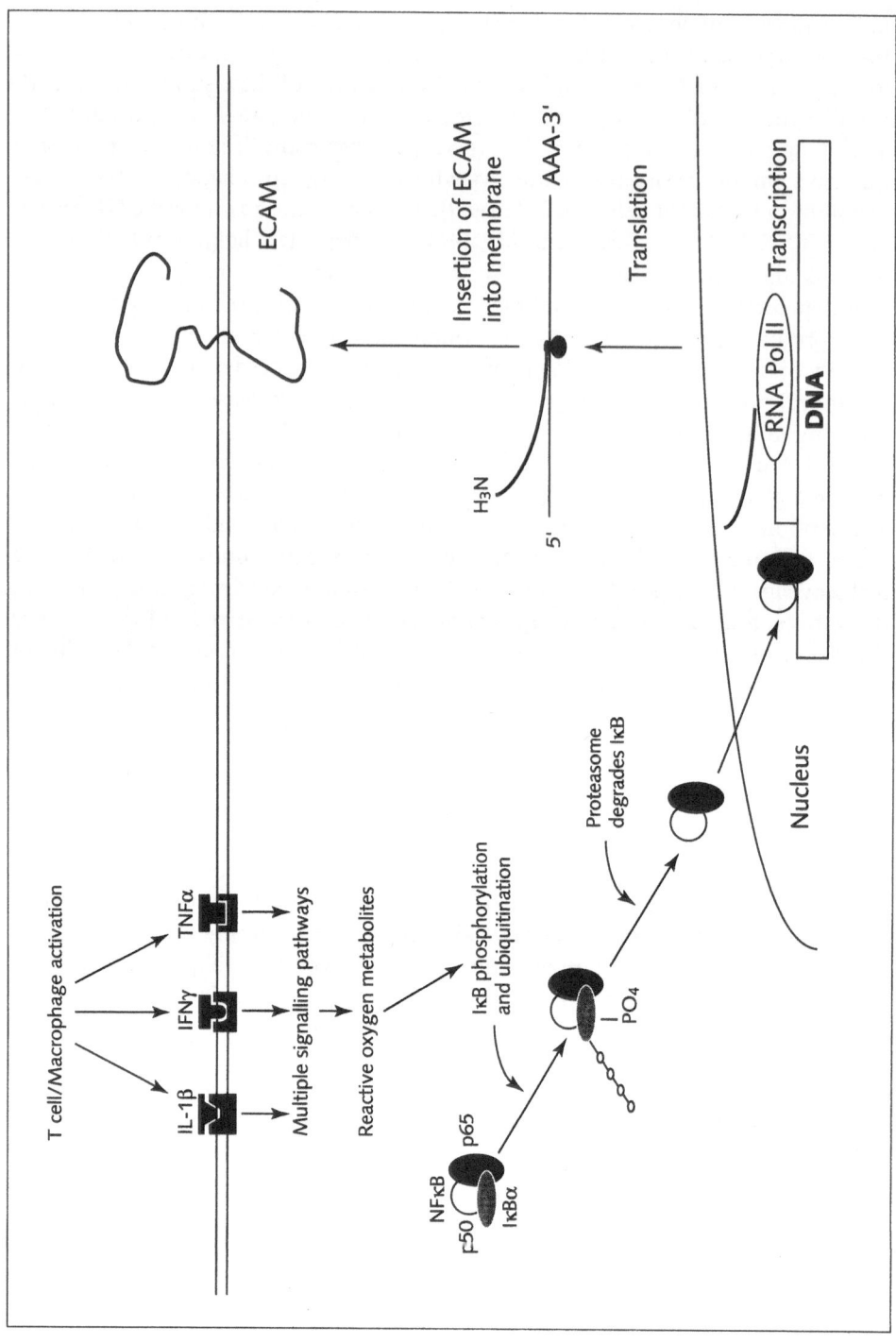

inhibitor; $K_i = 0.6$ nM) p.o daily beginning 7 days following the induction of arthritis. Arthritic symptoms were monitored throughout the course of the study and were quantified using the total arthritis index score and measurement of paw volume. Twenty-eight days following the induction of arthritis, animals were sacrificed and inflamed organs (liver and paws) were retrieved for histological and biochemical analysis. In a first series of experiments, we found that PS-341 inhibited, in a dose-dependent manner, the TNF-induced activation of NF-κB in human endothelial cells (HUVECs) *in vitro*. In addition, we found that certain antioxidants or PS-341 significantly inhibited the TNF-induced surface expression of ICAM-1, E-selectin and VCAM-1 in HUVECs as well as inhibited the PG/PS-induced upregulation of iNOS in a murine macrophage cell line *in vitro*. We also found that oral administration of PS-341 attenuated polyarthritis induced by the intraperitoneal injection of PG/PS as assessed by significant reduction in the total arthritis and average hind paw volume [81]. Histologically, drug treatment attenuated the cellular infiltration, synovial thickening and pannus formation as well as the bone and cartilage erosion typical of PG/PS induced arthritis. This inhibition of polyarthritis correlated with significant reductions in plasma levels of nitrate and nitrite and IL-6 compared to vehicle treated controls. The gross liver inflammation score was also attenuated by drug treatment. Furthermore, PG/PS-induced upregulation of liver inducible nitric oxide synthase and VCAM-1 was significantly attenuated by therapeutic treatment with PS-341 [81]. This same proteasome inhibitor has been shown to attenuate the chronic granulomatous inflammation observed in experimental inflammatory bowel disease [63]. We conclude that the 26S proteasome and thus NF-κB play important roles in regulating the acute and chronic inflammation responses *in vivo*. These data also suggest that the anti-adhesive and anti-inflammatory properties of antioxidants, free radical scavengers and proteasome inhibitors may be due to their abilities to inhibit the activation of NF-κB and the subsequent upregulation of ECAM expression on the endothelium.

Nitric oxide as a modulator of leukocyte-endothelial cell interactions: anti-inflammatory, pro-inflammatory or both

Numerous studies have demonstrated that chronic joint inflammation is associated with the sustained overproduction of NO˙ [82-86]. There is increasing evidence to

Figure 2

Proposed mechanism for cytokine-induced transcriptional activation of endothelial cell adhesion molecule (ECAM) expression in the synovial microvasculature. NF-κB, IκB and RNA Pol II represent nuclear transcription factor κ B, inhibitor protein κ B-α and RNA polymerase II, respectively.

suggest that NO$^{\cdot}$, is very effective at modulating leukocyte-endothelial cell interactions *in vitro* and *in vivo*. For example, it has been demonstrated that NO$^{\cdot}$ attenuates the adhesion and recruitment of leukocytes in postcapillary venules exposed to different acute inflammatory stimuli such as ischemia and reperfusion, oxidized low density lipoproteins, or reactive oxygen metabolites [87–89]. One explanation that has been offered to explain the anti-adhesion properties of NO$^{\cdot}$ relates to the ability of this molecule to rapidly interact with and decompose superoxide ($O_2^{\cdot-}$). Since $O_2^{\cdot-}$ reacts with NO$^{\cdot}$ three times faster than with superoxide dismutase [90], it has been proposed that NO$^{\cdot}$ may act as a physiological scavenger of $O_2^{\cdot-}$. However, depending upon the relative fluxes of each radical, NO$^{\cdot}$ may inhibit or enhance oxidant production via the degradation or synthesis of peroxynitrite ($ONOO^-$) [91, 92]. This possibility is supported by studies demonstrating that NO$^{\cdot}$ donors are only effective in inhibiting leukocyte-endothelial cell adhesion in models of inflammation wherein SOD is also anti-adhesive [93, 94). Furthermore, inhibition of NO$^{\cdot}$ synthase results in an oxidant stress in postcapillary venules [95]. A second mechanism by which NO$^{\cdot}$ may attenuate leukocyte adhesion during the acute inflammatory response involves modulation of ECAM expression. It was recently reported that an NO$^{\cdot}$ donor prevents the mobilization of preformed P-selectin that is observed within 30 min after reperfusion of the ischemic intestine [96]. Furthermore, it has been shown that exogenous NO$^{\cdot}$ donors induce the expression of and stabilize IκB thereby maintaining NF-κB in its inactive form bound to IκB [97]. Indeed, this is the mechanism proposed to account for the ability of NO$^{\cdot}$ to attenuate VCAM-1 surface expression on HUVECs *in vitro* [98,99].

Although we, as well as others, have shown potent anti-adhesive activity of NO$^{\cdot}$ *in vitro* and in acute inflammation *in vivo*, the role of NO$^{\cdot}$ in chronic joint inflammation may be much different. In fact, numerous studies have indicated that chronic joint inflammation may be attenuated by administration of a variety of NOS inhibitors indicating that NO$^{\cdot}$ may directly or indirectly promote rather than inhibit chronic inflammation [53–59, 85, 86]. Several groups have demonstrated that more selective iNOS inhibitors (e.g. aminoguanidine, L-NIL) are effective at inhibiting joint inflammation when administered prophylactically. Therapeutic administration of iNOS inhibitors have proven to be either less effective or inactive [86].

The mechanisms by which the sustained overproduction of iNOS-derived NO$^{\cdot}$ promotes chronic joint inflammation have not been clearly delineated, however, there are several possibilities. For example, it has been demonstrated that NO$^{\cdot}$ or NO$^{\cdot}$-derived metabolites may promote chemotaxis of some leukocytes *in vitro* [100, 101). Nitric oxide or NO$^{\cdot}$-derived metabolites may also promote leukocyte infiltration in an indirect manner by enhancing the production of proinflammatory mediators such as IL-8 or TNF [102, 103]. Furthermore, Lander and coworkers have demonstrated that NO$^{\cdot}$ or one of its auto-oxidation products activates lymphocytes to product TNF [103]. Finally, NO$^{\cdot}$ may rapidly interact with certain reactive oxygen species such as $O_2^{\cdot-}$ to yield the potent oxidant $ONOO^-$ [104]. Because of the large influx of phagocytic leukocytes such as PMNs, monocytes, macrophages and eosinophils, it is not unreasonable to suggest that iNOS-derived NO could promote chronic gut inflammation by reacting with leukocyte-derived $O_2\cdot^-$ to form $ONOO^-$ which in turn upregulate cytokine and/or ECAM expression and injure the tissue.

Conclusions

Leukocyte-endothelial cell adhesion is an early and rate-determining component of the microvascular and tissue dysfunction that accompanies chronic joint inflammation. It is modulated by $NO\cdot$, $O_2\cdot^-$ and possibly other radical species. The realization that leukocyte adhesion may be critical in the pathogenesis of RA has resulted in an intensive effort to define the molecular mechanisms which regulate ECAM expression *in vivo*. As a result of this effort, a large body of new information on the contribution of different glycoproteins to specific components of the leukocyte recruitment process, i.e. rolling, adherence and emigration has been generated. A by-product of this investigative effort is the availability of reagents that inhibit specific steps in the recruitment cascade, which may provide the opportunity for development of new drugs that may control as well as reverse the inflammatory response. Pharmacologic manipulation of free radical activity is one approach to achieving this. While the therapeutic potential of adhesion molecule inhibition is only just beginning, it appears likely that novel agents which target this component of the inflammatory response will be expanded in the clinical setting in the not too distant future.

Acknowledgments
Some of this work was supported by the Arthritis Center of Excellence at LSU Medical Center in Shreveport.

References

1   Kavanaugh AF, Davis LS, Nichols LA, Norris SH, Rothlein R, Scharschmidt LA, Lipsky PE (1994) Treatment of refractory rheumatoid arthritis with a monoclonal antibody to intercellular adhesion molecule 1. *Arthritis Rheum* 37: 992–999
2   Kavanaugh AF, Davis LS, Jain RI, Nichols LA, Norris SH, Lipsky PE (1996) A Phase I/II open label study of the safety and efficacy of an anti-ICAM-1 (intercellular adhesion molecule-1; CD54) monoclonal antibody in early rheumatoid arthritis. *J Rheumatol* 23: 1338–1344
3   Kavanaugh AF, Schulze-Koops H, Davis LS, Lipsky PE (1997) Repeat treatment of

rheumatoid arthritis patients with a murine anti-intercellular adhesion molecule 1 monoclonal antibody. *Arthritis Rheum* 40: 849–853

4   Schimmer RC, Schrier DJ, Flory CM, Dykens J, Tung DKL, Jacobson PB, Friedl HP, Conroy MC, Schimmer BB, Ward PA (1997) Streptococcal cell wall-induced arthritis. *J Immunol* 159: 4103–4108

5   Issekutz AC, Ayer L, Miyasaka M, Issekutz TB (1996) Treatment of established adjuvant arthritis in rats with monoclonal antibody to CD18 and very late activation antigen-4 integrins suppresses neutrophil and T-lymphocyte migration to the joints and improves clinical disease. *Immunol* 88: 569–576

6   Issekutz AC and Issekutz TB (1995) Monocyte migration to arthritis in rats utilizes both CD11/CD18 and very late activation antigen 4 integrin mechanisms. *J Exp Med* 181: 1197–1203

7   Kulka JP, Bocking D, Ropes MW (1955) Early joint lesions of rheumatoid arthritis. *Arch Pathol* 59: 129–150

8   Schumacher HR (1975) Synovial membrane and fluid morphologic alterations in early rheumatoid arthritis: Microvascular injury and virus-like particles. *Ann NY Acad Sci* 256: 39–64

9   Schumacher HR Jr (ed) (1993) *Primer on the rheumatic diseases*. Arthritis Foundation Printing, Atlanta, 86–89

10   Weyand CM, Goronzy JJ (1997) Pathogenesis of rheumatoid arthritis. *Adv Rheumatol* 81: 29–55

11   Firestein GS (1998) Rheumatoid synovitis and pannus. In: JH Klippel, PA Dieppe (eds): *Rheumatology*. Mosby, London, 513.1–513.24

12   Schulze-Koops H, Lipsky PE, Kavanaugh AF, Davis LS (1995) Elevated Th1- or Th0-like cytokine mRNA in peripheral circulation of patients with rheumatoid arthritis. *J Immunol* 155: 5029–5037

13   Odeh M (1997) Short analytical review: New insights into the pathogenesis and treatment of rheumatoid arthritis. *Clin Immunol Immunopathol* 83: 103–116

14   Lebsack ME, Paul CC, Bloedow DC (1991) Subcutaneous IL-1 receptor antagonist in patients with rheumatoid arthritis (abstract). *Arthritis Rheum* 34 (Supp 9): S45

15   Elliott MJ, Maini RN, Feldmann M, Kalden JR, Antoni C, Smolen JS, Leeb B, Breedveld FC, Macfarlane JD, Bilj H, Woody JN (1994) Randomized double-blind comparison of chimeric monoclonal antibody to tumor necrosis factor alpha (cA2) versus placebo in rheumatoid arthritis. *Lancet* 344: 1105–1110

16   Springer TA (1994) Traffic signals for lymphocyte recirculation and leukocyte emigration: the multistep paradigm. *Cell* 76: 301–314

17   Kishimoto TK (1991) A dynamic model for neutrophil localization to inflammatory sites. *J NIH Res* 3: 75–77

18   Schmid-Schonbein, GW, Usami, S, Skalak, T, Chien, S (1980) The interaction of leukocytes and erythrocytes in capillary and postcapillary vessels. *Microvasc Res* 19: 45–70

19   Granger DN (1997) Cell adhesion and migration. II. Leukocyte-endothelial cell adhesion in the digestive system. *Am J Physiol* 273: G982–G986

20   McEver RP (1991) GMP-140, a receptor that mediates interactions of leukocytes with activated platelets and endothelium. *Trends in Cardiovasc Med* 1: 152–156

21   McEver RP (1991) Selectins: novel receptors that mediate leukocyte adhesion during inflammation. *Thromb Haemostasis* 65: 223–228

22   Patel KD, Zimmerman GA, Prescott SM et al (1991) Oxygen radicals induce human endothelial cells to express GMP-140 and bind neutrophils. *J Cell Biol* 112: 749–759

23   Springer TA, Lasky LA (1991) Sticky sugars for selectins. *Nature* 349: 196–197

24   Picker LJ, Warnock RA, Burns AR et al (1991) The neutrophil selectin LECAM-1 presents carbohydrate ligands to the vascular selectins ECAM-1 and GMP-140. *Cell* 66: 921–933

25   Granger DN, Kubes P (1994) The microcirculation and inflammation: modulation of leukocyte-endothelial cell adhesion. *J Leuk Biol* 55: 662–675

26   Kishimoto TK, Jutila MA, Berg EL et al (1989) Neutrophil Mac-1 and MEL-14 adhesion proteins inversely regulated by chemotactic factors. *Science* 245: 1238–1241

27   Marlin SD, Springer TA (1987) Purified intercellular adhesion molecule-1 (ICAM-1) is a ligand for lymphocyte function-associated antigen 1 (LFA-1). *Cell* 51: 813–819

28   Smith CW, Marlin SD, Rothlein R et al (1989) Cooperative interactions of LFA-1 and MAC-1 with intercellular adhesion molecule-1 in facilitating adherence and transendothelial migration of human neutrophils *in vitro*. *J Clin Invest* 83: 2008–2017

29   Carlos TM, Harlan JM (1990) Membrane proteins involved in phagocyte adherence to endothelium. *Immunol Rev* 114: 5–28,

30   Larson RS, Springer TA (1990) Structure and function of leukocyte integrins. *Immunol Rev* 114: 181–217

31   Springer TA (1990) Adhesion receptors of the immune system. Nature 346: 425–434

32   Montefort S, Holgate ST (1991) Adhesion molecules and their role in inflammation. *Resp Med* 85: 91–99

33   Diamond MS, Staunton DE, Marlin SD et al (1991) Binding of the integrin Mac-1 (CD11b/CD18) to the third immunoglobulin-like domain of ICAM-1 (CD54) and its regulation by glycosylation. *Cell* 65: 961–971

34   Staunton DE, Dustin ML, Springer TA (1989) Functional cloning of ICAM-2, a cell adhesion ligand for LFA-1 homologous to ICAM-1. *Nature* 339: 61–64

35   De Fougerolles AR, Stacker SA, Schwarting R, Springer TA (1991) Characterization of ICAM-2 and evidence for a third counter-receptor for LFA-1. *J Exp Med* 174: 253–267

36   Butcher EC, Picker LJ (1996) Lymphocyte homing and homeostasis. *Science* 272: 60–66

37   Muller W, Seigi SA, Deng X et al (1993) PECAM-1 is required for transendothelial migration of leukocytes. *J Exp Med* 178: 449–460

38   Cronstein BN (1994) Adhesion molecules in the pathogenesis of rheumatoid arthritis. *Curr Opin Rheumatol* 6: 300–304

39   Tak PP, Thurkow EW, Daha MR, Kluin PM, Smeets TJM, Meinders AE, Breedveld FC (1995) Expression of adhesion molecules in early rheumatoid synovial tissue. *Clin Immunol Immunopathol* 77: 236–242

40   Ishikawa H, Hirata S, Andoh Y, Kubo H, Nakagawa N, Nishibayashi Y, Mizuno K

(1996) An immunohistochemical and immunoelectron microscopic study of adhesion molecules in synovial pannus formation in rheumatoid arthritis. *Rheumatol Int* 16: 53–60

41   Mellbye OJ, Shen Y, Hogasen K, Mollnes TE, Forre O (1996) Adhesion molecule expression and complement activation in vessel walls in synovial tissue from patients with chronic inflammatory joint disease. *Clin Rheumatol* 15: 441–447

42   Mulherin DM, Veale DJ, Belch JJF, Bresnihan B, Fitzgerald O (1996) Adhesion molecule in untreated inflammatory arthritis. *QJ Med* 89: 195–203

43   Oppenheimer-Marks N, Lipsky PE (1996) Short Analytical Review: Adhesion molecules as targets for the treatment of autoimmune diseases. *Clin Immunol Immunopathol* 79: 203–210

44   McMurray RW (1996) Adhesion molecules in autoimmune disease. *Sem Arth Rheum* 25: 215–233

45   Chapman ML, Rubin BR, Gracy RW (1989) Increased carbonyl content of proteins in synovial fluid from patients with rheumatoid arthritis. *J Rheumatol* 16: 15–18

46   Ialenti A, Moncada S, DiRosa M (1993) Modulation of adjuvant arthritis by endogenous nitric oxide. *Br J Pharmacol* 110: 701–706

47   Halliwell B (1995) Free Radicals and rheumatic disease. In: B Henderson, JCW Edwards, ER Pettipher (eds): *Mechanisms and models in rheumatoid arthritis.* Academic Press Ltd, London, 301–306

48   Skaleric U, Allen JB, Smith PD, Mergenhagen SE, Wahl SM (1991) Inhibitors of reactive oxygen intermediates suppress bacterial cell wall-induced arthritis. *J Immunol* 147: 2559–2564

49   Edwards SW, Hughes V, Barlow J and Bucknall R (1988) Immunological detection of myeloperoxidase in synovial fluid from patients with rheumatoid arthritis. *Biochem J* 250: 81–85

50   Dabbagh AJ, Blake DR and Morris CJ (1992) Effect of iron complexes on adjuvant arthritis in rats. *Ann Rheum Dis* 51: 516–521

51   Blake DR, Merry P, Stevens C, Dabbagh A, Sahinoglu T, Allen R, Morris C (1990) Iron free radicals and arthritis. *Proc Nutr Soc* 49: 239–245

52   Biemond P, Swaak AJG, Koster JF (1984) Protective factors against oxygen free radicals and hydrogen peroxide in rheumatoid arthritis synovial fluid. *Arthritis Rheum* 27: 760–765

53   Weinberg JB, Granger DL, Pisetsky DS, Seldin MF, Misukonis MA, Mason SN, Pippen AM, Ruiz P, Wood ER, Gilkeson GS (1994) The role of nitric oxide in the pathogenesis of spontaneous murine autoimmune disease: increased nitric oxide production and nitric oxide synthase expression in MRL-1pr/1pr mice, and reduction of spontaneous glomerulonephritis and arthritis by orally administered N^G-monomethyl-$_L$-arginine. *J Exp Med* 179: 651–660

54   Stefanovic-Racic M, Stadler J, Evans CH (1993) Nitric oxide and arthritis. *Arthritis Rheum* 36: 1036–1044

55   Stefanovic-Racic M, Meyers K, Meschter C, Coffey JW, Hoffman RA, Evans CH (1994)

N-monomethyl arginine, an inhibitor of nitric oxide synthase, suppresses the development of adjuvant arthritis in rats. *Arthritis Rheum* 37: 1062–1069

56 Connor JR, Manning PT, Settle SL, Moore WM, Jerome GM, Webber RK, Tjoeng FS, Currie MG (1995) Suppression of adjuvant-induced arthritis by selective inhibition of inducible nitric oxide synthase. *Eur J Pharm* 273: 15–24

57 Shingu M, Takahashi S, Ito M, Hamamatsu N, Suenaga Y, Ichibangase Y, Nobunaga M (1994) Anti-inflammatory effects of recombinant human manganese superoxide dismutase on adjuvant arthritis in rats. *Rheumatol Int* 14: 77–81

58 Cannon GW, Openshaw SJ, Hibbs JB Jr, Hoidal JR, Huecksteadt TP, Griffiths MM (1996) Nitric oxide production during adjuvant-induced and collagen-induced arthritis. *Arthritis Rheum* 39: 1677–1684

59 McCartney-Francis N, Allen JB, Mizel DE, Albina JE, Xie Q, Nathan CF, Wahl SM (1993) Suppression of arthritis by an inhibitor of nitric oxide synthase. *J Exp Med* 178: 749–754

60 Baeuerle PA, Henkle T (1994) Function and activation of NF-κB in the immune system. *Ann Rev Immunol* 58: 1–27

61 Collins T, Read MA, Neish AS et al (1995) Transcriptional regulation of endothelial cell adhesion molecules: NF-κB and cytokine-inducible enhancers. *FASEB J* 9: 899–909

62 Read MA, Neish AS, Luscinkas FW et al (1995) The proteasome pathway is required for cytokine-induced endothelial-leukocyte adhesion molecule expression. *Immunity* 2: 493–506

63 Conner EM, Brand S, Davis JM et al (1997) Proteasome inhibition attenuates nitric oxide synthase expression, VCAM-1 transcription and the development of chronic colitis. *J Pharm Exp Ther* 282: 1615–1622

64 Baeuerle PA, Baltimore D (1995) IκB: a specific inhibitor of NF-κB transcription factor. *Science* 268: 522–523

65 Schreck R, Rieber P, Baeuerle PA (1991) Reactive oxygen intermediates as apparently widely used messengers in the activation of NF-κB transcription factor and HIV-1. *Embo J* 10: 2247–2258

66 Schreck R, Meier B, Mannel DN et al (1992) Dithiocarbamates as potent inhibitors of nuclear factor κB activation in intact cells. *J Exp Med* 175: 11810

67 Schreck R, Albermann K, Baeuerle PA (1992) NF-κB: an oxidative stress-responsive transcription factor of eukaryotic cells. *Free Rad Res Comm* 17: 221–237

68 Schmidt KN, Amstad P, Cerutti P et al (1995) The roles of hydrogen peroxide and superoxide as messengers in the activation of transcription factor NF-κB. *Chem Biol* 2: 13–22.

69 Sen CK, Packer L (1996) Antioxidant and redox regulation of gene transcription. *FASEB J* 10: 709–720

70 Munroe DG, Wang EY, MacIntyre P et al (1995) Novel intracellular signaling function of prostaglandin H synthase-1 in NF-κB activation. *J Inflamm* 45: 260–268

71 Weber C, Erl W, Pietsch A et al (1994) Antioxidants inhibit monocyte adhesion by suppressing nuclear factor-κB mobilization and induction of vascular cell adhesion mole-

cule-1 in endothelial cells stimulated to generate radicals. *Arterioscler Thromb* 14: 1665–1673

72 Suzuki Y, Wang W, Vu TH et al (1992) Effect of NADPH oxidase inhibition on endothelial cell ELAM-1 mRNA expression. *Biochem Biophys Res Comm* 184: 1339– 1343

73 Schulze-Osthoff K, Beyaert R, Vandervoorde V et al (1993) Depletion of the mitochondrial electron transport abrogates the cytotoxic and gene-inductive effects of TNF. *EMBO J* 12: 3095–3104

74 Blackwell TS, Blackwell TR, Holden EP et al (1996) In vivo antioxidant treatment suppresses nuclear factor-kappa B activation and neutrophilic lung inflammation. *J Immunol* 157: 1630

75 Ye SF, Malik AB (1997) *In vivo* inhibition of nuclear factor-kB activation prevents inducible nitric oxide synthase expression and systemic hypotension in a rat model of septic shock. *J Immunol* 159: 3976–3983

76 Handel ML, McMorrow LB, Gravallese EM (1995) Nuclear factor-κB in rheumatoid synovium. *Arthritis Rheum* 38: 1762–1770

77 Mercurio F, Zhu H, Murray BW et al (1997) IKK-1 and IKK-2: Cytokine-activated IκB Kinases essential for NF-κB activation. *Science* 278: 860–866

78 Woronicz JD, Gao X, Cao Z et al (1997) IκB Kinase-β: NF-κB activation and complex formation with IκB kinase-α and NIK. *Science* 278: 866–869

79 Goldberg AL (1995) Functions of the proteasome: the lysis at the end of the tunnel. *Science* 268: 522–523

80 Palombella VJ, Rando OJ, Goldberg AL et al (1994) The ubiquitin-proteasome pathway is required for processing the NF-κB1 precursor protein and the activation of NF-κB. *Cell* 78: 773–785

81 Palombella VJ, Conner EM, Fuseler JW, Destree A, Davis JM, Laroux FS, Wolf RE, Huang J, Brand S, Elliott PJ et al (1998) Role of the proteasome and NF-kappaB in streptococcal cell wall-induced polyarthritis. *Proc Natl Acad Sci USA* 95: 15671–15676

82 Evans CH, Stefanovic-Racic M, Lancaster J (1995) Nitric oxide and its role in orthopaedic disease. *Clin Ortho Rel Res* 275–294

83 Cochran FR, Selph J, Sherman P (1996) Insights into the role of nitric oxide in inflammatory arthritis. *Med Res Rev* 16: 547–563

84 Anbar M, Gratt BM (1997) Role of nitric oxide in the physiopathology of pain. *J Pain Symptom Manage* 14: 225–254

85 Salvemini D, Wang Z-Q, Wyatt PS, Bourdon DM, Marino MH, Manning PT, Currie MG (1996) *Brit J Pharmacol* 118: 829–838

86 Fletcher DS, Widmer WR, Luell S, Christen A, Orevillo C, Shah S, Visco D (1998) Therapeutic administration of a selective inhibitor of nitric oxide synthase does not ameliorate the chronic inflammation and tissue damage associated with adjuvant-induced arthritis in rats. *J Pharmacol Exp Therapeutics* 284: 714–721

87 Kurose I, Wolf R, Grisham MB et al (1994) Modulation of ischemia/reperfusion-induced microvascular dysfunction by nitric oxide. *Circ Res* 74: 376–382

88   Gaboury J, Woodman RC, Granger DN et al(1993) Nitric oxide prevents leukocyte adherence: role of superoxide. *Am J Physiol* 265: H862–H867

89   Liao, L, Granger, DN (1995) Modulation of oxidized low-density lipoprotein-induced microvascular dysfunction by nitric oxide. *Am J Physiol* 268: H1643–1650

90   Huie RE, Padmaja S (1993) The reaction of NO with superoxide. *Free Rad Res Comm* 18: 195–199

91   Miles AM, Bohle DS, Glassbrenner PA et al (1996) Modulation of superoxide-dependent oxidation of hydroxylation reactions by nitric oxide. *J Biol Chem* 271: 40–47

92   Wink DA, Cook JA, Kim SY et al (1997) Superoxide modulates the oxidation and nitrosation of thiols by nitric oxide-derived reactive intermediates. *J Biol Chem* 272: 11147–11151

93   Kurose I, Wolf R, Grisham MB et al (1994) Modulation of ischemia/reperfusion-induced microvascular dysfunction by nitric oxide. *Circ Res* 74: 376–382

94   Gaboury J, Woodman RC, Granger DN et al (1993) Nitric oxide prevents leukocyte adherence: role of superoxide. *Am J Physiol* 265: H862–H867

95   Suematsu M, Tamatani T, Delano FA et al (1994) Microvascular oxidative stress preceding leukocyte activation elicited by *in vivo* nitric oxide suppression. *Heart Circ Physiol* 35: H2410–H2415

96   Gauthier TW, Davenpeck KL, Lefer AM (1994) Nitric oxide attenuates leukocyte-endothelial interaction via P-selectin in splanchnic ischemia-reperfusion. *Am J Physiol* 267: G562–G568

97   Peng HB, Libby P, Liao JK (1995) Induction and stabilization of IkBx by nitric oxide mediates inhibition of NF-κB. *J Biol Chem* 270: 14214–14219

98   DeCaterina R, Libby P, Peng HB et al (1995) Nitric oxide decreases cytokine-induced endothelial cell activation: Nitric oxide selectively reduces endothelial cell expression of adhesion molecules and proinflammatory cytokines. *J Clin Invest* 96: 60–68

99   Khan BV, Harrison DG, Olbrych MT et al (1996) Nitric oxide regulates vascular cell adhesion molecule 1 gene expression and redox-sensitive transcriptional events in human vascular endothelial cells. *Proc Nat Acad Sci USA* 93: 9114–9119

100 Kaplan SS, Billiar T, Curran RD et al (1989) Inhibition of chemotaxis with N^G-monomethyl-L-arginine. A role for cyclic GMP. *Blood* 74: 1885–1887

101 Beauvais F, Michel L, Dubertret L (1995) Exogenous nitric oxide elicits chemotaxis of neutrophils *in vitro*. *J Cell Physiol* 165: 610–614

102 Villarete LH, Remick, DG (1995) Nitric oxide regulation of IL-8 expression in human endothelial cells. *Biochem Biophys Res Commun* 211: 671–676

103 Lander HM, Jacovina AT, Davis RJ et al (1996) Differential activation of mitogen-activated protein kinases by nitric oxide-related species. *J Biol Chem* 271: 19705–19709

104 Grisham MB, Granger DN, Lefer, DJ (1998) Modulation of leukocyte-endothelial interactions by reactive metabolites of oxygen and nitrogen: relevance to ischemic heart disease. *Free Rad Biol Med* 25: 404–433

Role of thioredoxin in the redox regulation of gene expression in inflammatory diseases

Takashi Okamoto and Toshifumi Tetsuka

Department of Molecular Genetics, Nagoya City University Medical School, 1 Kawasumi, Mizuho-cho, Mizuho-ku, Nagoya 467, Japan

Introduction

Oxygen is an essential molecule to generate energy for all aerobic life forms including humans. However, while oxygen is indispensable for such cells to obtain the essential chemical energy as a form of adenosine triphosphate (ATP), which is called respiration, incomplete reduction of oxygen generates highly active, as well as toxic, forms called radical oxygen intermediates (ROI). In addition to being produced as physiological side-products of electron transfer reactions using oxygen as an electron acceptor, ROI are produced in the cell by various environmental stimuli such as infection of microbes (viruses, bacteria, etc.), ionizing and UV irradiation, and pollutants (i.e. oxidants), which are collectively called "oxidative stress". These ROI are highly reactive with biological macromolecules, producing lipid peroxides (which are often radicals), inactivating proteins and mutating DNA (by producing 8-hydroxy-deoxy-guanosine, 8-OH-dG, or breaking nucleic acid chains).

Therefore, cells must have acquired multiple endogenous anti-oxidant systems which have been a prerequisite for the maintenance of a stable form of life under such harmful conditions. These defense mechanisms include reducing enzyme systems for reduction such as glutaredoxin and thioredoxin [1, 2]. However, recent studies have revealed that actions of these reducing enzymes together with the limited oxidation of protein molecules, so far reported, by ROI are involved in cell signaling [1–4]. The term "redox regulation" has thus been proposed indicating the active role of oxido-reductive modifications of proteins in regulating their activities. In other words, oxidation and reduction of biomolecules are considered to be "signals" in certain instances and are utilized for the maintenance of cellular homeostasis.

Cellular defense mechanism against oxidative stress

A major component of the first line defense system is GSH. GSH is present in the cell at millimolar levels. GSH reduces peroxides in the presence of glutathione per-

Free Radicals and Inflammation, edited by P. G. Winyard, D. R. Blake and C. H. Evans

oxidase and the oxidized GSH (GSSG) is enzymatically restored by NADPH-dependent reduction of GSH reductase. Other antioxidant molecules in the cell include nutrients such as tocopherol (vitamin E) and ascorbate (vitamin C) and anti-oxidant enzymes that detoxify ROI such as SODs and catalase.

The second line defense system is to repair the oxidized macromolecules. It is known that thioredoxin (Trx) not only reacts with ROI but also has an activity to repair the oxidized protein by reducing protein disulfides through oxidation of its redox reactive cysteins (Trp-Cys-Gly-Pro-Cys). Likewise, glutaredoxin, which contains a similar conserved active-site sequence of Cys-Pro-Tyr-Cys with Trx, also reduces protein disulfides. It appears that while GSH is directly involved in scavenging ROI, Trx appears to participate in this cascade by repairing the oxidized proteins through its reducing activity. This reversible oxidation and reduction of a functional protein determines its activity. Therefore, GSH itself may not be directly involved in the redox signaling but the intensity of the oxidative signal may be determined by the internal GSH level. Thus, total GSH/GSSG content could be a useful indicator for the responsiveness of the cellular redox signaling. This redox regulatory pathway is clearly illustrated in the NF-κB activation pathway [5–9].

Transcription factor NF-κB and its involvement in various pathologies

NF-κB regulates expression of a wide variety of cellular and viral genes (see [5–8] for reviews). These genes include cytokines such as IL-2, IL-6, IL-8, GM-CSF and TNF, cell adhesion molecules such as ICAM-1 and E-selectin, inducible nitric oxidase synthase (iNOS) and viruses such as human immunodeficiency virus (HIV) and cytomegalovirus [10–20]. Since NF-κB is responsible for transcriptional induction of these genes, it is considered to be causally involved in the currently intractable diseases such as acquired immunodeficiency syndrome (AIDS), hematogenic cancer cell metastasis and rheumatoid arthritis (RA). Although the genes induced by NF-κB are variable according to the context of cell lineage and are also under the control of other transcription factors, NF-κB plays a major role in regulation of expression of these genes and thus contributes a great deal to the pathophysiological processes. The following are some examples:

Acquired immunodeficiency syndrome (AIDS)

Among the cellular transcription factors that bind to cis-regulatory elements within the viral promoter region (long terminal repeat; LTR), NF-κB is known to play an indispensable role in the HIV life cycle especially in the virus reactivation process within the latently infected cells. After activation through intracellular signaling pathways such as those elicited by T cell receptor antigen complex or by receptors for IL-1 or TNF, NF-κB initiates HIV gene expression by binding to the target DNA element within LTR [11, 20–22]. Then, the virus-encoded trans-activator Tat is produced and triggers explosive viral replication [23–25]. Since activation of HIV gene expression by cellular transcription factors conceptually precedes the production of Tat, NF-κB is regarded as a critical determinant of the maintenance and breakdown of the viral latency. Various attempts including the use of antioxidants have been suggested to be effective in preventing the clinical development of AIDS by blocking HIV replication [26–28].

Inflammation and cancer metastasis

Since NF-κB regulates expression of cell adhesion molecules (CAMs), it is considered to play a role in inflammation and hematogenic cancer cell metastasis [29]. NF-κB induces E-selectin on the surface of vascular endothelial cells [30–31] as well as ICAM-1 and VCAM-1. Since most leukocytes and some cancer cells constitutively express a ligand for E-selectin, called sialyl-Lewis^x antigen, on their cell surface, induction of E-selectin is considered to be a rate determining step of cell-cell interaction in the endothelium [32, 33]. We and others have demonstrated that interfering with the induction of these CAMs by various compounds known to block NF-κB, such as N-acetylcysteine, aspirin and pentoxyphillin, eventually prevented these interactions [29].

Rheumatoid arthritis (RA)

Similarly, accumulating evidence suggests the involvement of NF-κB in the pathogenesis of rheumatoid arthritis (RA) [34–36]. In fact, Handel et al. [37] have demonstrated the presence of NF-κB subunit proteins, p65 and p50, in the nuclei of synovial lining cells of fresh synovial tissue obtained from patients with RA indicating activation of NF-κB *in situ*. Because of its regulatory role in gene expression of IL-1, TNF, IL-2, IL-6, IL-8, GM-CSF, chemokines such as RANTES and MIP-1α, ICAM-1, E-selectin and iNOS that are known to be overexpressed in the rheumatoid synovium, NF-κB is considered to be a major regulator in the expansion and maintenance of the chronic inflammatory response in affected joints. For example, sustained NF-κB activation would induce production of cytokines and thus activate maturation of B lymphocytes to produce antibodies while GM-CSF and chemokine production together with overexpression of cell adhesion molecules would support recruitment of leukocytes from blood stream, thus augmenting the local inflammatory response. Additionally, some of the effective anti-rheumatic drugs including corticosteroids, aspirin and gold compounds, are now known to block the NF-κB cascade. Since these features of inflammatory responses are not specific for RA and are found in other chronic inflammatory processes irrespective of the affected organs or tissues, pathologic roles of NF-κB are probably universal. Therefore, clinical applicability of anti-rheumatic drugs should be further evaluated in other pathologies where NF-κB plays a role.

Signal transduction pathway for NF-κB activation as a basis of signal transduction therapy

NF-κB consists of two subunit molecules, p65 and p50, and usually exists as a molecular complex with an inhibitory molecule, IκB, in the cytosol [19, 20, 38–42]. Upon stimulation of the cells such as by proinflammatory cytokines, IL-1 and TNF, IκB is dissociated and NF-κB is translocated to the nucleus and activates expression of target genes (Fig. 1). In addition to these physiological stimuli, this NF-κB activation cascade is also triggered by ionizing and UV irradiation and oxidative reagents such as hydrogen peroxide [43–45]. It is noted that NF-κB is the first eukaryotic transcription factor shown to respond to oxidative stress.

Activation of NF-κB by the kinase cascade

There are at least two biochemically independent steps in the NF-κB activation cascade: kinase pathways and a redox-signaling pathway. However, these two distinct pathways are involved in the NF-κB activation cascade in a coordinate fashion, which may contribute to a fine tune, as well as fail-safe, regulation of NF-κB activity. At least two distinct types of kinase pathways are known to be involved in NF-κB activation: NF-κB kinase and IκB kinase (Fig. 1). Downstream of adaptor molecules of TNF and IL-1 receptors, TRAF2 and TRAF6 respectively, NF-κB-inducing

Figure 1

Signal transduction pathways for NF-κB activation. The first step involves kinase pathways such as by NF-κB and IκB kinases. The second step involves "redox regulation" by thioredoxin (TRX). After the stimulation of the cells by TNF or IL-1, for example, radical oxygen intermediates (ROI) are produced. ROI not only induces activation of kinase cascade but also production of thioredoxin (Trx). TRAF is known to be associated with the TNF receptor and is known to stimulate NF-κB activation. Similarly, IRAK (IL-1 receptor associated kinase) is considered to participate in the NF-κB activation through its ability to phosphorylate IkB. Phosphorylation of NF-κB or IκB will release NF-κB. However, NF-κB must go through the Trx-mediated reduction of the "redox-sensitive" cysteine to recognize the target DNA sequence (κB site). The phosphorylated IκB will be ubiquitinated and then degraded by proteasome or other proteases.

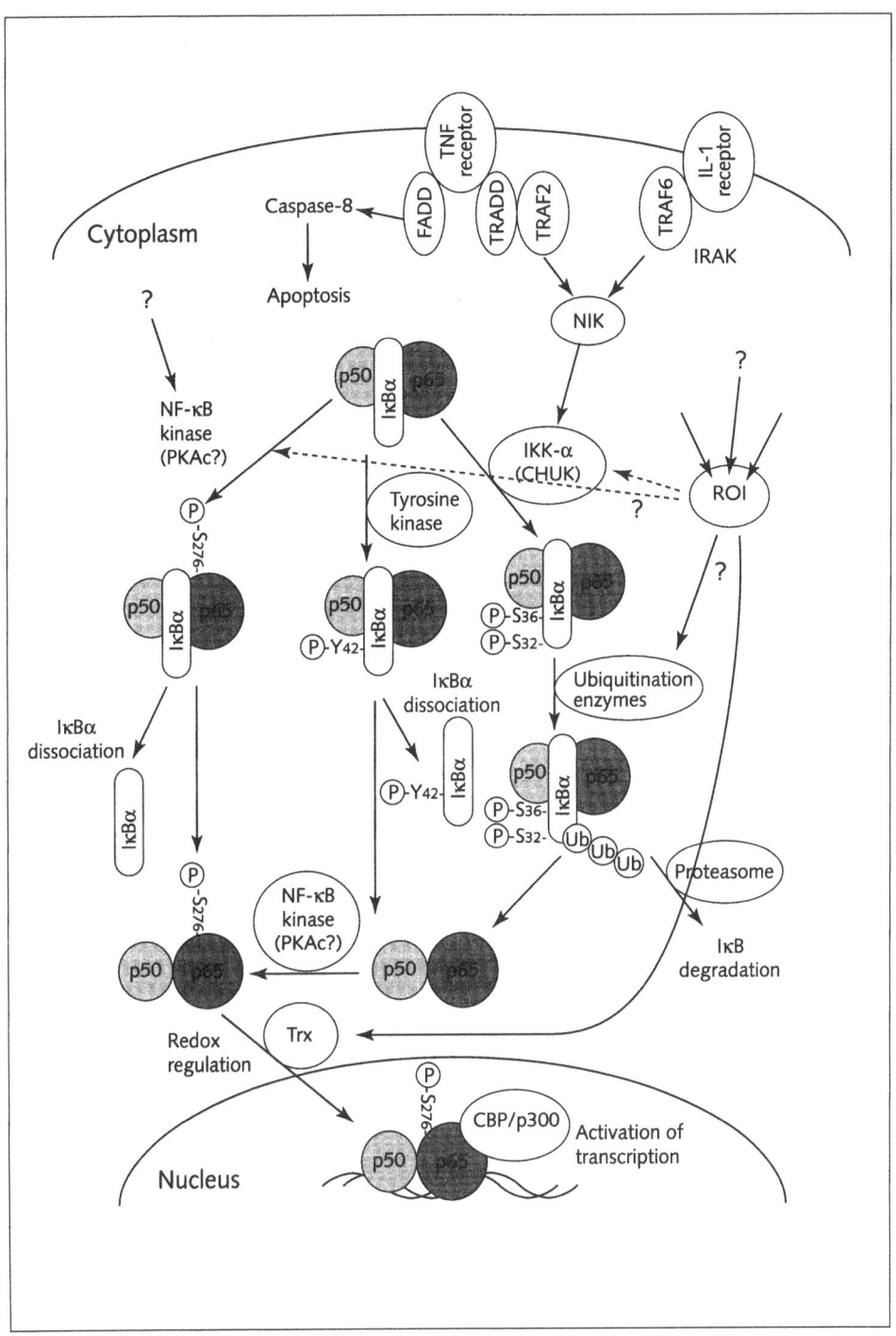

kinase (NIK) has been identified [49]. Recent two-hybrid screen has identified a kinase previously known as CHUK [50], which has turned out to be a specific kinase for IκB, IKK-α [51, 52]. Since it has been shown that IKK-α directly interacts with IκB, identification of all the necessary, though not sufficient yet, components for the NF-κB-activation cascade has been completed at least in part. There is other evidence suggesting the presence of kinase cascade(s) that phosphorylate NF-κB. We found a 43 kD serine kinase, named NF-κB kinase, that is associated with NF-kB [53]. This kinase phosphorylates the subunits, particularly p65, of NF-κB and dissociates it from IκB. Similar findings were reported by others [54–56]. Consistent with these findings, NF-κB was shown to be phosphorylated in some cell lines [54–56] and IκB was phosphorylated in others in response to stimulation with TNF or IL-1 [57, 58]. However, while there is a report indicating the presence of the catalytic subunit of protein kinase A (PKAc) in the NF-κB/IκB complex as an activator of this cascade [59], we and others were not able to demonstrate that PKAc was responsible for activation [56, 60]. There is still some controversy regarding the kinase responsible for p65 phosphorylation.

Trx-mediated redox regulation of the DNA-binding activity of NF-κB

After dissociation from IκB, however, NF-κB must go through redox regulation by the cellular reducing catalyst, thioredoxin (Trx) [62–63] in order to recognize the target DNA sequence and induce transcription. Trx is a cellular reducing catalyst and is known to participate in redox reactions through reversible oxidation of its active center dithiol to a disulfide (Fig. 2). Interestingly, human Trx has been initially identified as a factor responsible for induction of the α subunit of IL-2 receptor which has been revealed to be under the control of NF-κB [64]. We and others have demonstrated *in vitro* that NF-κB cannot bind to the κB DNA sequence of the target genes until it is reduced [62, 63, 65–66]. Based on the estimate of a high local pI value near one of the conserved cysteine residues, we have assigned the cysteine residue at the 62nd amino acid position of the p50 subunit as a target of the redox regulation [63] which was confirmed by a site-directed mutagenesis study by others [67] in which the cysteine 62 substitution abolished the DNA binding activity. Similarly, a possible redox-sensitive cysteine residue is located within the p65 subunit.

Structural basis for the Trx-mediated redox regulation of NF-κB

Structural biological approaches have provided physical evidence supporting the molecular mechanism of the redox regulation of NF-κB by Trx. Crystallographic examination have demonstrated the three-dimensional structure of the NF-κB subunit p50 homodimer associated with the target DNA [68, 69]. NF-κB appears to

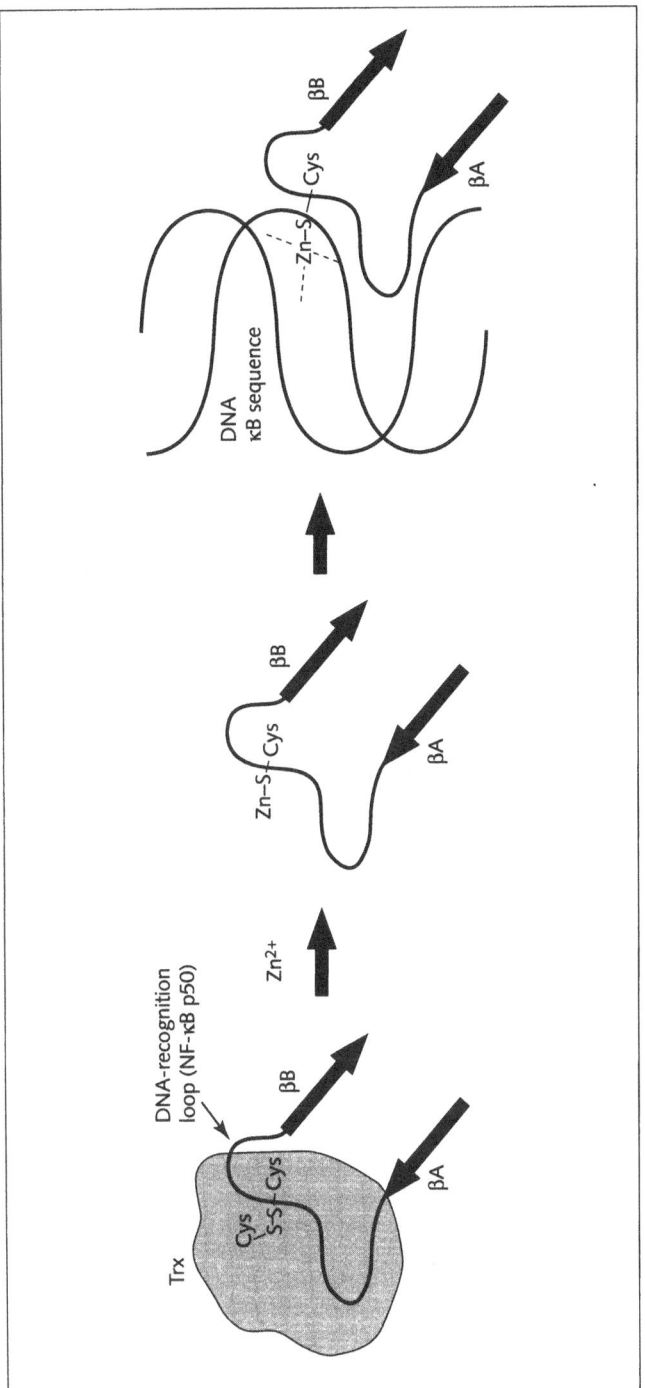

Figure 2

Redox regulation of the DNA-binding activity of NF-κB by Trx. A boot-shaped hollow on the surface of Trx, also containing the redox-sensitive cysteines, could stably recognize the DNA-binding loop of p50 and reduce the oxidized cysteine by donating protons in a structure-dependent way (based on the 3-D structure of Trx molecule with the DNA-binding loop peptide of p50 [70]). Zinc is required to make NF-κB competent for the DNA-binding [71]. When zinc dissociates with NF-κB, Trx may be dissociated from NF-κB.

have a novel DNA-binding structure called the β-barrel, a group of beta sheets stretching toward the target DNA. There is a loop in the tip of the β-barrel structure that intercalates with the target nucleotide bases and is considered to make a direct contact with the DNA. This DNA-recognition loop of p50 contains the residue corresponding to cysteine 62 that we predicted to be the target of redox regulation, although in both studies this cysteine was replaced with alanine (presumably because of technical reasons) for crystallization [62, 63]. Furthermore, another group has solved the 3-D structure of the Trx molecule that is associated with the DNA-binding loop of p50 by using NMR [70]. A boot-shaped hollow on the surface of Trx containing the redox-active cysteines could stably recognize the DNA-binding loop of p50 [68, 69] and is likely to reduce the oxidized cysteine on p50 by donating protons in a structure-dependent fashion. Therefore, the reduction of NF-κB by Trx is considered to be specific and dependent on the structural compatibility between the target protein and Trx. However, the inter-molecular disulfide bridge formation between Trx and NF-κB might be transient since the binding of Trx to the NF-κB DNA-binding loop would block the recognition of the DNA moiety because of the apparent competition of the same cysteine residue. In favor of this model, we have demonstrated that NF-κB and Trx concomitantly migrated to the nucleus in rheumatoid synovial cells during the first phase of the NF-κB activation process and that Trx was relocated in the cytoplasm after 30 min of stimulation while the NF-κB nuclear predominance was still observed for several hours.

In addition to the above findings, our *in vitro* binding study has demonstrated that zinc is required for the DNA binding activity of NF-κB as well as the reduction of the redox-sensitive cysteine [63, 70, 71]. We therefore concluded that zinc ions might be a necessary component of active NF-κB and that addition of monovalent gold ions could efficiently block its activity by oxidizing the redox-active cysteines on NF-κB. Since monovalent gold did not appear to replace zinc [71], it is likely that the gold ion oxidizes these thiolate anions on NF-κB into disulfides and thus abrogates the DNA-binding activity because of its higher oxidation potential relative to the zinc ion. It is notable that gold compounds have been successfully used for the treatment of RA [72, 73]. Our finding could explain why gold is effective in RA and suggests that NF-κB might have a crucial role in the disease process [37, 74]. It may be that gold compounds are potentially effective in other diseases where NF-κB plays a pathological role.

Signal transduction therapy for the diseases associated with aberrant NF-κB activation

Involvement of ROI is suggested at least in one of the essential steps of the NF-κB activation pathway, since the signaling was efficiently blocked by pretreatment of the cells with antioxidants such as N-acetyl-L-cysteine (NAC) or α-lipoic acid [26,

27, 28, 43–48]. Therefore, anti-oxidants are considered to be effective NF-κB inhibitors. Moreover, we found that NAC could also block the induction of Trx [61]. Therefore, anti-NF-κB actions of antioxidants are considered to be two-fold: (1) blocking the signaling immediately downstream of the signal elicitation, and (2) suppression of induction of the redox effector Trx. Further elucidation of kinase cascade(s) involved in the NF-κB-activation process, such as tissue-specific distribution and specific inhibitors, should provide us with more information to develop disease-specific therapeutic strategies for blocking aberrant NF-κB activation.

References

1 Holmgren A (1985) Thioredoxin. *Ann Rev Biochem* 54: 237–271

2 Holmgren A (1989) Thioredoxin and glutaredoxin systems. *J Biol Chem* 264: 13963–13966.

3 Ziegler DM (1985) Role of reversible oxidation-reduction of enzyme thios-disulfides in metabolic regulation. *Ann Rev Biochem* 54: 305–329

4 Allen JF (1993) Redox control of transcription: sensors, response regulators, activators and repressors. *FEBS Lett* 332: 203–207

5 Gilmore TD (1990) NF-kappa B, KBF-1, dorsal and related matters. *Cell* 62: 841–843

6 Baeuerle PA (1991) The inducible transcription activator NF-kappa B: regulation by distinct protein subunits. *Biochim Biophys Acta* 1072: 63–80

7 Baeuerle PA, Henkel T (1994) Function and activation of NF-kappa B in the immune system. *Ann Rev Immunol* 12: 141–179

8 Thanos D, Maniatis T (1995) NF-kappa B: a lesson in family values. *Cell* 80: 529–532

9 Maekawa T, Itoh F, Okamoto T, Kurimoto M, Imamoto F, Ishii S (1989) Identification and purification of the enhancer-binding factor of human immunodeficiency virus-1. Multiple proteins and binding to other enhancers. *J Biol Chem* 264: 2826–2831

10 Schindler U, Baichwal VR (1994) Three NF-kappa B binding sites in the human E-selectin gene required for maximal tumor necrosis factor alpha-induced expression. *Mol Cell Biol* 14: 5820–5831

11 Okamoto T, Matsuyama T, Mori S, Hamamoto Y, Kobayashi N, Yamamoto N, Josephs SF, Wong-Staal F, Shimotohno K (1989) Augmentation of human immunodeficiency virus type 1 gene expression by tumor necrosis factor alpha. *AIDS Res Hum Retrovir* 5: 131–138

12 Stade BG, Messer G, Riethmuller G, Johnson JP (1990) Structural characteristics of the 5' region of the human ICAM-1 gene. *Immunobiol* 182:79–87

13 Mukaida N, Mahe Y, Matsushima K (1990) Cooperative interaction of nuclear factor-kappa B- and cis-regulatory enhancer binding protein-like factor binding elements in activating the interleukin-8 gene by pro-inflammatory cytokines. *J Biol Chem* 265: 21128–21133

14 Roebuck KA, Rahman A, Lakshminarayanan V, Janakidevi K, Malik AB (1995) H_2O_2

and tumor necrosis factor-alpha activate intercellular adhesion molecule 1 (ICAM-1) gene transcription through distinct cis-regulatory elements within the ICAM-1 promoter. *J Biol Chem* 270: 18966–18974

15 Donnelly RP, Crofford LJ, Freeman SL, Buras J, Remmers E, Wilder RL, Fenton MJ (1993) Tissue-specific regulation of IL-6 production by IL-4. Differential effects of IL-4 on nuclear factor-kappa B activity in monocytes and fibroblasts. *J Immunol* 151: 5603–5612

16 Schreck R, Baeuerle PA (1990) NF-kappa B as inducible transcriptional activator of the granulocyte-macrophage colony-stimulating factor gene. *Mol Cell Biol* 10:1281–1286

17 Staynov DZ, Cousins DJ, Lee TH (1995) A regulatory element in the promoter of the human granulocyte-macrophage colony-stimulating factor gene that has related sequences in other T-cell-expressed cytokine genes. *Proc Natl Acad Sci USA* 92: 3606–3610

18 Xie Q-W, Kashiwabara Y, Nathan C (1994) Role of transcription factor NF-kappa B/Rel in induction of nitric oxide synthase. *J Biol Chem* 269: 4705–4708

19 Sen R, Baltimore D (1986) Inducibility of kappa immunoglobulin enhancer-binding protein NF-kappa B by a posttranslational mechanism. *Cell* 46: 705–716

20 Nabel G, Baltimore D (1987) An inducible transcription factor activates expression of human immunodeficiency virus in T cells. *Nature* 326: 711–713

21 Bohnlein E, Lowenthal JW, Siekevitz M, Ballard DW, Franza BR, Greene WC (1988) The same inducible nuclear proteins regulates mitogen activation of both the interleukin-2 receptor-alpha gene and type 1 HIV. *Cell* 53: 827–836

22 Okamoto T, Benter T, Josephs S F, Sadaie M R, Wong-Staal F (1990) Transcriptional activation from the long-terminal repeat of human immunodeficiency virus *in vitro*. *Virology* 177: 606–614

23 Arya SK, Guo C, Josephs SF, Wong-Staal F (1985) Trans-activator gene of human T-lymphotropic virus type III (HTLV-III). *Science* 229: 69–73.

24 Sodroski J, Patarca R, Rosen C (1985) Location of the trans-activating region on the genome of human T-cell lymphotropic virus type III. *Science* 229: 74–77

25 Okamoto T, Wong-Staal F (1986) Demonstration of virus-specific transcriptional activator(s) in cells infected with HTLV-III by an *in vitro* cell-free system. *Cell* 47: 29–35

26 Roederer M, Staal FJT, Raju PA, Ela SW, Herzenberg LA, Herzenberg LA (1990) Cytokine-stimulated human immunodeficiency virus replication is inhibited by N-acetyl-Lcysteine. *Proc Natl Acad Sci USA* 87: 4884–4888

27 Suzuki YJ, Aggarwal BB, Packer L (1992) Alpha-lipoic acid is a potent inhibitor if NF-kappa B activation in human T cells. *Biochem Biophys Res Commun* 189: 1709–1715

28 Merin JP, Matsuyama M, Kira T, Baba M, Okamoto T (1996) α-Lipoic acid blocks HIV-1 LTR-dependent expression of hygromycin resistance in THP-1 stable transformants. *FEBS Lett* 394:9–13Æ

29 Tozawa K, Sakurada S, Kohri K, Okamoto T (1995) Effects of anti-nuclear factor kappa B reagents in blocking adhesion of human cancer cells to vascular endothelial cells. *Cancer Res* 55: 4162–4167

30 Montgomery KF, Osborn L, Hession C, Tizard R, Goff D, Vassallo C, Tarr PI, Bomsz-
    tyk K, Lobb R, Harlan JM, Pohlman TH (1991) Activation of endothelial-leukocyte
    adhesion molecule 1 (ELAM-1) gene transcription. *Proc Natl Acad Sci USA* 88:
    6523–6527

31 Whelan J, Ghersa P, Huijsduijnen RH, Gray J, Chandra G, Talabot F, DeLamarter JF
    (1991) An NF kappa B-like factor is essential but not sufficient for cytokine induction
    of endothelial leukocyte adhesion molecule 1 (ELAM-1) gene transcription. *Nucl Acid
    Res* 19: 2645–2653

32 Dejana E, Bertocci F, Bortolami MC, Regonesi A, Tonta A, Breviario F, Giavazzi R
    (1988) Interleukin 1 promotes tumor cell adhesion to cultured human endothelial cells.
    J Clin Invest 82: 1466–1470

33 Takada A, Ohmori K, Yoneda T, Tsuyuoka K, Hasegawa A, Kiso M, Kannagi R (1993)
    Contribution of carbohydrate antigens sialyl Lewis A and sialyl Lewis X to adhesion of
    human cancer cells to vascular endothelium. *Cancer Res* 53: 354–361

34 Alvaro-Gracia JM, Zvaifler NJ, Brown CB, Kaushansky K, Firestein GS (1991)
    Cytokines in chronic arthritis. VI. Analysis of the synovial cells involved in granulocyte
    macrophage colony-stimulating factor production and gene expression in rheumatoid
    arthritis and its regulation by IL-1 and TNF-α. *J Immunol* 146: 3365–3372.

35 Ulfgren AK, Lindblad S, Klareskog L, Andersson J, Andersson U (1995) Detection of
    cytokine producing cells in the synovial membrane from patients with rheumatoid
    arthritis. *Ann Rheum Dis* 54: 654–659

36 Arend WP, Dayer JM (1995) Inhibition of the production and effects of interleukin-1
    and tumor necrosis factor α in rheumatoid arthritis. *Arthritis Rheum* 38: 151–157

37 Handel ML, McMorrow LB, Gravallese EM (1996) Nuclear factor-κB in rheumatoid
    synovium. Localization of p50 and p60. *Arthritis Rheum* 38: 1762–1770

38 Baeuerle PA, Baltimore D (1988) Activation of DNA-binding activity in an apparently
    cytoplasmic precursor of the NF-kappa B transcription factor. *Cell* 53: 211–217

39 Baeuerle PA, Baltimore D (1988) I-kappa B: a specific inhibitor of the NF-kappa B tran-
    scription factor. *Science* 242: 540–546

40 Ghosh S, Gifford AM, Riviere LR, Tempst P, Nolan GP, Baltimore D (1990) Cloning of
    the p50 DNA binding subunit of NF-kappa B: homology to Rel and dorsal. *Cell* 62:
    1019–1029

41 Ghosh S, Baltimore D (1990) Activation *in vitro* of NF-kappa B by phosphorylation of
    its inhibitor I-kappa B. *Nature* 344: 678–682

42 Read MA, Whitley MZ, Williams AJ, Collins T (1994) The proteasome pathway is
    required for cytokine-induced endothelial-leukocyte adhesion molecule expression. *J
    Exp Med* 179: 503–512

43 Schreck R, Albermann K, Baeuerle PA (1992) Nuclear factor kappa B: An oxidative
    stress-responsive transcription factor of eukaryotic cells (a review). *Free Rad Res
    Comms* 17: 221–237

44 Schreck R, Rieber P, Baeuerle PA (1991) Reactive oxygen intermediates as apparently

widely used messengers in the activation of the NF-kappa B transcription factor and HIV-1. *EMBO J* 10: 2247–2258

45 Meyer M, Schreck R, Baeuerle PA (1993) H_2O_2 and antioxidants have opposite effects on activation of NF-kappa B and AP-1 in intact cells: AP-1 as secondary antioxidant-responsive factor. *EMBO J* 12: 2005–2015

46 Biswas DK, Dezube BJ, Ahlers CM, Pardee AB (1993) Pentoxifylline inhibits HIV-1 LTR-driven gene expression by blocking NF-kappa B action. *J AIDS* 6: 778–786

47 Suzuki YJ, Packer L (1994) Signal transduction for nuclear factor-kappa B activation. Proposed location of antioxidant-inhibitable step. *J Immunol* 153: 5008–5015

48 Packer L, Witt EH, Tritschler HJ (1995) α-Lipoic acid as a biological antioxidant. *Free Rad Biol Med* 19: 227–250

49 Malinin NL, Boldin MP, Kovalenko AV, Wallach D (1997) MAP3K-related kinase involved in NF-kappa B induction by TNF, CD95 and IL-1. *Nature* 385: 540–544

50 Connelly MA, Marcu KB (1995) CHUK, a new member of the helix-loop-helix and leucine zipper families of interacting proteins, contains a serine-threonine kinase catalytic domain. *Cell Mol Biol Res* 41: 537–549

51 Regnier CH. Song HY. Gao X. Goeddel DV. Cao Z. Rothe M (1997) Identification and characterization of an IkappaB kinase. *Cell* 90: 373–383

52 DiDonato JA, Hayakawa M, Rothwarf DM, Zandi E, Karin M (1997) A cytokine-responsive IkappaB kinase that activates the transcription factor NF-kappaB. *Nature* 388: 548–54

53 Hayashi T, Sekine T, Okamoto T (1993) Identification of a new serine kinase that activates NF-kappa B by direct phosphorylation. *J Biol Chem* 826: 26790–26795

54 Naumann M, Scheidereit C (1994) Activation of NF-kappa B *in vivo* is regulated by mutiple phosphorylations. *EMBO J* 13: 4597–4607

55 Li C-CH, Dai R-M, Chen E, Longo DL (1994) Phosphorylation of NF-κB1-p50 is involved in NF-kappa B activation and stable DNA binding. *J Biol Chem* 269: 30089–30092

56 Ollivier V, Parry GCN, Cobb RR, de Prost D, Mackman N (1996) Elevated cyclic AMP inhibits NF-kappaB-mediated transcription in human monocytic cells and endothelial cells. *J Biol Chem* 271: 20828–20835

57 Brown K, Gerstberger S, Carlson L, Franzoso G, Siebenlist U (1995) Control of I-kappa B-alpha proteolysis by site-specific, signal-induced phosphorylation. *Science* 267: 1485–1488

58 Chen ZJ, Parent L, Maniatis T (1996) Site-specific phosphorylation of IκBα by a novel ubiquitination-dependent protein kinase activity. *Cell* 84: 853–862

59 Zhong H, SuYang H, Erdjument-Bromage H, Tempst P, Ghosh S (1997) The transcriptional activity of NF-kappaB is regulated by the IkappaB-associated PKAc subunit through a cyclic AMP-independent mechanism. *Cell* 89: 413–424

60 Neumann M, Grieshammer T, Chuvpilo S, Kneitz B, Lohoff M, Schimpl A, Franza BR Jr, Serfling E (1995) RelA/p65 is a molecular target for the immunosuppressive action of protein kinase A. *EMBO J* 14: 1991–2004

61   Sachi Y, Hirota K, Masutani H, Toda K, Okamoto T, Takigawa M, Yodoi J (1995) Induction of ADF/TRX by oxidative stress in keratinocytes and lymphoid cells. *Immunol Lett* 44: 189–193

62   Okamoto T, Ogiwara H, Hayashi T, Mitsui A, Kawabe T, Yodoi J (1992) Human thioredoxin/adult T cell leukemia-derived factor activates the enhancer binding protein of human immunodeficiency virus type 1 bt thiol redox control mechanism. *Int Immunol* 4: 811–819

63   Hayashi T, Ueno Y, Okamoto T (1993) Oxidoreductive regulation of nuclear factor kappa B. Involvement of a cellular reducing catalyst thioredoxin. *J Biol Chem* 268: 11380–11388

64   Tagaya Y, Maeda Y, Mitsui A, Kondo N, Matsui H, Hamuro J, Brown J, Arai K I, Yokota T, Wakasugi H, Yodoi J (1989) ATL-derived factor (ADF), an IL-2 receptor/Tac inducer homologous to thioredoxin; possible involvement of dithiol-reduction in the IL-2 receptor induction. *EMBO J* 8: 757–764

65   Molitor JA, Ballard DW, Greene WC (1991) Kappa-B-specific DNA binding proteins are differentially inhibited by enhancer mutations and biological oxidation. *New Biol* 3: 987–996

66   Toledano MB, Leonard WJ (1991) Modulation of transcription factor NF-kappa B binding activity by oxidation-reduction *in vitro*. Proc Natl Acad Sci USA 88: 4328–4332

67   Matthews JR, Wakasugi N, Virelizier J-L, Yodoi J, Hay RT (1992) Thioredoxin regulates the DNA binding activity of NF-kappa B by reduction of a disulfide bond involving cystein 62. *Nucleic Acids Res* 20: 3821–3830

68   Ghosh G, Van Duyne G, Ghosh S, Sigler PB (1995) Structure of NF-kappa B p50 homodimer bound to a kappa B site. *Nature* 373: 303–310

69   Müller CW, Rey FA, Sodeoka M, Verdine GL, Harrison SC (1995) Structure of the NF-kappa B p50 homodimer bound to DNA. *Nature* 373: 311–317

70   Qin J, Clore GM, Kennedy WMP, Huth JR, Gronenborn AM (1995) Solution structure of human thioredoxin in a mixed disulfide intermediate complex with its target peptide from the transcription factor NF-kappa B. *Structure* 3: 289–297

71   Yang JP, Merin JP, Nakano T, Kato T, Kitade Y, Okamoto T (1995) Inhibition of the DNA-binding activity of NF-kappa B by gold compounds *in vitro*. *FEBS Lett* 361: 89–96

72   Skosey JL (1993) Treatment of rheumatoid arthritis. In: DJ McCarty, WJ Koopman (eds): *Arthritis and allied conditions*. Lea & Febiger, Philadelphia, 603–614

73   Insel PA (1996) Analgesic-antipyretic and anti-inflammatory agents and drugs employed in the treatment of gout. In: JG Hardman et al (eds): *The pharmacological basis of therapeutics*. Macmillan, New York, 670–681

74   Sakurada S, Kato T, Okamoto T (1996) Induction of cytokines and ICAM-1 by proinflammatory cytokines in primary rheumatoid synovial fibroblats and infibition by N-acetyl-L-cysteine and aspirin. *Int Immunol* 8: 1483–1493

Reactive oxygen species and the regulation of metalloproteinase expression

Yvonne Y.C. Lo[1], Johnson M. S. Wong[2], Wing-Fai Cheung[1] and Tony F. Cruz[1]

[1]Connective Tissue Research Group, Samuel Lunenfeld Research Institute, Mount Sinai Hospital, Toronto, Ontario M5G 1X5 and Department of Cellular and Molecular Pathology, University of Toronto, Ontario M5S 1A8, Canada; [2]Banting and Best Department of Medical Research and Department of Molecular and Medical Genetics, University of Toronto, Toronto, Ontario M5G 1L6, Canada

Introduction

Irreparable degradation of articular cartilage is a characteristic feature of arthritic diseases and much of this degradation occurs as a result of increased levels of matrix metalloproteinases (MMPs) such as collagenase and stromelysin [1–6]. The elevated levels of degradative enzymes are due to increased synthesis by cells in joint tissue such as chondrocytes and synoviocytes, as well as invading cells, such as macrophages and neutrophils [7–9]. Thus, depending on the type of joint disease, several cell types may be involved in promoting cartilage destruction. In osteoarthritic cartilage, there is a marked depletion of matrix around the chondrocyte suggesting that this cell plays a key role in cartilage degradation. In inflammatory arthritis, both resident cells, synoviocytes and chondrocytes, as well as invading inflammatory cells are involved.

While it has been difficult to assess definitively the contribution of each cell type to the overall production of MMPs, the role of proinflammatory mediators in the induction of MMPs in arthritic joints has become clear. Cytokines such as interleukin-1 (IL-1) and tumour necrosis factor (TNF) are elevated in arthritic joints and are able to stimulate matrix metalloproteinase production by a variety of cell types in culture and *in vivo* [10–13]. Both of these cytokines play an important role in cartilage destruction. For example, IL-1 induces the loss of proteoglycans in cartilage explant cultures [14–16] and when administered intraarticularly *in vivo* [17, 18]. The breakdown of cartilage components correlates with increased levels of MMPs. Considerable attention is now focused on the production of MMPs as a major cause of cartilage destruction in arthritis.

Although cytokines have been implicated for the increase in MMP production in arthritic joints, little is known on the signalling mechanisms transduced following cytokine binding to its receptor which may serve as potential therapeutic targets.

Free Radicals and Inflammation, edited by P. G. Winyard, D. R. Blake and C. H. Evans
© 2000 Birkhäuser Verlag Basel/Switzerland

Since cytokine induction of *c-fos* and *c-jun* expression and activator protein-1 (AP-1) activation are required events for the induction of MMP expression, considerable efforts from a number of laboratories have focused on the identification of cytokine induced signalling mechanisms regulating the expression and activation of these two transcription factors [19]. Recently, we have demonstrated that IL-1 induced reactive oxygen species (ROS) are involved in the induction of *c-fos*, *c-jun* and collagenase expression. Suppression of ROS levels with antioxidants (e.g. N-acetylcysteine, NAC) or with inhibitors of ROS production (e.g. diphenyleneiodonium, DPI) inhibited IL-1 induction of *c-fos* and collagenase expression by chondrocytes [20–22]. These data indicate that IL-1 induced ROS production may be a key signalling event responsible for the induction of early response genes. The general objective of this chapter is to summarize the underlying mechanisms mediating the involvement of ROS in cytokine induced AP-1 activation and MMP expression.

Role of matrix metalloproteinases

MMP activity in arthritis

Matrix metalloproteinases (MMPs) are zinc- and calcium-dependent enzymes capable of degrading various components of the extracellular matrix. Based on structural and functional studies, the MMPs can be classified into three main subfamilies, collagenases, gelatinases and stromelysins [23, 24]. MMPs differ from each other significantly in substrate specificity. Of relevance to arthritis is the collagenase and stromelysin subfamilies of MMPs. The collagenase subgroup, which can degrade collagen II, the major collagen fiber in cartilage, is comprised of three members: interstitial collagenase (collagenase-1, MMP-1), neutrophil collagenase (MMP-8) and collagenase-3 (MMP-13). Recently, collagenase-3 (MMP-13), a new member, was found to preferentially cleave type II collagen with much higher efficiency than collagenase-1 [25]. Stromelysins do not have the ability to degrade matrix collagen II; however, collagens III, IV, V, X, proteoglycans and fibronectins are efficient substrates. The MMPs are involved in tissue remodeling processes during normal development and in pathological processes accompanying tumor invasion and arthritis. Evidence has been obtained showing overexpession of collagenase-1 and -3 in osteoarthritic and rheumatic joints, in agreement with their role as key players in the process of joint destruction [25–33]. Moreover, synovial lining and cartilage are both rich sources of these MMPs [25, 26, 28, 31, 32]. Because of the important enzymatic activity of MMPs, their production is highly regulated through transcriptional control [34]. The activity of MMPs is also tightly controlled as they are secreted as latent proenzymes that need to be activated by other proteinases and can be inactivated by complexing with tissue inhibitors of metalloproteinases (TIMPs) [23, 24].

Regulation of MMP gene expression

The process of gene expression is orchestrated by the concerted actions of multiple transcription factors which bind to their cognate sequences in the promoter region. Except for the gelatinase A (MMP-2) promoter, AP-1 sites have been found in all the MMP promoters studied [35–38]. AP-1 site is also known as TPA response element for its role in conferring stimulating responses to phorbol esters. The importance of the AP-1 site, recognized by Fos and Jun heterodimers, in MMP expression has been demonstrated for human collagenase-1 and -3 and stromelysin [37, 39, 40]. However, the most extensively studied promoter is that of the collagenase-1 gene. Antisense oligonucleotides directed against the *c-fos* gene and mutation in the AP-1 site completely blocked phorbol ester induction of collagenase [39, 41]. Moreover, in cell lines that do not express *c-jun*, collagenase expression was severely impaired [42]. Given its importance in regulating collagenase expression, the AP-1 site itself is nevertheless not sufficient for full induction. At least two other elements are known to functionally cooperate with the AP-1 site. A PEA3/Ets site acts synergistically with the AP-1 site to achieve maximum induction by phorbol ester, serum or various oncogenes [43, 44]. Ets/PEA3 site is also present in the promoters of collagenase-3 and stromelysin-1 genes, suggesting a common regulatory mechanism of transcription for these genes [38, 45]. Interestingly, Chamberlain et al. identified another AP-1-like sequence, deletion of which resulted in substantial reduction of phorbol ester responsiveness [46]. Protein-protein interaction without DNA binding offers another way of regulating gene expression. The demonstration that AP-1 can physically interact with the transcription factor NF-κB resulting in enhanced DNA binding [47] raises the possibility that collagenase expression may also be controlled by NF-κB.

Reactive oxygen species in arthritis

Nature and sources of ROS

In recent years, a growing body of evidence implicates a class of small molecules termed reactive oxygen species (ROS) in contributing to joint destruction in arthritis. Reactive oxygen species is a collective term to include not only free radicals, but also some potentially dangerous non-radical derivatives of oxygen such as hydrogen peroxide (H_2O_2), singlet oxygen and hypochlorous acid [48, 49]. The biologically relevant free radicals derived from oxygen are the superoxide anion and hydroxyl radical. Among different ROS, the hydroxyl radical is the most reactive and short-lived and thus capable of doing significant damage to biological molecules in its vicinity. Hydroxyl radical is produced in living organisms by the Fenton reaction in which trace amounts of metal ions, primarily ferrous ions, react with hydrogen peroxide. Superoxide radical is much less reactive than hydroxyl radical and its toxic effect is mainly the result of secondary formation of other radicals. For instance, superoxide reacts with nitric oxide (NO), a radical with an unpaired electron delocalized between the two atoms, to form peroxynitrite [50]. As well, superoxide can undergo spontaneous dismutation to yield hydrogen peroxide, a reaction that can also be catalyzed by the ubiquitous superoxide dismutase. Hydrogen peroxide itself is even less reactive than superoxide and thus longer-lived. Moreover, because of its membrane permeability, hydrogen peroxide can be released into the extracellular space and diffuses into neighboring cells. Since various types of ROS can be interconverted by enzymatic and chemical reactions, more reactive species can be derived from relatively less reactive ones such as superoxide and hydrogen peroxide.

Several enzyme systems are responsible for the generation of ROS. Phagocytic cells including neutrophils, monocytes and macrophages, when stimulated, undergo a respiratory burst to generate both superoxide and hydrogen peroxide, the latter as the product of superoxide dismutation [51, 52]. The source of superoxide generation in these cells is a membrane-bound NADPH oxidase which remains dormant until activated by a complex cascade of signal transduction [53]. A similar enzyme complex also appears to exist in nonphagocytic cells including fibroblasts, smooth muscle cells and chondrocytes [20, 54–56]. In these cases, ROS generated are released inside the cell and thus have the potential to serve as intracellular second messengers. ROS can also be generated within mitochondria during respiration as a result of electron leakage and during the catalytic steps of other enzyme systems including cytochrome P-450 reductase, cyclooxygenase and lipoxygenase. In addition to cell-derived ROS, synovial fluid in inflamed joints appears to contain sufficient free iron to catalyze the Fenton reaction which generates the highly toxic hydroxyl radicals [57]. Finally, the process of ischemia-reperfusion in which hypoxic tissue undergoing reoxygenation generates significant amounts of ROS has been suggested to occur in chronic joint inflammation [58]. According to this hypothesis, daily activities and rest can produce cycles of ischemia and reperfusion within the joint leading to ROS formation.

In view of the potentially damaging effects of various ROS, eukaryotic cells contain many specialized enzymes such as superoxide dismutase and catalases devoted to the removal of ROS. In addition, many small molecules have the ability to neutralize oxidants. Examples of these antioxidant molecules include glutathione and the vitamins ascorbic acid and α-tocopherol [59]. Thus, the endogenous ROS levels represent a dynamic state dictated by their combined rates of generation and elimination. Hence, deficiencies of antioxidants or increased formation of ROS can produce oxidative stress, one of the many pathologies seen in inflammatory joint diseases. Interestingly, the levels of ascorbic acid and α-tocopherol had been shown to be significantly lower in sera of rheumatoid arthritic patients than in normal controls [60].

ROS and cartilage destruction

ROS play a significant role in the process of joint destruction by directly acting on cartilage components, activating proteolytic enzymes and inhibiting cartilage repair (Fig. 1). Superoxide may affect the integrity of cartilage by inhibiting collagen gelation and stimulating hyaluronic acid depolymerization [61, 62]. Hypochlorous acid produced from neutrophils can degrade proteoglycans [63] whereas exposure of purified proteoglycan to hydrogen peroxide led to its depolymerization and impaired interactions with hyaluronic acid and link proteins [64]. Hydrogen peroxide can also derive its damaging effects indirectly by inhibiting proteoglycan and hyaluronic acid synthesis [65–67]. Moreover, ROS have also been shown to activate human neutrophil procollagenase, thus initiating degradation of cartilage during inflammation of the joint [68].

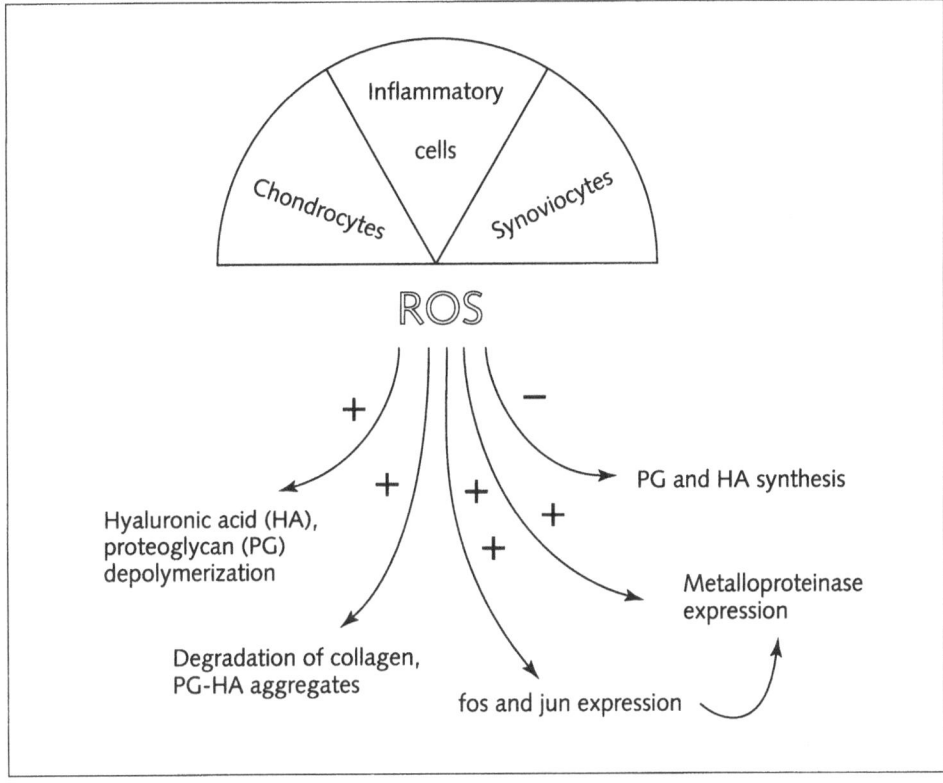

Figure 1
Mechanism of ROS-mediated cartilage destruction.

Nitric oxide (NO) is another free radical secreted in large amounts by inflammatory cells and cytokine-stimulated synoviocytes and chondrocytes [20, 69, 70]. Consistent with the above, nitrate and nitrite concentrations in human synovial fluid were shown to be higher in arthritic patients [71]. Importantly, large amounts of NO could upset the normal joint physiology by suppressing the synthesis of proteoglycan and glycosaminoglycan [72, 73] and preventing chondrocyte proliferation [74]. Furthermore, NO can cause cartilage degradation by stimulating the production and activation of cartilage-degrading metalloproteinases [22, 75].

ROS as signaling molecules

Apart from the direct effects of ROS on joint components and cartilage cellular physiology, recent findings strongly implicate a role of ROS as second messengers mediating the deleterious effects of cytokines (Fig. 1). ROS fulfil many prerequisites as messenger molecules: they are small, diffusible and ubiquitous, can be produced rapidly and have very short half-lives. Also, enzyme systems that have the capacity to generate and eliminate ROS exist in many, if not all cell types. Furthermore, like classical second messengers, ROS can exert pleiotropic effects on cellular events including changes in gene expression, increased DNA synthesis and cellular proliferation [20, 76–78]. More recently, a role for ROS in growth factor action was first delineated from our studies on basic fibroblast growth factor stimulation of *c-fos* expression in chondrocytes [20]. Subsequently, Toren Finkel's group demonstrated that platelet-derived growth factor (PDGF) treatment of smooth muscle cells induces production of intracellular H_2O_2 which are required for DNA synthesis and chemotaxis [78].

In addition to growth factors, cytokines such as TNF and IL-1 have been demonstrated to stimulate ROS release in many cell types including chondrocytes and synoviocytes [20, 22, 79–81]. Furthermore, the endogenously produced ROS may serve as common signaling molecules regulating the activity of the transcription factor NF-κB in response to cytokines and other stimuli. Experimental evidence came from the observation that various antioxidants block the activation of NF-κB by all stimuli tested [82]. Moreover, hydrogen peroxide but not other ROS potently activated NF-κB in many cell types [83, 84]. Oxidants can also stimulate transcription of other transcription factor genes such as *c-jun*, *c-fos* and *c-myc* in various cell types [20, 21, 77]. ROS may also regulate other cellular components other than transcription factors. For instance, NO can directly activate guanylyl cyclase and modulate the activity of iron responsive element binding protein [85]. Recently, the small GTP-binding protein Ras is also found to be subject to redox regulation, with nitrosylation of a critical cysteine residue acting as a switch to induce Ras signaling activity [86].

Regulation of AP-1 by ROS

Transcriptional regulation by ROS

Pro-inflammatory cytokines IL-1 and TNF mediate their effects through signal transduction cascades that culminate in a nuclear response characterized by activation of transcriptional regulators including NF-κB and AP-1. Hence, genes with an AP-1 binding site, such as those encoding collagenase and stromelysin, are direct targets for the two cytokines. Studies from our laboratory have implicated the involvement of ROS in TNF- and IL-1-mediated upregulation of *c-fos* and *c-jun* gene expression in bovine chondrocytes [20–22]. Not only were antioxidants shown to inhibit cytokine induction of both genes, their induction could also be brought about by exogenous addition of hydrogen peroxide (Fig. 2) [20, 21].

Since *c-fos* and *c-jun* genes are early response genes mainly regulated at the transcriptional level, the underlying mechanisms whereby ROS regulate their expression

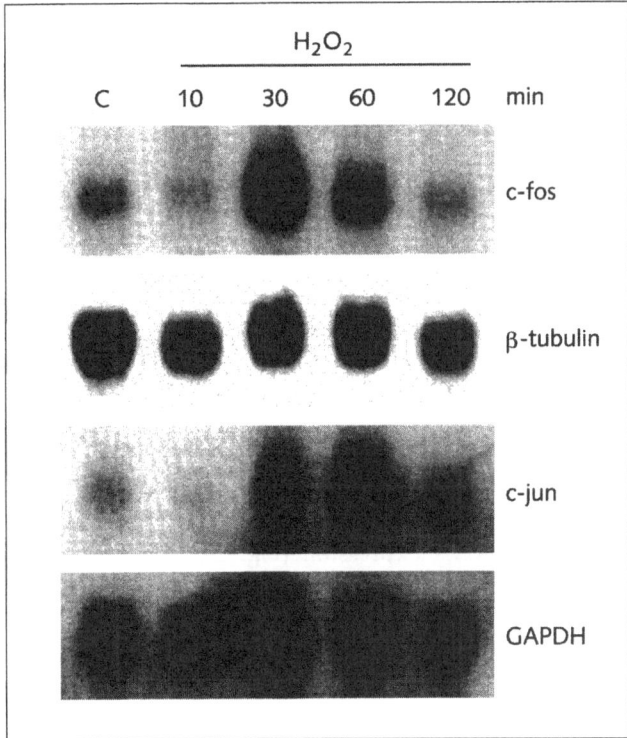

Figure 2
Hydrogen peroxide stimulates c-fos and c-jun gene expression in chondrocytes.

are likely to be transcriptional as well. Studies analyzing the *c-fos* gene promoter revealed that the serum response element (SRE) is a critical sequence determinant regulating *c-fos* expression [87]. The SRE is in fact a composite element consisting of a binding site for the serum response factor (SRF) and an Ets motif. Binding by SRF results in the recruitment of ternary complex factor (TCF) which is comprised of members of the Ets family of transcriptional regulators. Elk-1 is one of the TCFs that forms at the *c-fos* promoter whose phosphorylation stimulates *c-fos* promoter activity. Kinases known to phosphorylate TCF have been identified as the ERK group of the MAP kinase family [87, 88]. Consistent with this, ERK activation leads to elevated AP-1 activity via *c-fos* induction [88]. Although ERK activity can be stimulated by ROS [89–91], cytokine stimulation usually only modestly stimulates ERK activity [92, 93]. In agreement with others, we observed only minimal stimulation (two to three-fold) of ERKs upon cytokine or H_2O_2 treatment of chondrocytes or synoviocytes (unpublished data). The same treatment, however, resulted in significant activation of the JNK group of MAP kinases (see below). Since recent data showed that JNK can also efficiently phosphorylate Elk-1 [94], cytokine and ROS induction of *c-fos* expression is probably largely the result of JNK activation with only a minor contribution from the ERKs.

The *c-jun* gene promoter contains two AP-1-like sequences termed JUN1 and JUN2, each of which is bound by a heterodimer of Jun in association with another transcription factor, ATF2 [95, 96]. Hence, the *c-jun* promoter is autoregulated by its own gene product. Activation of the *c-jun* promoter involves phosphorylation of the prebound c-Jun-ATF2 heterodimers by c-Jun NH_2-terminal kinases/stress-activated protein kinases (JNKs/SAPKs) [97]. Phosphorylation by JNKs of the activation domains of c-Jun and ATF2 increases their activation potential [97–99]. These findings, along with our observations that *c-jun* gene expression is modulated by ROS led us to hypothesize that JNKs might also be regulated by cytokines with ROS as activating intermediates. Indeed, IL-1 and TNF potently activated JNK activity in chondrocytes (Fig. 3A) [21] and synoviocytes (Fig. 3B). More importantly, pretreatment with antioxidants, ascorbic acid and N-acetylcysteine, antagonized the stimulating effects of cytokine on c-Jun kinase activity, indicating that *in vivo* ROS production plays a role in the signaling process (Fig. 3A and B). Exogenous addition of hydrogen peroxide also dramatically activated JNK activity (Fig. 3A and B) [21], correlating with the effect on *c-jun* mRNA expression (Fig. 2). Both JNK1 and JNK2 isoforms contribute to the ROS-mediated cytokine stimulation of c-Jun kinase activity, since activation of both kinases were markedly inhibited by antioxidant [21]. JNK is also a molecular target for NO whose production is significantly enhanced by cytokines. NO-donating agent (S-nitroso-N-acetylpenicillamine, SNAP) can stimulate Jun kinases but the effect is modest when compared to that by hydrogen peroxide (Fig. 3A and B) [21]. We have also evaluated the role of p38, which can efficently phosphorylate and activate ATF2 [100], in the induction of *c-jun*. In general, activation of p38 by cytokines and ROS is significant but weaker

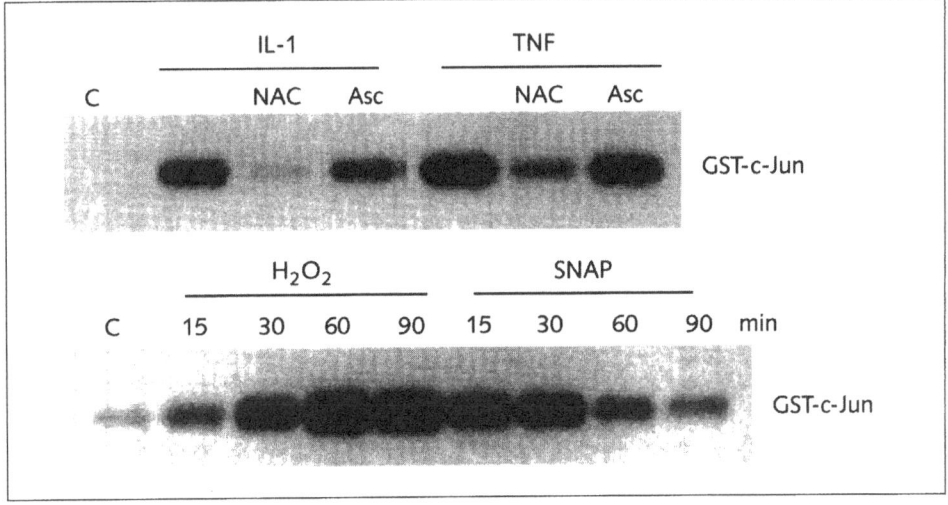

Figure 3A
JNK activation in chondrocytes
Top: Antioxidants inhibit cytokine activation of JNK activity; bottom: H_2O_2 and NO (SNAP)
stimulate JNK activity.

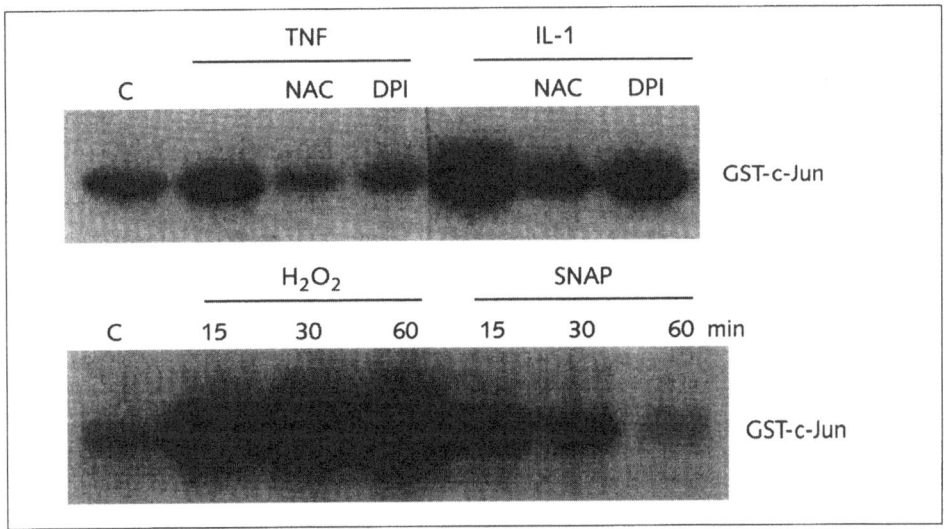

Figure 3B
JNK activation in synoviocytes
Top: NAC and DPI inhibit cytokine activation of JNK activity; bottom: H_2O_2 and NO (SNAP)
stimulate JNK activity.

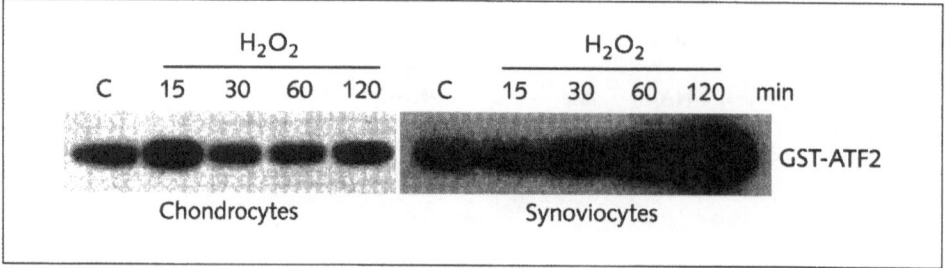

Figure 3C
Stimulation of p38 activity by hydrogen peroxide in chondrocytes and synoviocytes.

than that of JNKs (unpublished data and Fig. 3C), arguing that p38 kinase also contributed to *c-jun* induction.

The exact pathway from ROS release to JNK activation has yet to be characterized. The inhibitory effect of diphenyleneiodonium (DPI) on JNK activation implicates the involvement of flavonoid-containing enzymes such as NADPH oxidase and nitric oxide synthase (Fig. 3B) [21]. Since Rac1, a component of the NADPH oxidase associated with nonphagocytic cells (101), has been shown to be an upstream regulator of JNK [93], it is conceivable that Rac1 stimulates JNK by increasing ROS levels through activation of the oxidase complex. On the other hand, the cellular mechanism of ROS sensing and the identity of the direct sensor molecules remain to be characterized. JNKs themselves do not appear to be the direct targets of ROS (unpublished data). Conceivably, ROS can inhibit a critical phosphatase that normally downregulates the MAP kinase cascade, indirectly leading to an overall increase in kinase activity. Indeed, hydrogen peroxide is a potent inhibitor of tyrosine phosphatases [102, 103]. The recent identification of a phosphatase selective for the JNK pathway [104] also suggests that specific stimulation of only one MAP kinase cascade could occur if various phosphatases exhibit differential sensitivity to inhibition by ROS. Furthermore, direct stimulation of a kinase pathway by ROS may also occur and this form of redox regulation of oxidant sensor molecules has recently been demonstrated for the protooncogene Ras. In this case, direct modification by NO of a key cysteine residue inhibits the GTPase activity, maintaining the Ras protein in the active configuration [86]. It remains to be determined if NO stimulation of JNK is mediated by similar nitrosylation of other small GTP-binding, Ras-related proteins such as Cdc42 and Rac known to be upstream regulators of JNKs [93].

Analysis of the expression of the collagenase gene which is under the control of AP-1 yields a picture consistent with a requirement for new protein synthesis of critical factors such as that of c-Fos and c-Jun. As expected, agents blocking the release

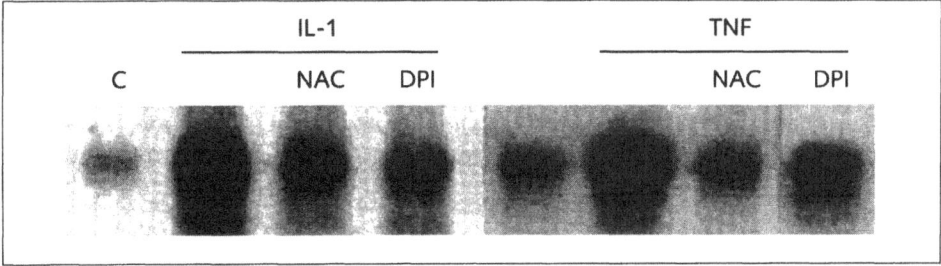

Figure 4
NAC and DPI inhibit IL-1 and TNF induction of collagenase mRNA levels in chondrocytes.

or actions of ROS inhibited cytokine-stimulated collagenase gene expression, probably as the direct consequence of blocking mRNA induction of *c-fos* and *c-jun*
(Fig. 4) [22]. When the role of NO in collagenase expression was assessed using a
NO synthase inhibitor, only a partial reduction of IL-1-induced collagenase mRNA
levels was observed [22]. This is in agreement with the ability of SNAP, a NO-
donating agent, to stimulate collagenase mRNA expression [22] although significantly weaker than IL-1. Hence, NO might contribute to the progression of arthritis not only by directly activating metalloproteinase activity [75], but also by acting
as inducers of collagenase gene expression. The relationship between cytokines,
ROS and gene expression with respect to MMP production is summarized in Figure 5.

Post-translational regulation by ROS

The DNA binding activity of Fos and Jun is subject to an unusual post-translational regulation involving reduction-oxidation (redox) of a single conserved cysteine
residue [105]. This cysteine residue is required to be in the reduced –SH form to per-
mit DNA binding. A nuclear protein, identified as a DNA repair enzyme known as
Ref-1, acts as the redox factor and enhances AP-1 DNA binding by maintaining the
critical cysteine residues in the reduced form [106]. Redox regulation is not unique
to AP-1 as Ref-1 is also capable of enhancing DNA binding of other transcription
factors, including Myb and NF-κB [106]. This, coupled with the finding that AP-1
can physically associate with NF-κB [47], raises the possibility that the collagenase
promoter may also be regulated by NF-κB via a redox-sensitive pathway.

The observation that *in vitro* DNA binding of AP-1 and NF-κB is markedly
decreased by oxidation [105, 106] creates a dilemma with the findings of ROS being
inducers of activity of the same two factors. This conflicting data can be reconciled

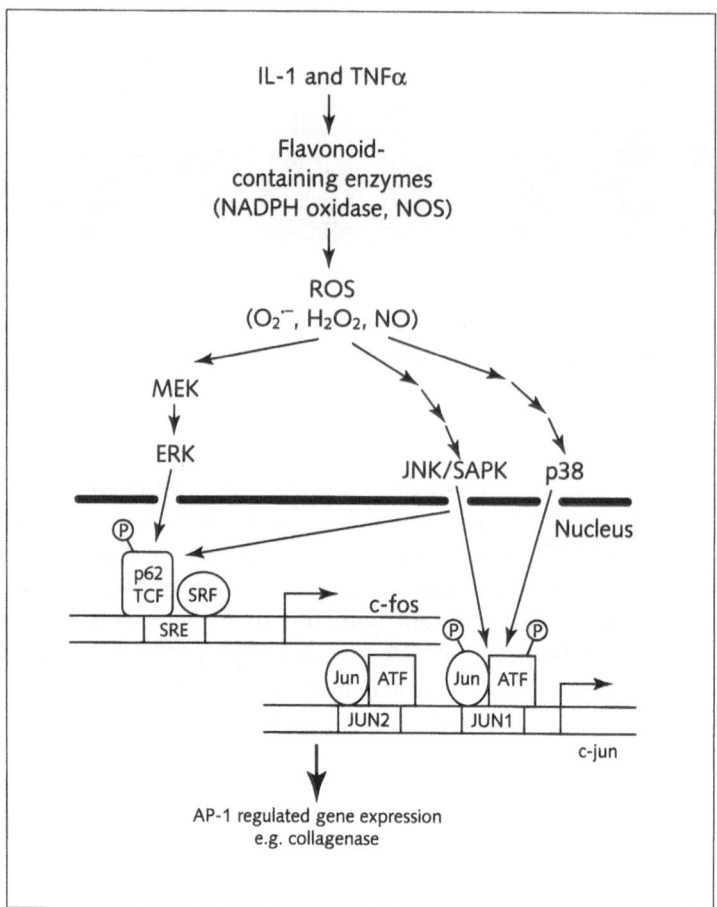

Figure 5
Model for ROS regulation of fos, jun and metalloproteinase expression.

if one takes into account the fact that a eukaryotic cell is compartmentalized, with different proteins confined to either the cytosol or the nucleus. Activation of NF-κB by ROS likely involves stimulating nuclear translocation of the transcription factor by enhancing dissociation of NF-κB from its cytosolic inhibitor protein IκB. Similarly, JNKs normally reside in the cytosol until they are activated by phosphorylation by upstream kinases. Hence, stimulation of JNKs by ROS also occurs in the cytosol regardless of whether ROS inhibit a phosphatase or directly activate the kinase cascade. On the other hand, Ref-1 is localized in the nucleus where it counteracts the oxidation inactivation process of transcription factors.

Therapeutic considerations

The finding that blocking ROS production can inhibit AP-1 and collagenase and stromelysin expression suggests that antioxidant therapy may be useful in the treatment of arthritis, perhaps by impeding the rate of cartilage degradation. Clinical trials have shown that intraarticular injection of superoxide dismutase ameliorated the symptoms of inflammatory joint diseases [107, 108]. However, this therapeutic treatment which requires local injection of the affected joints is not an ideal approach for long-term palliative care of arthritic patients. A better strategy is to test antioxidants that have yielded clinical success in other diseases to see if they also exert beneficial effects in arthritis. Very recently, oral intake of the powerful antioxidant probucol was shown to prevent restenosis after balloon coronary angioplasty [109] and to lower LDL cholesterol levels in patients with heart diesease [110]. Further, there is growing evidence that antioxidants enriched in red wines reduce or prevent heart disease. The exact mechanisms responsible for their action are not known [111]. However, considering the similarities in pathology between restenosis and arthritis, including increased cytokine and MMP levels, increased cell proliferation and inflammatory cell infiltration, it is possible that antioxidants inhibit these diseases by suppressing AP-1 regulated genes such as MMPs.

Combination therapy, conceptually analogues to the cocktail approach used in AIDS treatment, may hold promise to treat arthritis. It seems likely that new pharmacological agents directed at reducing intracellular ROS levels will emerge in the near future. For example, the realization that the radical NO contributes to the overall oxidative burden in inflamed joints has led to animal studies aiming at treating arthritis with inhibitors of NO synthesis; many of these studies have yielded promising results [112, 113]. Perhaps, combining NO synthase inhibitors and antioxidants with established clinical effects such as N-acetylcysteine [114, 115] represents a viable combination therapy that might give higher efficacy in arthritis treatment. Certainly, as our understanding of ROS in signal transduction and pathophysiology increases, parallel advances in effective antioxidant therapy should also take place.

Conclusion

The existing literature and the latest development in the area of ROS and arthritis research, as summarized in this review, strongly argue for a causative role of ROS in joint destruction. Hence, there is a sound rationale for the therapeutic use of antioxidants in the treatment of arthritis. Antioxidant therapy may not be the cure for arthritis, but it may help slow down the degenerative changes in the inflamed joints. Since the development of joint diseases involves a complex interplay between numerous cellular responses, anti-inflammatory drugs alone are clearly not sufficient to block disease progression. Combining antioxidants, many of which have good tolerance records, and other new or established anti-arthritic drugs may provide a new approach to treat arthritis.

References

1 Howell DS (1986) Pathogenesis of osteoarthritis. *Am J Med* 80 (suppl 4B): 24–28

2 Pujol JP, Loyau G (1987) Interleukin-1 and osteoarthritis. *Life Sci* 41: 1187-1198

3 Shinmei M, Okada Y, Masuda K, Naramatsu M, Kikuchi T, Harigai M, Shimomura Y (1990) The mechanism of cartilage degradation in osteoarthritic joints. *Semin Arthritis Rheum* 19 (suppl 1): 16–20

4 Pelletier J-P, Mineau F, Faure M-P, Martel-Pelletier J (1990) Imbalance between the mechanisms of activation and inhibition of metalloproteases in the early lesions of experimental osteoarthritis. *Arthritis Rheum* 33: 1466–1476

5 Woessner JF Jr, Gunja-Smith Z (1991) Role of metalloproteinases in human osteoarthritis. *J Rheumatol* 18 (suppl 27): 99–101

6 Vincenti MP, Clark IM, Brinckerhoff CE (1994) Using inhibitors of metalloproteinases to treat arthritis. Easier said than done? *Arthritis Rheum* 37: 1115–1126

7 Konttinen YT, Honkanen VEA (1988) Future trends in the treatment of rheumatoid arthritis in the light of current etiopathogenetic theories Scand. *J Rheumatol* 74: 7–17

8 Shiozawa S, Shiozawa K (1988) A review of the histopathological evidence on the pathogenesis of cartilage destruction in rheumatoid arthritis Scand. *J Rheumatol* 74: 65–72

9 Arend WP, Dayer J-M (1990) Cytokines and cytokine inhibitors or antagonists in rheumatoid arthritis. *Arthritis Rheum* 33: 305–315

10 Gowen M, Wood DD, Ihrie EJ, McGuire MKB, Russell RGG (1983) An interleukin-1-like factor stimulates bone resorption *in vitro*. *Nature* 306: 378–380

11 Kandel RA, Pritzker K, Mills G, Cruz TF (1990) Fetal bovine serum inhibits collagenase production in chondrocyte cultures: Interleukin-1 reverses this effect. *Biochim Biophys Acta* 1053: 130–134

12 Kandel RA, Petelycky M, Dinarello CA, Minden M, Pritzker KPH, Cruz TF (1990) Comparison of the effect of interleukin-6 and interleukin-1 on collagenase and proteoglycan production by chondrocytes. *J Rheumatol* 17: 953–957

13 Verschure PJ, Van Noorden CJ (1990) The effects of interleukin-1 on articular cartilage destruction as observed in arthritic diseases, and its therapeutic control. *Clin Exp Rheumatol* 8:303–313

14 Arner EC, Pratta MA (1989) Independent effects of interleukin-1 on proteoglycan breakdown, proteoglycan synthesis, and prostaglandin E2 release from cartilage in organ culture. *Arthritis Rheum* 32: 288–297

15 Morales TI, Hascall VC (1989) Effects of interleukin-1 and lipopolysaccharides on pro-

tein and carbohydrate metabolism in bovine articular cartilage organ cultures. *Connect Tissue Res* 19: 255–275

16 Martel-Pelletier J, Zafarullah M, Kodama S, Pelletier J-P (1991) *In vitro* effects of inter-leukin 1 on the synthesis of metalloproteases, TIMP, plasminogen activators and inhibitors in human articular cartilage. *J Rheumatol* 18 (suppl 27): 80–84

17 Dingle JT, Page Thomas DP, King B, Bard DR (1987) *In vivo* studies of articular tissue damage mediated by catabolin/interleukin 1. *Ann Rheum Dis* 46: 527–533

18 Staite ND, Richard KA, Aspar DG, Franz KA, Galinet LA, Dunn CJ (1990) Induction of an acute erosive monarticular arthritis in mice by interleukin-1 and methylated bovine serum albumin. *Arthritis Rheum* 33: 253–260

19 Karin M (1995) The regulation of AP-1 activity by mitogen-activated protein kinases. *J Biol Chem* 270: 16483–16486

20 Lo YYC, Cruz TF (1995) Involvement of reactive oxygen species in cytokine and growth factor induction of c-fos expression in chondrocytes. *J Biol Chem* 270: 11727–11730

21 Lo YYC, Wong JMS, Cruz TF (1996) Reactive oxygen species mediate cytokine activa-tion of c-Jun NH2-terminal kinases. *J Biol Chem* 271: 15703–15707

22 Lo YYC, Conquer JA, Grinstein S, Cruz TF (1998) Interleukin-1β induction of c-fos and collagenase expression in articular chondrocytes: Involvement of reactive oxygen species. *J Cell Biochem* 69: 19–29

23 Woessner JF Jr (1991) Matrix metalloproteinases and their inhibitors in connective tis-sue remodeling. *FASEB J* 5: 2145–2154

24 Kleiner DE Jr, Stetler-Stevenson WG (1993) Structural biochemistry and activation of matrix metalloproteases. *Curr Opin Cell Biol* 5: 891–897

25 Mitchell PG, Magna HA, Reeves LM, Lopresti-Morrow LL, Yocum SA, Rosner PJ, Geoghegan KF, Hambor JE (1996) Cloning, expression, and type II collagenolytic activ-ity of matrix metalloproteinase-13 from human osteoarthritic cartilage. *J Clin Invest* 97: 761–768

26 Dean DD, Azzo W, Martel-Pelletier J, Pelletier JP, Woessner JF Jr (1987) Levels of met-alloproteases and tissue inhibitor of metalloproteases in human osteoarthritic cartilage. *J Rheumatol* 14: 43–51

27 Brinckerhoff CE (1991) Joint destruction in arthritis: Metalloproteinases in the spot-light. *Arthritis Rheum* 34: 1073–1075

28 Gravallese EM, Darling JM, Ladd L, Katz JN, Gilmcher LH (1991) *In situ* hybridiza-tion studies of stromelysin and collagenase messenger RNA expression in rheumatoid synovium. *Arthritis Rheum* 34: 1076–1084

29 Clark IM, Powell LK, Ramsey S, Hazelman BL, Cawston TE (1993) The measurement of collagenase, tissue inhibitor of metalloproteinases (TIMP), and collagenase-TIMP complex in synovial fluids from patients with osteoarthritis and rheumatoid arthritis. *Arthritis Rheum* 36: 372–379

30 Lohmander LS, Hoerrner LA, Lark MW (1993) Metalloproteinases, tissue inhibitor, and proteoglycan fragments in knee synovial fluid in human osteoarthritis. *Arthritis Rheum* 36: 181–189

31   Wolfe GC, MacNaul KL, Buechel FF, McDonnell J, Hoerrner LA, Lark MW, Moore VL, Hutchinson NI (1993) Differential *in vivo* expression of collagenase messenger RNA in synovium and cartilage. *Arthritis Rheum* 36: 1540–1547

32   Wernicke D, Seyfert C, Hinzmann B, Gromnica-Ihle E (1996) Cloning of collagenase 3 from the synovial membrane and its expression in rheumatoid arthritis and osteoarthritis. *J Rheumatol* 23: 590–595

33   Moldovan F, Pelletier JP, Hambor J, Cloutier JM, Martel-Pelletier J (1997) Collagenase-3 (matrix metalloprotease 13) is preferentially localized in the deep layer of human arthritis cartilage *in situ*: *in vitro* mimicking effect by transforming growth factor beta. *Arthritis Rheum* 40: 1653–1661

34   Borden P, Heller RA (1997) Transcriptional control of matrix metalloproteinases and the tissue inhibitors of matrix metalloproteinases. *Crit Rev Eukaryot Gene Expr* 7: 159–178

35   Gaire M, Magbanua Z, McDonnell S, McNeil L, Lovett DH, Martrisian LM (1994) Structure and expression of the human gene for the matrix metalloproteinase matrilysin. *J Biol Chem* 269: 2032–2040

36   Schorpp M, Mattei MG, Herr I, Gack S, Schaper J, Angel P (1995) Structural organization and chromosomal localization of the mouse collagenase type I gene. *Biochem J* 308: 211–217

37   Borden P, Solymar D, Sucharczuk A, Lindman B, Cannon P, Heller RA (1996) Cytokine control of interstitial collagenase and collagenase-3 gene expression in human chondrocytes. *J Biol Chem* 271: 23577–23581

38   Tardif G, Pelletier JP, Dupuis M, Hambor JE, Martel-Pelletier J (1997) Cloning, sequencing and characterization of the 5'-flanking region of the human collagenase-3 gene. *Biochem J* 323: 13–16

39   Angel P, Imagawa M, Chiu R, Stein B, Imbra RJ, Rahmsdorf HJ, Jonat C, Herrlich P, Karin M (1987) Phorbol ester-inducible genes contain a common cis element recognized by a TPA-modulated trans-acting factor. *Cell* 49: 729–739

40   Buttice G, Quinones S, Kurkinen M (1991) The AP-1 site is required for basal expression but is not necessary for TPA-response of the human stromelysin gene. *Nucleic Acids Res* 19: 3723–3731

41   Schonthal A, Herrlich P, Rahmsdorf HJ, Ponta H (1988) Requirement for fos gene expression in the transcriptional activation of collagenase by other oncogenes and phorbol esters. *Cell* 54: 325–334

42   Marshall-Heyman H, Engel G, Ljungdahl S, Shoshan MC, Svensson C, Wasylyk B, Linder S (1994) Tumorigenic and metastatic properties of two ras-oncogene transfected rat fibrosarcoma cell lines defective in c-jun. *Oncogene* 9: 3655–3663

43   Gutman A, Wasylyk B (1990) The collagenase gene promoter contains a TPA and oncogene-responsive unit encompassing the PEA3 and AP-1 binding sites. *EMBO J* 9: 2241–2246

44   Auble DT, Brinckerhoff CE (1991) The AP-1 sequence is necessary but not sufficient for phorbol ester induction of collagenase in fibroblasts. *Biochemistry* 30: 4629–4635

45 Buttice G, Kurkinen M (1993) A polyomavirus enhancer A-binding protein-3 site and Ets-2 protein have a major role in the 12-O-tetradecanoyl phorbol-13-acetate response of the human stromelysin gene. *J Biol Chem* 268: 7196–7204

46 Chamberlain SH, Hemmer RM, Brinckerhoff CE (1993) Novel phorbol ester response region in the collagenase promoter binds Fos and Jun. *J Cell Biochem* 52: 337–351

47 Stein B, Baldwin AS Jr, Ballard DW, Greene WCI, Angel P, Herrich P (1993) Cross-coupling of the NF-kappa B p65 and Fos/Jun transcription factors produces potentiated biological function. *EMBO J* 12: 3879–3891

48 Fischer AB (1988) Intracellular production of oxygen derived free radicals. In: B Halliwell (ed): Oxygen radicals and tissue injury. The Upjohn Co, Bethesda, MD, 34–42

49 Halliwell B, Gutteridge JMC (1989) *Free radicals in biology and medicine*, 2nd ed. Clarendon Press, Oxford

50 Wink DA, Hanbauer I, Grisham MB, Laval F, Nims RW, Laval J, Cook J, Pacelli R, Liebmann J, Krishna M, Ford PC, Mitchell JB (1996) Chemical biology of nitric oxide: regulation and protective and toxic mechanisms. *Curr Top Cellu Regul* 34: 159–187

51 Babior BM (1984) The respiratory burst of phagocytes. *J Clin Invest* 73: 599–601

52 Bellavite P (1988) The superoxide forming enzymatic system of phagocytes. *Free Rad Biol Med* 4: 225–261

53 Bokoch GM (1994) Regulation of the human neutrophil NADPH oxidase by the Rac GTP-binding proteins. *Curr Opin Cell Biol* 6: 212–218

54 Griendling KK, Minieri CA, Ollerenshaw JD, Alexander RW (1994) Angiotensin II stimulates NADH and NADPH oxidase activity in cultured vascular smooth muscle cells. *Circ Res* 74: 1141–1148

55 Jones SA, Wood JD, Coffey MJ, Jones OTG (1994) The functional expression of p47-phox and p67-phox may contribute to the generation of superoxide by an NADPH oxidase-like system in human fibroblasts. *FEBS Lett* 355: 178–182

56 Thannickal VJ, Fanburg BL (1995) Activation of an H_2O_2-generating NADH oxidase in human lung fibroblasts by transforming growth factor beta 1. *J Biol Chem* 270: 30334–30338

57 Buettner GR, Chamulitrat W (1990) The catalytic activity of iron in synovial fluid as monitored by the ascorbate free radical. *Free Rad Biol Med* 8: 55–56

58 Blake DR, Merry P, Kidd BL, Unsworth J, Outhwaite JM, Ballard R, Morris CJ, Gray L, Lunec J (1989) Hypoxic-reperfusion injury in the inflamed human joint. *Lancet* 1: 289–293

59 Sies H (1993) Oxidative stress: oxidants and antioxidants. *Exp Physiol* 82: 291–295

60 Situnayake RD, Thurnham DI, Kootathep S, Chirico S, Lunec J, Davis M, McCornkey B (1991) Chain breaking antioxidant status in rheumatoid arthritis: clinical and laboratory correlates. *Ann Rheum Dis* 50: 81–86

61 Greenwald RA, Moy WW (1979) Inhibition of collagen gelation by action of the superoxide radical. *Arthritis Rheum* 22: 251–259

62 Greenwald RA, Moy WW (1980) Effect of oxygen-derived free radicals on hyaluronic acid. *Arthritis Rheum* 23: 455–463

63   Kowanko IC, Bates EJ, Ferrante A (1989) Mechanisms of human neutrophil mediated cartilage damage *in vitro*: the role of lysosomal enzymes, hydrogen peroxide and hypochlorous acid. *Immunol Cell Biol* 67: 321–329

64   Roberts CR, Roughley PJ, Mort JS (1989) Degradation of human proteoglycan aggregate induced by hydrogen peroxide. *Biochem J* 259: 805–811

65   Bates EJ, Johnson CC, Lowther DA (1985) Inhibition of proteoglycan synthesis by hydrogen peroxide in cultured bovine articular cartilage. *Biochim Biophys Acta* 838: 221–228

66   Bates EJ, Lowther DA, Johnson CC (1985) Hyaluronic acid synthesis in articular cartilage: an inhibition by hydrogen peroxide. *Biochem Biophys Res Commun* 132: 714–720

67   Schalwijk J, van den Berg WB, van de Putte LB, Joosten LAB (1985) Hydrogen peroxide suppresses the proteoglycan synthesis of intact articular cartilage. *J Rheumatol* 12: 205–210

68   Saari H, Sorsa T, Lindy O, Suomalainen K, Halinen S, Konttinen YT (1992) Reactive oxygen species as a regulator of human neutrophil and fibroblast interstitial collagenases. *Int J Tissue React* 14: 113–120

69   Murrell GAC, Dolan MM, Jang D, Szabo C, Warren RF, Hannafin JA (1996) Nitric oxide – an important articular free radical. *J Bone Joint Surg (Am)* 78: 265–274

70   Stefanovic-Racic M, Meyers K, Meschter C, Coffey J W, Hoffman RA, Evans CH (1994) N-monomethyl arginine, an inhibitor of nitric oxide synthase, suppresses the development of adjuvant arthritis in rats. *Arthritis Rheum* 37: 1062–1069

71   Ueki Y, Miyake S, Tominaga Y, Eguchi K (1996) Increased nitric oxide levels in patients with rheumatoid arthritis. *J Rheumatol* 23: 230–236

72   Hauselmann HJ, Oppliger L, Michel BA, Stefanovic-Racic M, Evans CH (1994) Nitric oxide and proteoglycan biosynthesis by human articular chondrocytes in alginate culture. *FEBS Lett* 352: 361–364

73   Jarvinen TAH, Moilanen T, Jarvinen TLN, Moilanen E (1995) Nitric oxide mediates interleukin-1 induced inhibition of glycosaminoglycan synthesis in rat articular cartilage. *Mediat Inflamm* 4: 107–111

74   Blanco FJ, Lotz M (1995) IL-1-induced nitric oxide inhibits chondrocyte proliferation via PGE2. *Exp Cell Res* 218: 319–325

75   Murrell GAC, Jang D, Williams RJ (1995) Nitric oxide activates metalloprotease enzymes in articular cartilage. *Biochem Biophys Res Commun* 206: 15–21

76   Murrell GA, Francis MJ, Bromley L (1990) Modulation of fibroblast proliferation by oxygen free radicals. *Biochem J* 265: 659–665

77   Rao GN, Berk BC (1992) Active oxygen species stimulate vascular smooth muscle cell growth and proto-oncogene expression. *Circ Res* 70: 593–599

78   Sundaresan M, Yu ZX, Ferrans VJ, Irani K, Finkel T (1995) Rquirement for generation of H_2O_2 for platelet-derived growth factor signal transduction. *Science* 270: 296–299

79   Iwasaki Y, Matsubara T, Hirohata K (1988) A mechanism of cartilage destruction in

immunologically-mediated inflammation: increased superoxide anion release from chondrocytes in response to interleukin-1 and interferons. *Orthop Trans* 12: 438–444

80 Rathakrishnan C, Tiku K, Raghavan A, Tiku ML (1992) Release of oxygen radicals by articular chondrocytes: a study of luminol-dependent chemiluminescence and hydrogen peroxide secretion. *J Bone Miner Res* 7: 1139–1148

81 Tawara T, Shingu M, Nobunaga M, Naono T (1991) Effects of recombinant human IL-1β on production of prostaglandin E₂, leukotriene B₄, NAG and superoxide by human synovial cells and chondrocytes. *Inflammation* 15: 145–157

82 Schreck R, Meier B, Mannel DN, Droge W, Baeuerle PA (1992) Dithio-carbamates as potent inhibitors of nuclear factor kappa B activation in intact cells. *J Exp Med* 175: 1181–1194

83 Schreck R, Albermann K, Baeuerle PA (1992) Nuclear factor kappa B: an oxidative stress-responsive transcription factor of eukaryotic cells (a review). *Free Rad Res Comms* 17: 221–237

84 Kaul N, Forman HJ (1996) Activation of NF kappa B by the respiratory burst of macrophages. *Free Rad Biol Med* 21: 401–405

85 Stamler JS (1994) Redox signaling: Nitrosylation and related target interactions of nitric oxide. *Cell* 78: 931–936

86 Lander HM (1997) An essential role for free radicals and derived species in signal transduction. *FASEB J* 11: 118–124

87 Price MA, Hill C, Treisman R (1996) Integration of growth factor signals at the c-fos serum response element. *Phil Trans Royal Soc Lond-Series B*: Biological Sciences 351: 551–559

88 Price MA, Cruzalegui FH, Treisman R (1996) The p38 and ERK Map kinase pathways cooperate to activate ternary complex factors and c-fos transcription in response to UV light. *EMBO J* 15: 6552–6563

89 Fialkow L, Chan CK, Rotin D, Grinstein S, Downey GP (1994) Activation of the mitogen-activated protein kinase signaling pathway in neutrophils. *J Biol Chem* 269: 31234–31242

90 Stevenson MA, Pollock SS, Coleman CN, Calderwood SK (1994) X-irradiation, phorbol esters and H2O2 stimulate mitogen-activated protein kinase activity in NIH-3T3 cells through the formation of reactive oxygen intermediates. *Cancer Res* 54: 12–15

91 Guyton KZ, Liu Y, Gorospe M, Xu Q, Holbrook NJ (1996) Activation of mitogen-activated protein kinase by H2O2 Role in cell survival following oxidant injury. *J Biol Chem* 271: 4138–4142

92 Kyriakis JM, Banerjee P, Nikolakaki E, Dai T, Rubie EA, Ahmad MF, Avruch J, Woodgett JR (1994) The stress-activated protein kinase subfamily of c-Jun kinases. *Nature* 369: 156–160

93 Denhardt DT (1996) Signal-transducing protein phosphorylation cascades mediated by Ras/Rho proteins in the mammalian cell: the potential for multiplex signalling. *Biochem J* 318: 729–747

94 Whitmarsh AJ, Shore P, Sharrocks AD, Davis RJ (1995) Integration of MAP kinase signal transduction pathways at the serum response element. *Science* 269: 403–407

95 Devary Y, Gottlieb RA, Lau LF, Karin M (1991) Rapid and preferential activation of the c-jun gene during the mammalian UV response. *Mol Cell Biol* 11: 2804–2811

96 van Dam H, Duyndam M, Rottier R, Bosch A, de Vries-Smits L, Herrlich P, Zantema A, Angel P, van der Eb AJ (1993) Hetreodimer formation of c-Jun and ATF-2 is responsible for induction of c-jun by the 243 amino acid adenovirus E1A protein. *EMBO J* 12: 479–487

97 Wilhelm D, van Dam H, Herr I, Baumann B, Herrlich P, Angel P (1995) Both ATF-2 and c-Jun are phosphorylated by stress-activated protein kinases in response to UV irradiation. *Immunobiol* 193: 143–148

98 Smeal T, Binetruy B, Mercola DA, Birrer M, Karin M (1991) Oncogenic and transcriptional cooperation with Ha-Ras requires phosphorylation of c-Jun on serines 63 and 73. *Nature* 354: 494–496

99 van Dam H, Wilhelm D, Herr I, Steffen A, Herrlich P, Angel P (1995) ATF-2 is preferentially activated by stress-activated protein kinases to mediate c-jun induction in response to genotoxic agents. *EMBO J* 14: 1798–1811

100 Raingeaud J, Whitmarsh AJ, Barrett T, Derijard B, Davis RJ (1996) MKK3- and MKK6-regulated gene expression is mediated by the p38 mitogen-activated protein kinase signal transduction pathway. *Mol Cell Biol* 16: 1247–1255

101 Sundaresan M, Yu ZX, Ferrans VJ, Sulciner DJ, Gutkind JS, Irani K, Goldschmidt-Clermont PJ, Finkel T (1996) Regulation of reactive-oxygen-species generation in fibroblasts by Rac1. *Biochem J* 318: 379–382

102 Hecht D, Zick Y (1992) Selective inhibition of protein tyrosine phosphatase activities by H_2O_2 and vanadate *in vitro*. *Biochem Biophys Res Commun* 188: 773–779

103 Sullivan SG, Chiu DTY, Errasfa M, Wang JM, Qi JS, Stern A (1994) Effects of H_2O_2 on protein tyrosine phosphatase activity in HER 14 cells. *Free Rad Biol Med* 16: 399–403

104 Muda M, Theodosiou A, Rodrigues N, Boschert U, Camps M, Gillieron C, Davies K, Ashworth A, Arkinstall S (1996) The dual specificity phosphatases M3/6 and MKP-3 are highly selective for inactivation of distinct mitogen-activated protein kinases. *J Biol Chem* 271: 27205–27208

105 Abate C, Patel L, Rauscher FJ III, Curran T (1990) Redox regulation of Fos and Jun DNA-binding activity *in vitro*. *Science* 249: 1157–1162

106 Xanthoudakis S, Miao G, Wang F, Pan YC, Curran T (1992) Redox activation of Fos-Jun DNA binding activity is mediated by a DNA repair enzyme. *EMBO J* 11: 3323–3335

107 Flohe L (1988) Superoxide dismutase for therapeutic use: clinical experience, dead ends and hopes. *Mol Cell Biochem* 84: 123–131

108 McIlwain H, Silverfield JC, Cheatum DE, Poiley J, Taborn J, Ignaczak T, Multz CV (1989) Intra-articular orgotein in osteoarthritis of the knee: a placebo-controlled efficacy, safety and dosage comparison. *Am J Med* 87: 295–300

109 Tardif JC, Cote G, Lesperance J, Bourassa M, Lambert J, Doucet S, Bilodeau L, Nattel S, de Guise P (1997) Probucol and multivitamins in the prevention of restenosis after coronary angioplasty. Multivitamins and Probucol Study Group. *N Engl J Med* 337: 365–372

110 Anderson TJ, Meredith IT, Yeung AC, Frei B, Selwyn AP, Ganz P (1995) The effect of cholesterol-lowering and antioxidant therapy on endothelium-dependent coronary vasomotion. *N Engl J Med* 332: 488–493

111 Soleas GJ, Diamandis EP, Goldberg DM (1997) Wine as a biological fluid: History, production, and role in disease prevention. *J Clin Lab Anal* 11: 287–313

112 McCartney-Francis N, Allen JB, Mizel DE, Albina JE, Xie QW, Nathan CF, Wahl SM (1993) Suppression of arthritis by an inhibitor of nitric oxide synthase. *J Exp Med* 178: 749–754

113 Stefanovic-Racic M, Stadler J, Georgescu HI, Evans CH (1994) Nitric oxide synthesis and its regulation by rabbit synoviocytes. *J Rheumatol* 21: 1892–1898

114 De Flora S, Cesarone CF, Balansky RM, Albini A, D'Agostini F, Bennicelli C, Bagnasco M, Camoirano A, Scatolini L, Rovida A et al (1995) Chemopreventive properties and mechanisms of N-Acetylcysteine. The experimental background. *J Cell Biochem* 22: 33–41

115 De Flora S, Grassi C, Carati L (1997) Attenuation of influenza-like symptomatology and improvement of cell-mediated immunity with long-term N-acetylcysteine treatment. *Eur Respir J* 10: 1535–1541

Nitric oxide and inflammatory joint diseases

Chris H. Evans[1] and Maja Stefanovic-Racic[2]

[1]Center for Molecular Orthopaedics, Harvard Medical School, 221 Longwood Avenue, Boston, MA 02115, USA; [2]Department of Orthopaedic Surgery, University of Pittsburgh School of Medicine, 200 Lothrop Street, Room C-313 PUH, Pittsburgh, PA 15213, USA

Introduction

Inflammation of joints occurs as a result of injury or disease and imposes considerable suffering and economic loss. Despite the existence of numerous anti-inflammatory drugs, treatment of inflammatory joint conditions remains unsatisfactory, especially when the inflammation is chronic, as in rheumatoid arthritis (RA). Evidence that nitric oxide (NO) is generated in inflamed joints has raised hopes of improving treatment by modulating the intra-articular activity of NO (reviewed in [1]).

Moveable joints typically contain a cavity or space, known as the joint space, within which the ends of the long bones articulate. A small volume of synovial fluid serves a lubricating function. The articulating surfaces are covered by a smooth, resilient tissue known as articular cartilage. This is avascular, aneural and alymphatic, and contains a relatively sparse population of articular chondrocytes embedded within an abundant extracellular matrix. The major macromolecular components of this matrix are collagens and proteoglycans. Certain joints, such as the knee, contain additional cartilaginous stabilizing structures known as menisci; the meniscal cartilage has important biochemical differences from articular cartilage. All non-cartilaginous surfaces within the joint are covered by a lining known as the synovium. This is a thin structure containing two types of resident synoviocytes, the type A cells that resemble macrophages, and the type B cells that are fibroblastic. The underlying sub-synovium is highly vascularized and well innervated. The biology of cartilage and synovium has been reviewed recently in [2].

Inflammation of synovial joints usually includes a synovitis and a large increase in the volume and cellularity of the synovial fluid. The inflamed synovium is thickened due to hyperplasia of the resident type B synoviocytes, influx of inflammatory leukocytes and enhanced deposition of matrix. Greater permeability of the capillaries underlying the synovium contributes to the increased volume of the synovial fluid which, during acute inflammation, can contain very high concentrations of polymorphonuclear leukocytes.

Free Radicals and Inflammation, edited by P. G. Winyard, D. R. Blake and C. H. Evans
© 2000 Birkhäuser Verlag Basel/Switzerland

The cartilages of the inflamed joint, in contrast, do not become colonized by leukocytes. This partly reflects the lack of a blood supply and the inability of inflammatory cells to adhere to the cartilaginous matrix. Nevertheless, during joint inflammation there is a loss of the cartilaginous matrix due to the catabolic activities of chondrocytes which have become stimulated in response to soluble factors released from the inflamed synovium and synovial fluid leukocytes. Among these soluble factors interleukin-1 (IL-1) is particularly potent. IL-1 and a limited number of other cytokines, such as tumor necrosis factor (TNF), also inhibit the synthesis of matrix macromolecules, and are therefore particularly damaging to cartilage.

A variety of events, ranging from sports injuries to arthritis, can trigger joint inflammation. In many cases, the acute inflammation following trauma to joints spontaneously resolves whereas in several forms of arthritis the inflammation persists chronically. NO may be involved in both acute and chronic inflammation, as well as in the loss of cartilage that accompanies these conditions. This chapter reviews the evidence for such involvements.

Arthritis

Textbooks on arthritis make reference to a hundred or so varieties of arthritis, the word itself being derived from the Greek for "inflamed joint". The inflammation is at its most persistent and damaging in RA.

RA is an inflammatory arthropathy that is thought by many to result from autoimmune reactions to certain as yet unidentified intraarticular antigens. These reactions provoke major synovial alterations. The tissue becomes enormously thickened due to increased cellularity and increased deposition of extracellular matrix. Unlike normal synovium, the rheumatoid synovium is heavily infiltrated with leukocytes, particularly CD4+ lymphocytes (T helper lymphocytes) and macrophages. Cytokines produced locally by activated macrophages and resident synoviocytes are thought to be particularly important mediators of intraarticular disease activity (reviewed in [4]).

Rheumatoid synovium forms a distinctive structure, known as pannus, which attaches to and invades the adjacent cartilage, as well as the underlying subchondral bone. These erosive activities are particularly damaging, leading to distortion and destruction of the joints which, in many cases, is uncontrollable and leaves patients with total joint replacement surgery as their only clinical recourse.

RA typically affects many joints on the same patient, particularly the knuckle, wrist and knee joints, and may be accompanied by systemic manifestations such as fever and the formation of subcutaneous "rheumatoid" nodules. Osteoarthritis (OA), in contrast, usually involves only a few joints, such as the hips and knees, and is not accompanied by major systemic or extraarticular associations. The degree of synovial inflammation in OA is much lower than in RA, and is not associated with the formation of pannus.

The major pathological lesion in OA is a focal loss of articular cartilage. Unlike RA, where the cartilage is lost in a centripetal fashion as the pannus progressively invades from the edges, cartilage loss in OA usually starts centrally in areas subjected to the highest mechanical loading. The size of these ulcerated areas increases both in width and depth, eventually denuding the articulating osseous surfaces of their cartilaginous covering.

Other rheumatic conditions with joint involvement include Lyme arthritis, which follows infection by the spirochaete *Borrelia burgdorferi*, and systemic lupus erythematosus (SLE; lupus), a generalized autoimmune condition. Although the joints of patients with lupus become inflamed, erosions are usually absent. The various forms of arthritis are described more fully in [3].

From this brief orientation, it is clear that for NO to be an important mediator in the pathophysiology of one or more arthritides it should be a key component in immunity, inflammation or cartilage loss. The evidence on this matter will now be reviewed.

Production of NO in arthritis

There is good evidence of elevated NO production in several animal models of arthritis (Tab. 1), as well as in human RA, OA and lupus (Tab. 2). In all cases, elevated levels of NO_x have been measured in synovial fluids, blood, urine, monocytes or macrophages. Nitrotyrosine, an indicator of peroxynitrite formation, has been found in human synovial fluids recovered from patients with RA, but not OA [30]. *In situ* techniques have confirmed the expression of iNOS in synovium and articular cartilage recovered from joints of patients with RA and OA, as well as in synovium, lymph nodes, spleen and liver of rodents with experimental RA [14].

According to the data of Sakurai et al., [30] most of the human synovial cells that express iNOS are type A synoviocytes and endothelial cells, with lower expression in infiltrating mononuclear cells and type B synoviocytes. McInnes et al., [33] in contrast, suggest that the majority of the iNOS-positive cells within synovium are type B synoviocytes; according to Grabowski et al. [31] macrophages, fibroblasts and vascular smooth muscle cells are all iNOS+ in human rheumatoid synovium. Expression of iNOS does not necessarily mean that the cells are producing large amounts of NO, and it is well known that the synthesis of NO by human macrophages, at least under *in vitro* conditions, is modest. Rabbit synovial fibroblasts produce large amounts of NO in response to certain cytokines [36]. Human synovial fibroblasts, in contrast, do not produce NO *in vitro* when stimulated with IL-1, TNF or leukemia inhibitory factor [37], but they have been reported to do so when stimulated with mixtures of cytokines that include γ-interferon [38]. When

Table 1 - Evidence for increased production of nitric oxide in animal models of arthritis

Tissue/Fluid	Species	Model	Reference
Synovium	Rat	SCW	[5]
Synovial fluid	Rabbit	AIA	[6]
Blood	Rat	Adjuvant	[7, 8]
	Mouse	K_3CrO_8	[9]
	Mouse	Septic	[10]
Urine	Rat	Adjuvant	[11–14]
	Rat	CIA	[14]
	Mouse	Lyme	[15]
	Mouse	Lupus	[16]
Macrophages	Rat	Adjuvant	[17, 18]

AIA, antigen-induced arthritis; CIA, collagen-induced arthritis; SCW, streptococcal cell wall-induced arthritis; K_3CrO_8, potassium peroxochromate. Under physiological conditions, this releases free radicals and hydrogen peroxide, while inhibiting glutathione reductase. When injected into the footpads of mice it produces rapidly an inflammation that persists for several weeks.
Septic arthritis was produced by infection with Staphylococcus aureus.
Murine lyme arthritis was produced by infection with Borrelia burgdorferi.
Murine lupus occurs spontaneously in the MRL-lpr/lpr strain of mice.

human rheumatoid synovium is explanted, it generates NO spontaneously although the amounts produced are quite modest [30, 33]. Leukocytes recovered from the synovial fluid of patients with RA do not spontaneously produce detectable amounts of NO [38].

The other potential major source of NO in the inflamed joint is the articular cartilage. There is little doubt that articular chondrocytes produce large quantities of NO when activated *in vitro* with IL-1 [39] and certain other stimuli, such as IL-17 [40] and TNF [37]. *Ex vivo* analysis of human articular cartilage recovered at the time of joint replacement surgery has confirmed the presence of mRNA and protein that is recognized by probes for iNOS in both RA and OA [30–32]. It has been suggested that the NOS present in articular cartilage recovered from patients with OA is not standard iNOS but either a dysregulated form of nNOS [32] or a novel isoform, "OA-NOS" [41].

Despite such strong evidence of NO production in arthritic joints, it is still unclear to what degree NO is a mediator of disease, a protective molecule or a neutral bystander. Ueki et al. [24] noted correlations between serum levels of nitrite and a variety of measurements of disease activity, as well as serum levels of TNF and IL-6.

Table 2 - *Evidence compatible with nitric oxide production in human arthritis*

Observation	Disease	References
NO_2^-/NO_3^- in serum and/or synovial fluid	RA, OA, lupus spondyloarthropathy[1], various rheumatic diseases	[19–26]
S-nitrosoproteins in serum, synovial fluid	RA, OA	[27]
Hydroxyarginine in serum[2]	RA, lupus	[28]
Nitrotyrosine in serum, synovial fluid	RA	[29]
NOS mRNA +/or protein in synovium +/or cartilage	RA, OA	[30–33]
NO production by synovium +/or cartilage *ex vivo*	RA, OA	[30, 32, 33]
iNOS in blood monocytes	RA	[34]
NO in exhaled air	lupus	[35]

[1]*Spondyloarthropathies are an interrelated group of rheumatic disorders affecting the spine, peripheral joints and tissues surrounding the joints.*
[2]*Hydroxyarginine is an intermediate in the synthesis of NO from arginine by NOS.*

However, in a separate study rheumatoid patients were treated with prednisolone which dramatically ameliorated disease activity without having major effects on urinary nitrate concentrations [20]. Nevertheless, levels of S-nitrosoproteins were reported to decrease significantly in parallel with clinical improvement in response to pulse methylprednisolone treatment [27]. The nitrate concentrations present in sera obtained from patients with spondyloarthropathies were elevated only in cases of active disease; when the disease was inactive, serum nitrate levels were indistinguishable from normal controls [22]. This might implicate NO in disease "flares", rather than in the underlying chronic disease process.

Effects of NOS inhibitors

The role of NO in arthritis has been evaluated experimentally by introducing NOS inhibitors into animal models of disease. Many, but not all, studies have shown a prophylactic effect of NOS inhibitors on the development of rodent models of RA (Tab. 3). There are, however, many inconsistencies. Adjuvant induced arthritis is, for instance, susceptible to NAME, NMA and NIL, but not to aminoguanidine. Collagen-induced arthritis in mice is not susceptible to inhibitors of NOS, and the iNOS "knockout" mouse remains vulnerable to c.i.a. A murine equivalent of Lyme arthri-

Table 3 - Responsiveness of animal models of arthritis to prophylactic treatment with inhibitors of NOS

Susceptible to NOS inhibitors			Resistant to NOS inhibitors		
Model	Inhibitor	Ref.	Model	Inhibitor	Ref.
Rat, adjuvant	NAME, NMA, NIL	[7, 11, 17]	Rat, adjuvant	AG	[7, 42]
Rat, SCW	NAME	[5]	Mouse, CIA	iNOS$^{-/-}$	[43]
Mouse, lupus	NMA	[16]	Mouse, lupus	iNOS$^{-/-}$	[44]
Rabbit, AIA	NAME	[6]	Mouse, Lyme	iNOS$^{-/-}$	[15]
Dog, OA	NIL	[45]			

iNOS$^{-/-}$, mice in which the iNOS has been disrupted (iNOS "knockout"); AG, aminoguanidine; for other definitions see legend to Tab. 1

tis, in which mice are infected with *B. burgdorferi*, is resistant to NOS inhibition. However, NIL has been recently reported to prevent the onset of experimental OA in a canine model involving transaction of the anterior cruciate ligament (ACL).

There are two published studies in which NOS inhibitors have been added to animals therapeutically, rather than prophylactically (Tab. 4). In none of these was a therapeutic effect noted, despite the ability of the inhibitors to normalize NO production in these animals.

It is difficult to know what to make of these findings. At face value they suggest that NO is important to the initiation of arthritis in many animal models of disease, but that inhibition of NO alone is not therapeutic. One weakness of most of these studies is that they rely upon the use of NOS inhbitors delivered systemically. Such reagents have properties in addition to those of inhibiting NOS and, when administered parenterally, potentially affect many different organ systems. These shortcomings are well illustrated by studies of the MRL-1pr/1pr mouse which spontaneously develops a form of murine lupus. Treatment of these animals with NMA retards disease development and inhibits the accompanying synovial inflammation [16]. In iNOS deficient mice, however, synovial inflammation is no different from that in iNOS$^+$ mice, even though rheumatoid factor levels and renal vasculitis are reduced in the iNOS$^-$ mice [44].

It is possible that inhibition of iNOS alone will not prove to have a reliable anti-inflammatory effect in joints, but that dual inhibition of iNOS and additional inflammatory components will. For example, Miesel et al. [9] produced a powerful anti-inflammatory effect in rat paws by inhibiting both NOS and NADPH oxidase.

Table 4 - Effects of NOS inhibitors on animal models of established RA

Model	Inhibitor	Effect	Reference
Rat, adjuvant	NMA	None	[42]
Rat, adjuvant	AG	None; some exacerbation	[42]
Rat, adjuvant	NIL	None	[8]
Rat, SCW	NIL	None	unpublished, cited in [8]

NO and cartilage metabolism

As described earlier, in OA the major pathological lesions occur in the articular cartilage. As articular chondrocytes are capable of producing large amounts of NO, this radical has been implicated in the pathophysiology of OA especially as NOS is induced in articular cartilage during the development of human OA [30–32].

Depletion of the cartilaginous matrix by chondrocytes can occur in two ways, viz by increasing its catabolism or decreasing its synthesis. Breakdown of the cartilaginous matrix is proteolytic. There is evidence that matrix metalloproteinases (MMPs) mediate at least some aspects of the extracellular, proteolytic degradation of the matrix. The role of NO in matrix breakdown remains a controversial subject. Two groups have independently claimed that NO increases MMP production and thus enhances matrix breakdown [46, 47]. However, several other studies have failed to identify NO as a catabolic mediator suggesting instead that, if anything, NO is protective and inhibits MMP production [48–50]. Controversy also surrounds the effects of NO on the synthesis of prostaglandin E_2 (PGE_2) by chondrocytes. Two reports claim that NO inhibits PGE_2 production [51, 52], while others show the opposite [39, 53, 54]. These matters await clarification. NO inhibits the production of IL-6, IL-8, IL-1Ra [54, 55] and TGF-β_1 [56] by chondrocytes. The effects, if any, on matrix metabolism of IL-6 and IL-8 are not known; IL-1Ra and TGF-β_1, however, should be protective.

Data concerning the effect of NO on matrix synthesis are more consistent and collectively suggest that, in general, NO suppresses the synthesis of both proteoglycan and collagen by cartilage [49, 50, 57–60]. However, several issues remain to be addressed. Proteoglycan synthesis by bovine cartilage, for example, does not appear to be inhibited by NO [48]. Moreover, the responsiveness of rabbit articular cartilage to NO may decline dramatically with age [61]. In humans, proteoglycan synthesis by chondrocytes obtained from the deep layers of cartilage is strongly inhibited by endogenously produced NO while proteoglycan synthesis by superficial chondrocytes is far less responsive to NO [50].

The mechanism through which NO inhibits proteoglycan production is not known, but our preliminary data indicate an effect on the synthesis of the core protein rather than on glycosaminoglycan synthesis [62]. There is evidence that this occurs indirectly via an inhibitory effect of NO on TGF-β synthesis [56]. NO also inhibits collagen synthesis, possibly by inhibiting the important processing enzyme prolyl hydroxylase [60].

In addition to its effects on matrix synthesis, NO inhibits the ability of chondrocytes to adhere and migrate, via an affect on actin assembly [63]. This, in conjunction with inhibition of matrix synthesis, might interfere with the ability of chondrocytes to repair cartilage lesions that occur as a result of arthritis or injury.

Finally, it has been reported that endogenously produced NO has the potential to kill articular chondrocytes by apoptosis or to protect them from the necrotising effects of other oxygen-derived free radicals [64]. Lotz and co-workers have postulated that after a chondrocyte undergoes apoptosis in response to NO, the residual debris becomes a matrix vesicle which promotes mineralization [65]. This series of events could link NO both to the reduced cellularity and increased mineralization of osteoarthritic cartilage. NO and cartilage metabolism has been reviewed in [66].

NO and traumatically induced inflammation

Traumatic insults to the joint frequently damage intraarticular structures such as ligaments, menisci and articular cartilage while provoking acute, often self-resolving inflammatory reactions. In a preliminary study of synovial fluids aspirated from human joints following acute rupture of the anterior cruciate ligament (ACL), we were surprised to find no evidence that NO_2^- levels were increased (our unpublished data). This is despite the fact that concentrations of TNF, IL-6 and a number of other inflammatory cytokines were elevated and there was evidence of loss of proteoglycan from the cartilaginous matrix [67].

NO could, however, be produced and consumed locally within damaged intraarticular tissues where it may help explain the puzzling observation that these tissues heal poorly. As noted in the previous section, endogenously produced NO alters the behavior of articular chondrocytes in ways which are incompatible with efficient healing. Chondroid cells within the menisci of rabbit [68] and human (our unpublished data) knee joints are also capable of generating considerable quantities of NO which reduce the synthesis of matrix molecules.

Recent studies of rabbit ACL also suggest a role for endogenously produced NO in suppressing healing. In particular, damage to the ACL induced the synthesis of NO which inhibited matrix production, a key component of healing. Of significance was the observation that the medial collateral ligament (MCL), which is able to heal following injury, produced far less NO and was less sensitive to the effects of exogenous NO [69].

Conclusions

NO is produced in elevated amounts in RA, OA and probably other forms of arthritis. Both intra- and extra-articular cells have the potential to contribute to this. Despite early promising data from interventional studies in animal models, it remains unclear whether NO is critically involved in RA or other conditions producing joint inflammation. For NO antagonists to be useful anti-inflammatory or immunosuppressive agents of use in treating inflammatory and autoimmune diseases, they would need to be much cheaper or more efficacious than existing drugs of this nature. The latter restriction does not apply to a possible chondroprotective function for NO agonists or antagonists, as no such drugs pre-exist. If NO can be manipulated to modulate chondrocyte metabolism in the appropriate manner, this would have far reaching consequences for the treatment of OA as well as enhancing the repair of cartilage and, in an analogous fashion, other intraarticular tissues.

Acknowledgements
Supported, in part, by NIH grant RO1AR42025. Mrs. Lou Duerring kindly typed the manuscript.

References

1   Evans CH, Stefanovic-Racic M (1997) Nitric oxide in arthritis: it's probably there, but what's it doing? In: JR Lancaster, JF Parkinson (eds): *Nitric oxide, cytochromes P450, and sexual steroid hormones.* Springer, Berlin, 181–204

2   Evans CH (1999) Cartilage and Synovium. In: ME Baratz, AD Watson, JE Imbriglia, (eds): *Orthopaedic surgery: the essentials.* Thieme, New York, 33–48

3   Schumacher RH (ed) (1993) *Primer on the rheumatic diseases*, 10th edition. Arthritis Foundation, Atlanta

4   Feldmann M, Brennan FM, Maini RN (1996) Rheumatoid arthritis. *Cell* 85: 307–310

5   McCartney-Frances N, Allen JB, Mizel DE, Albina Q, Xie W, Nathan CF, Wohl SM (1993) Suppression of arthritis by an inhibitor of nitric oxide synthase. *J Exp Med* 178: 7540

6   Verissimo de Mello SB, Novaes GS, Laruindo IMM, Muscara MN, de Barros Maciel FM, Cossernelli W (1997) Nitric oxide synthase inhibitor influences prostaglandin and interleukin-1 production in experimental arthritic joints. *Inflamm Res* 46: 72–77

7   Connor JR, Manning PT, Settle SL, Moore WM, Jerome GM, Webber RK, Tjoeng FS, Currie MG (1995) Suppression of adjuvant-induced arthritis by selective inhibition of inducible nitric oxide synthase. *Eur J Pharmacol* 273: 15–24

8   Fletcher DS, Widmer WR, Luell S, Christen A, Orevillo C, Shah S, Visco D (1998) Therapeutic administration of a selective inhibitor of nitric oxide synthase does not ameliorate the chronic inflammation and tissue damage associated with adjuvant-induced arthritis in rats. *J Pharmacol Exp Ther* 284: 714–721

9   Miesel R, Kurprisz M, Kröger H (1996) Suppression of inflammatory arthritis by simultaneous inhibition of nitric oxide synthase and NADPH oxidase. *Free Rad Biol Med* 20: 75–81

10   Sakiniene E, Bremell T, Tarkowski A (1996) Addition of corticosteroids to antibiotic treatment ameliorates the course of experimental Staphylococcus aureus arthritis. *Arthritis Rheum* 39: 1596–1605

11   Stefanovic-Racic M, Meyers K, Meschter C, Coffey JW, Hoffman RA, Evans CH (1994) N-monomethylarginine an inhibitor of nitric oxide synthase, suppresses the onset of adjuvant arthritis in rats. *Arthritis Rheum* 37: 1062–1069

12   Stichtenoth DO, Gutzki FM, Tsikas D, Selve N, Bode-Böger SM, Böger RH, Frölich JC (1994) Increased urinary nitrate excretion in rats with adjuvant arthritis. *Ann Rheum Dis* 53: 547–549

13   Cannon GW, Remmers EF, Wilder RL, Hibbs JB, Griffiths MM (1995) Nitric oxide production during adjuvant-induced arthritis is associated with tumor necrosis factor genotype. *Transplant Proc* 27: 1543–1544

14   Cannon GW, Openshaw SJ, Hibbs JB, Hoidal JR, Hueckstead TP, Griffiths MM (1996) Nitric oxide production during adjuvant-induced and collagen-induced arthritis. *Arthritis Rheum* 39: 1677–1684

15   Seiler KP, Vavrin Z, Eichwald E, Hibbs JB, Weiss JJ (1995) Nitric oxide production during murine lyme disease: lack of involvement in host resistance or pathology. *Infect Immunol* 63: 3886–3895

16   Weinberg JB, Granger DL, Pisetsky DS, Seldin MF, Misukonis MA, Mason SN, Pippen AM, Ruiz P, Wood ER, Gilkeson GS (1994) The role of nitric oxide in the pathogenesis of spontaneous murine autoimmune disease: increased nitric oxide production and nitric oxide synthase expression in MRL-1pr/1pr mice, and reduction of spontaneous nephritis and arthritis by orally administered N^G-monomethyl-L-arginine. *J Exp Med* 179: 651–660

17   Ialenti A, Moncada S, Di Rosa M (1993) Modulation of adjuvant arthritis by endogenous nitric oxide. *Brit J Pharmacol* 110: 701–706

18   Zidek Z, Frankova D, Otava B (1995) Lack of causal relationship between inducibility/severity of adjuvant arthritis in the rat and disease associated changes in production of nitric oxide by macrophages. *Ann Rheum Dis* 54: 325–327

19   Farrell AJ, Blake DR, Palmer RMF, Moncada S (1992) Increased concentration of nitrite in synovial fluid and serum samples suggest increased nitric oxide synthesis in rheumatic diseases. *Ann Rheum Dis* 51: 1219–1222

20 Stichtenoth DO, Fauler J, Zeidler H, Frolich JC (1995) Urinary nitrate excretion is increased in patients with rheumatoid arthritis and reduced by prednisolone. *Ann Rheum Dis* 54: 820–824

21 Miesel R, Zuber M (1993) Reactive nitrogen intermediates, antinuclear antibodies and copper-thionein in serum of patients with rheumatic diseases. *Rheumatol Int* 13: 95–102

22 Stichtenoth DO, Wollenhaupt J, Andersone D, Zeidler H, Frolich JC (1995) Elevated serum nitrate concentrations in active spondyloarthropathies. *Br J Rheumatol* 34: 616–619

23 Grabowski PS, England AJ, Dykhuizen R, Copland M, Benjamin N, Reid DM, Ralston SH (1996) Elevated nitric oxide production in rheumatoid arthritis. Detection using the fasting urinary nitrate: creatinine ratio. *Arthritis Rheum* 39: 643–647

24 Ueki Y, Miyake S, Tominaga Y, Eguchi K (1996) Increased nitric oxide levels in patients with rheumatoid arthritis. *J Rheumatol* 23: 230–236

25 Renoux M, Hilliquin P, Galoppin L, Florentin I, Menkes CJ (1996) Release of mast cell mediators and nitrites into knee joint fluid in osteoarthritis – comparison with articular chondrocalcinosis and rheumatoid arthritis. *Osteoarthritis Cart* 4: 175–179

26 Belmont HM, Levartovsky D, Goel A, Amin A, Giorno R, Rediske J, Skovron ML, Abramson AB (1997) Increased nitric oxide production accompanied by the up-regulation of inducible nitric oxide synthase in vascular endothelium from patients with systemic lupus erythematosus. *Arthritis Rheum* 40: 1810–1816

27 Hilliquin P, Borderie D, Hernuann A, Menkes CJ, Ekindjian OG (1997) Nitric oxide as S-nitrosoproteins in rheumatoid arthritis. *Arthritis Rheum* 40: 1512–1517

28 Wigand R, Meyer J, Busse R, Hecker M (1997) Increased serum N^G-hydroxy-L-arginine in patients with rheumatoid arthritis and systemic lupus erythematosus as an index of an increased nitric oxide synthase activity. *Ann Rheum Dis* 56: 330–332

29 Kaur H, Halliwell B (1994) Evidence for nitric oxide-mediated oxidative damage in chronic inflammation. Nitrotyrosine in serum and synovial fluid form rheumatoid patients. *FEBS Lett* 350: 9–12

30 Sakurai H, Kohsaka H, Liu MF, Higashiyama H, Hirata Y, Kanno K, Saito I, Miyasaka N (1995) Nitric oxide synthase expression in inflammatory arthritides. *J Clin Invest* 96: 2357–2363

31 Grabowski PS, Wright PK, Van't Hot RJ, Helfrich MH, Ohshima H, Ralston SH (1997) Immunolocalization of inducible nitric oxide synthase in synovium and cartilage in rheumatoid arthritis and osteoarthritis. *Br J Rheumatol* 36: 651–655

32 Amin AR, DiCesare PE, Vyas P, Attur M, Tzeng E, Billiar TR, Stuchin SA, Abramson SB (1995) The expression and regulation of nitric oxide synthase in human osteoarthritis-affected chondrocytes: evidence for up-regulated neuronal nitric oxide synthase. *J Exp Med* 182: 2097–2102

33 McInnes IB, Leung BP, Field M, Wei XQ, Huang FP, Sturrock RD, Kinninmonth A, Weidner J. Mumford R, Liew FY (1996) Production of nitric oxide in the synovial membrane of rheumatoid and osteoarthritis patients. *J Exp Med* 184: 1519–1524

34 St. Clair EW, Wilkinson WE, Lang T, Sanders L, Misukonis MA, Gilkeson GS, Pisetsky

DS, Granger DL, Weinberg JB (1996) Increased expression of blood mononuclear cell nitric oxide synthase type 2 in rheumatoid arthritis patients. *J Exp Med* 184: 1173–1178

35   Rolla G, Brussino L, Bertero MT, Colagrande P, Converso M, Bucca C, Polizzi S, Caligaris-Cappio F (1997) Increased nitric oxide in exhaled air of patients with systemic lupus erythematosus. *J Rheumatol* 24: 1066–1071

36   Stefanovic-Racic M, Stadler J, Georgescu HI, Evans CH (1994) Nitric oxide synthesis and its regulation by rabbit synoviocytes. *J Rheumatol* 21: 1892–1898

37   Rediske JJ, Koehne CF, Zhang B, Lotz M (1994) The inducible production of nitric oxide by articular cell types. *Osteoarthritis Cart* 2: 199–206

38   Grabowski PS, MacPherson HM, Ralston SH (1996) Nitric oxide production in cells derived from the human joint. *Br J Rheumatol* 35: 207–213

39   Stadler J, Stefanovic-Racic M, Billiar TR, Curran RD, McIntyre LA, Georgescu HI, Simmons RL, Evans CH Articular chondrocytes synthesize nitric oxide in response to cytokines and lipopolysaccharide. *J Immunol* 147: 3915–3920

40   Lotz M, Bober L, Narula S, Dudler J (1996) IL-17 promotes cartilage degradation. *Arthritis Rheum* 39 (suppl): S120 abstract 559

41   Amin AR, Attur M, Vyas P, DiCesare PE, Patel P, Patel RN, Steiner G, Abramson SB (1996) Non-steroidal anti-inflammatory drugs inhibit the activity of COX-2 and nitric oxide synthase expressed in osteoarthritis-affected cartilage. *Arthritis Rheum* 39 (suppl): S81 abstract 326

42   Stefanovic-Racic M, Meyers K, Meschter C, Coffey JW, Hoffman RA, Evans CH (1995) Comparison of the nitric oxide synthase inhibitors methylarginine and aminoguanidine as prophylactic and therapeutic agents in rat adjuvant arthritis. *J Rheumatol* 22: 1922–1928

43   Visco DM, Fletcher DS, Orevillo CJ, Christen AJ, Shen CF, Widmer WR, Ronan J, Chartrain N, Mudgett JS (1997) NOS 2 deficient mice are susceptible to collagen-induced arthritis. *Trans Orthop Res Soc* 43: 416

44   Gilkeson GS, Mudgett JS, Seldin MF, Ruiz P, Alexander AA, Misukonis MA, Pisetsky DS, Weinberg JB (1997) Clinical and serologic manifestations of autoimmune disease in MRL-1pr/1pr mice lacking nitric oxide synthase type 2. *J Exp Med* 186: 365–373

45   Pelletier JP, Jovanovic D, Fernandes JC, Geng C, Manning P, Connor JR, DiBattista J, Martel-Pelletier J (1997) Selective inhibition of nitric oxide synthase reduces *in vivo* the progression of expermental osteoarthritic lesions and production of metalloproteinases and interleukin-1 (abstract). *Arthitis Rheum* 40 (suppl): S173 abstract 851

46   Murrell GAC, Jang D, Williams RJ (1995) Nitric oxide activates metalloprotease enzymes in articular cartilage. *Biochem Biophys Res Commun* 206: 15–21

47   Tamura T, Nakanishi T, Kimura Y, Hattori T, Sasaki K, Norimatsu H, Takahashi K, Takigawa M (1996) Nitric oxide mediates interleukin-1-induced matrix degradation and basic fibroblast growth factor release in cultured rabbit articular chondrocytes: a possible mechanism of pathological neovascularization in arthritis. *Endocrinol* 137: 3729–3737

48   Stefanovic-Racic M, Morales TI, Taskiran D, McIntyre LA, Evans CH (1996) The role

of nitric oxide in proteoglycan turnover by bovine articular cartilage organ cultures. *J Immunol* 156: 1213–1220

49 Stefanovic-Racic M, Möllers MO, Miller LA, Evans CH (1997) Nitric oxide and proteoglycan turnover in rabbit articular cartilage. *J Orthop Res* 15: 422–429

50 Häuselmann HJ, Stefanovic-Racic M, Michel BA, Evans CH (1998) Differences in nitric oxide production by superficial and deep human articular chondrocytes: implications for proteoglycan turnover in inflammatory joint diseases. *J Immunol* 160: 1444–1448

51 Blanco FJ, Lotz M (1995) IL-1-induced nitric oxide inhibits chondrocyte proliferation via PGE2. *Exp Cell Res* 218: 319–325

52 Marfield L, Jang D, Murrell GAC (1996) Nitric oxide enhances cyclooxygenase activity in articular cartilage. *Inflamm Res* 45: 254–258

53 Amin AR, Attur M, Patel RN, Thakker GD, Marshall PJ, Rediske J, Stuchin SA, Patel IR, Abramson SB (1997) Superinduction of cyclooxygenase-2 activity in human osteoarthritis-affected cartilage. *J Clin Invest* 99: 1231–1237

54 Evans CH, Oppliger L, Michel BA, Stefanovic-Racic M, Tsao M, Larkin LA, Häuselmann HJ (1994) Effect of nitric oxide on cytokine and prostaglandin synthesis by human articular cartilage. *Osteoarthritis Cart* 2 (suppl)1: 51

55 Pelletier JP, Mineau F, Ranger P, Tardif G, Martel-Pelletier J (1996) The increased synthesis of inducible nitric oxide inhibits IL-1Ra synthesis by human articular chondrocytes: possible role in osteoarthritic cartilage degradation. *Osteoarthritis Cart* 4: 77–84

56 Studer RK, Georgescu HI, Miller L, Evans CH (1999) Nitric oxide inhibits TGF-β production by chondrocytes: implications for matrix synthesis. *Arthritis Rheum* 42: 248–257

57 Taskiran D, Stefanovic-Racic M, Georgescu HI, Evans CH (1994) Nitric oxide mediates suppression of cartilage proteoglycan synthesis by interleukin-1. *Biochem Biophys Res Commun* 200: 142–142

58 Jarvinen TAK, Moilanen T, Jarvinen TLN, Moilanen E (1995) Nitric oxide mediates interleukin-1 induced inhibition of glycosaminoglycan synthesis in rat articular cartilage. *Med Inflamm* 4: 107–111

59 Häuselmann HJ, Oppliger L, Michel BA, Stefanovic-Razcic M, Evans CH (1994) Nitric oxide and proteoglycan biosynthesis by human articular chondrocytes in alginate culture. *FEBS Lett* 352: 361–364

60 Cao M, Westerhausen-Larson A, Niyibizi C, Kavalkovich K, Georgescu HI, Rizzo CF, Stefanovic-Racic M, Evans CH (1997) Nitric oxide inhibits the synthesis of type II collagen without altering Col2A1 mRNA abundance: prolyl hydroxylase as a possible target. *Biochem J* 324: 305–310

61 Spiroto S, Goldberg RL (1997) The ability of nitric oxide (NO) inhibitors to reverse an interleukin-1 (IL-1) induced depression of proteoglycan synthesis is age dependent. *Inflamm Res* 46 (suppl 2): S131–S132

62 Stefanovic-Racic M, Taskiran D, Hering TM, Georgescu HI, Evans CH (1998) Nitric oxide inhibits synthesis of aggrecan core protein without altering mRNA abundance. *Trans Orthop Res Soc* 23: 300

63   Frenkel SR, Clancy RM, Ricci JL, DiCesare PE, Rediske JJ, Abramson SB (1996) Effects of nitric oxide on chondrocyte migration, adhesion, and cytoskeletal assembly. *Arthritis Rheum* 39: 1905–1912

64   Blanco FJ, Ochs RL, Schwarz H, Lotz M (1995) Chondrocyte apoptosis induced by nitric oxide. *Am J Pathol* 146: 75–85

65   Hashimoto S, Ochs RL, Rosen F, Quach J, McCabe G, Solan J, Seeguiller JE, Teskeltaub R, Lotz M (1998) Chondrocyte-derived apoptotic bodies and calcification of articular cartilage. *Proc Natl Acad Sci USA* 95: 3094–3099

66   Evans CH, Watkins SC, Stefanovic-Racic M (1996) Nitric oxide and cartilage metabolism. *Meth Enzymol* 269: 75–88

67   Cameron M, Buchgraber A, Passler H, Vogt M, Thonar E, Fu FH, Evans CH (1997) The natural history of the anterior cruciate ligament-deficient knee. *Am J Sports Med* 25: 751–754

68   Cao M, Stefanovic-Racic M, Georgescu HI, Miller LA, Evans CH (1998) Generation of nitric oxide by lapine meniscal cells and its effect on matrix metabolism: stimulation of collagen production by arginine. *J Orthop Res* 16: 104–111

69   Cao M, Stefanovic-Racic M, Georgescu, HI, Fu FH, Evans CH (1998) Does nitric oxide explain the differential healing capacity of the anterior cruciate, posterior cruciate and medial collateral ligaments? *Am J Sports Med; in press*

Nitric oxide and bone destruction

Heather MacPherson and Stuart H. Ralston

Department of Medicine and Therapeutics, Foresterhill, Aberdeen AB25 2ZD, Scotland, UK

Background

Nitric oxide (NO) was identified as the moiety responsible for endothelium-derived smooth muscle relaxation activity in 1987 [1], but since then, it has been found to be responsible for a multitude of other physiological effects on several processes including platelet aggregation, cell adhesion, immune function and neurotransmission [2, 3]. Interest in the role of NO as a mediator of bone cell function began in 1991 when McIntyre and colleagues showed that NO gas and pharmacological NO donors exerted inhibitory effects on osteoclast activity and motility [4]. Although the physiological relevance of these findings were initially unclear, it has become apparent that NO is not only produced by bone cells and explant cultures in response to a variety of stimuli, but also that it exerts potent effects on cells of the osteoblast and osteoclast lineage. Here we review the factors which regulate NO production, the effects of NO on osteoblast and osteoclast activity, the physiological role of the L-arginine/NO pathway in bone and its potential as a therapeutic target in bone disease.

Synthesis of NO and regulation of NO production

NO is a short lived free radical that is generated physiologically by a group of enzymes known as the nitric oxide synthases (NOS) and by the action of gastric acid on dietary nitrite [5]. The NOS enzymes are oxido-reductases with homology to cytochrome P450 which produce NO by combining molecular oxygen with the terminal guanidino-nitrogen atom of the amino acid L-arginine [6], yielding L-citrulline as a co-product (Fig. 1). After its formation, NO is degraded rapidly to stable metabolites of nitrate and nitrite and these provide an indirect measure of rates of NO production both *in vivo* and *in vitro* [7]. Three isoforms of NOS have been identified which are conserved throughout species and share significant sequence homology with one another. They are endothelial NOS (ecNOS), neuronal NOS

Free Radicals and Inflammation, edited by P. G. Winyard, D. R. Blake and C. H. Evans
© 2000 Birkhäuser Verlag Basel/Switzerland

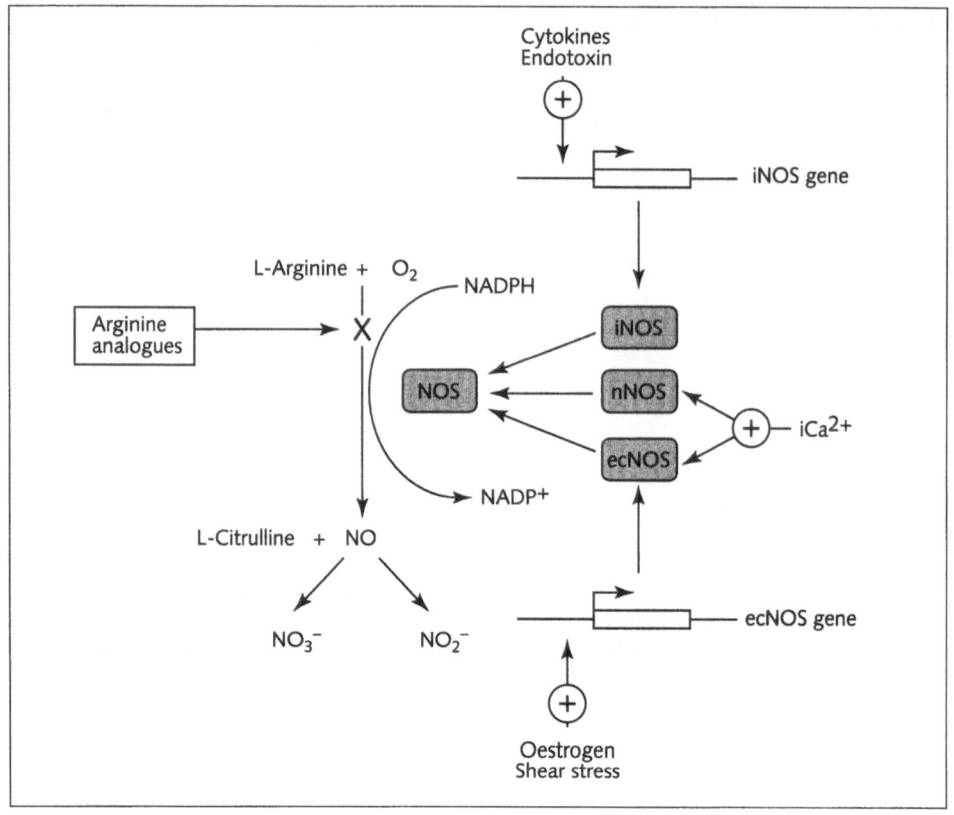

Figure 1
Synthesis and metabolism of nitric oxide
Nitric oxide is synthesised from L-arginine, by the nitric oxide synthase (NOS) enzymes. The
most important forms of NOS in bone are iNOS, which is induced by cytokines, and ecNOS
which is induced by mechanical strain and sex hormones.
Slightly modified from Ralston and van't Hof [57] and reproduced with the authors' permis-
sion (copyright Rapid Science Publishers).

(nNOS) and inducible NOS (iNOS). As the names suggest, the ecNOS and nNOS isoforms were first purified from vascular tissue and neuronal tissue respectively, whereas the iNOS isoform was first identified in macrophages [8–10]. It is now clear however, that all three NOS isoforms are expressed in other cells and tissues, including bone and bone derived cells. Both ecNOS and nNOS are constitutively expressed in their tissues of origin and because of this are often referred to as the "constitutive" NOS (cNOS) isoforms. Their activity is mainly regulated at the protein level by changes in intracellular Ca^{2+} [iCa^{2+}] concentrations, which together with calmodulin, binds to a recognition site in the NOS protein, causing a conformational change and enzyme activation. The cNOS pathway is characterised by rapid, but relatively short lived production of NO. Although it was initially considered that the amounts of NO which derive from cNOS activation are relatively small recent work in cultured osteocytes shows that these cells have the capacity to produce very high levels of NO, albeit for a short period of time [11]. Like cNOS, the iNOS enzyme has a calmodulin recognition site, but enzyme activity is largely independent of changes in [iCa^{2+}] since calcium and calmodulin are already tightly bound to the enzyme under physiological conditions. Rather, iNOS production is mainly regulated at the level of gene transcription. The most important stimuli for iNOS are pro-inflammatory cytokines such as interleukin-1 (IL-1), tumour necrosis factor (TNF), interferon-γ (IFNγ) and lipopolysaccharide (LPS). These factors cause activation of signalling pathways which culminate in activation of iNOS by interacting with various regulatory elements in the iNOS gene promoter (Fig. 1). Conversely, activation of iNOS is suppressed by glucocorticoids [12, 13] and anti-inflammatory cytokines such as IL-4, IL-10 and transforming growth factor β (TGFβ) [14–16]. Although the main effects of pro-inflammatory mediators is on iNOS transcription, LPS has also been shown to prolong the half-life of the iNOS mRNA. Furthermore, there is also some evidence to suggest that NO may directly inhibit enzyme activity thereby providing a feedback inhibitory loop [17, 18]. Finally, there is evidence in T cells that NO may auto-regulate its own production in an indirect way by inhibiting secretion of cytokines that stimulate iNOS transcription [19]. Unlike the cNOS enzymes, activation of the iNOS pathway occurs relatively slowly (hours), but after formation, catalytic activity continues for many days. In view of this, the iNOS pathway is generally considered to be capable of producing greater quantities of NO, over a longer time-frame, than the cNOS pathway.

Pharmacological inhibitors of NO production

Pharmacological inhibitors of NO production have been developed which take advantage of the fact that the NOS enzymes require several co-factors that are necessary for catalytic activity. The earliest inhibitors to be discovered were substituted analogues of arginine such as L-N-monomethyl arginine (L-NMMA), L-arginine-methyl ester (L-NAME), N-iminoethyl-L-ornithine (L-NIO) and aminoguanidine (AG). These substances bind to the enzyme in place of arginine and are capable of inhibiting the activity of all NOS isoforms to various degrees. Although arginine analogues are generally considered to be specific inhibitors of NOS they may exert non-specific effects on other arginine dependent enzyme systems [20]. Other compounds, such as the aromatic iodoniums, which inhibit flavoproteins such as FAD and FMN, also inhibit NOS activity, but these are relatively non-selective and could inhibit other enzymatic pathways at the same time [21]. Finally, NOS can be inhibited by compounds such as calcineurin and trifluoroperazine which bind to calmodulin, and compounds such as EGTA which chelate calcium. Although these substances are selective for the constitutive NOS as opposed to inducible NOS [22], they also inhibit other calcium-requiring enzymes, limiting their value as therapeutic agents. Strenuous efforts are being made by several pharmaceutical companies to develop isoform specific NOS inhibitors for clinical use, and some compounds have been identified which exhibit enhanced activity against the iNOS as opposed to cNOS enzymes, at least *in vitro*.

Molecular targets of NO

NO can act as an endocrine, autocrine or paracrine mediator of cellular activity. Although molecular NO has a short half life (3–5 s), it can bind reversibly to proteins such as albumin and exert effects in tissues distant from sites of production by releasing NO in target tissues [23]. The autocrine/paracrine actions of NO are facilitated by the fact that NO is a small molecule, which is lipid soluble and able to cross cell membranes readily to exert effects on intracellular targets. One of the best characterised molecular targets of NO is soluble guanylyl cyclase (sGC). NO binds to the heme moiety of sGC, resulting in a conformational change which causes enzyme activation. The resulting increase in intracellular cyclic guanine monophosphate (cGMP) is the main effector mechanism of NO action on vascular smooth muscle [24], although interestingly cGMP production is not thought to explain the effects of NO on osteoclasts [4, 25]. NO has also been shown to inhibit DNA synthesis and cell division via inactivation of the tyrosyl radical on the enzyme ribonucleotide reductase which is essential for the enzyme's catalytic activity. It has also been suggested that NO may also inhibit the activity of this enzyme by interacting with a non-heme iron atom associated with this protein [26]. NO can modify the structure and function of other proteins by reacting with sulphydryl residues and iron-sulphur centres. It is thought that the former action is responsible for the down-regulation of N-methyl-D-aspartate (NMDA) receptor activity, thus providing a neuroprotective effect [27]. The latter effect is thought to be responsible for the inhibitory actions of high NO concentrations on cell growth via the interaction with mitochondrial aconitase, a critical enzyme in the Krebs cycle [28]. Finally, NO can react with other free radicals such as superoxide to form the peroxynitrite anion and the hydroxyl radical. Production of these moieties may cause lipid peroxidation and protein nitrosylation and hence contribute to tissue damage that is a characteristic feature of an inflammatory response [29].

Expression and regulation of NOS isoforms in bone

The NOS enzymes were initially considered to have a relatively limited tissue distribution, but it is now known that all three isoforms are widely expressed outside their classical tissues of origin. Recent studies have shown that all three NOS isoforms can been detected in whole bone explants by reverse-transcriptase polymerase chain reaction (RT/PCR). More detailed localisation studies have shown the ecNOS isoform to be constitutively expressed by many bone-derived cells including osteoclasts, osteoblasts, osteocytes and bone marrow stromal cells. In contrast, iNOS is not expressed constitutively in adult bone or bone-derived cells, but can be induced by pro-inflammatory mediators and systemic inflammation. Osteoblasts, bone marrow macrophages and bone marrow stromal cells have all been shown to express iNOS upon cytokine stimulation [30], but data on osteoclast expression of iNOS is conflicting. Some workers have found evidence of iNOS in osteoclasts, whereas others have not [30]. Although nNOS mRNA has been detected in whole bone, there has been no convincing demonstration of nNOS protein in bone or bone-derived cells [30, 31], suggesting that nNOS may be confined to the nerves which innervate bone tissue.

Effects of NO on osteoclasts and bone resorption

NO has important effects on cells of the osteoclast lineage. High concentrations of NO exert an inhibitory effect on osteoclastic bone resorption *in vitro*, due to inhibition of osteoclast formation, osteoclast motility and resorptive function [32–34]. In keeping with these observations, NO donors have been shown to inhibit bone loss induced by ovariectomy and by corticosteroid treatment in rodents [35]. It is of interest that epidemiological data in man has shown an association between treatment with nitrates (NO donors) and bone mass which is again consistent with inhibitory effects of NO on bone resorption *in vivo* [36]. The molecular mechanisms by which NO inhibits the function of mature osteoclasts is not yet clear, but the inhibitory effects on osteoclast formation have been shown to be due in part, to NO-induced apoptosis of osteoclast progenitors. An interesting feature of this effect is that it seems to be highly dependent on a cytokine-induced co-stimulus, suggesting that the effects of NO on cells of the early osteoclast lineage may be dependent on an interaction between NO and signalling pathways which are activated by cytokines in bone. Although high levels of NO and NO donors inhibit bone resorption, constitutive NO production seems to be essential for normal osteoclast activity [37] and lower levels of NO have been found to enhance bone resorption stimulated by cytokines such as IL-1 and TNF [32, 33]. Interestingly, calciotropic hormones such as parathyroid hormone (PTH) and vitamin D metabolites do not

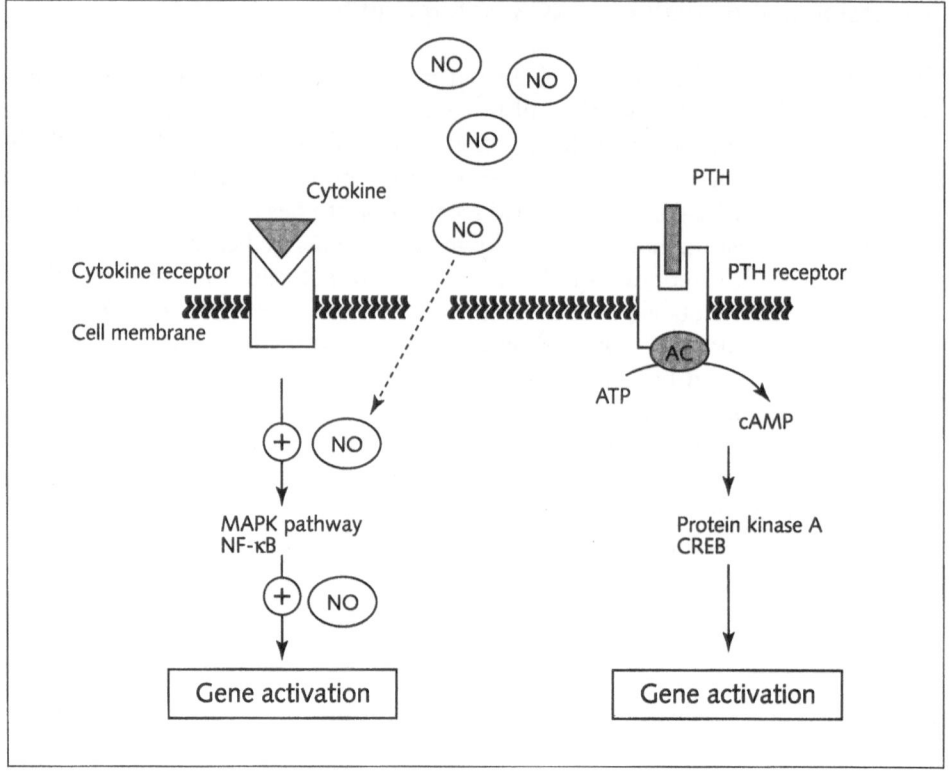

Figure 2
Nitric oxide and signal transduction pathways
Evidence from in vitro *experiments indicates that NO may interact with cytokine-induced,*
but not PTH-induced, signalling pathways in bone to modulate cellular activity [32, 41, 55,
56]. In this diagrammatic representation we speculate that NO diffuses across the cell mem-
brane to modify signalling proteins induced by cytokines such as the MAP kinases or NF-κB.
In contrast, the PTH induced adenylate cyclase-protein kinase A-CREB pathway seems not
be influenced by NO. The mechanisms by which NO exerts these effects are unclear, but
possibilities may include protein nitrosylation.

stimulate NO production in bone [33] and the resorption stimulated by these factors is uninfluenced by NO [33]. This suggests that NO may act principally as a
mediator of cytokine actions in bone and indicates that NO may modify cytokine
induced, but not calciotropic hormone-induced signalling pathways in bone cells
(Fig. 2). Although the *in vitro* data cited above suggest that basal NO production is
essential for normal osteoclast function, *in vivo* studies have shown that the NOS
inhibitor aminoguanidine (AG) increases bone resorption and accelerates bone loss

in normal and ovariectomised rats [38]. Other workers however, have found that the NOS inhibitor L-NAME does not accelerate bone loss in normal or ovariectomised rats [35, 39]. In view of this, it is possible that the effects of AG may have been a non-specific result due to inhibition of other enzyme systems such as those which are involved in production of polyamines [40]. Further studies in NOS knockout animals will be required to more clearly define the role of the L-arginine/NO pathway in regulating bone metabolism *in vivo*.

Effects of NO on osteoblasts and bone formation

The effects of NO on bone formation are less well characterised than those on bone resorption, but the available data suggests that, as in the case of osteoclasts, NO probably exerts biphasic effects on osteoblast activity. Cytokines are potent stimulators of NO production in cultured osteoblasts and several workers have shown that the inhibitory effects of cytokines on osteoblast growth are partly mediated by NO. While cytokine induced NO production in rodent osteoblasts causes cell death due to osteoblast apoptosis [41], this does not appear to be the case in human osteoblasts. The effects of NO on osteoblast differentiation are less clear. It has been shown that NO donors at high concentrations inhibit alkaline phosphatase (a marker of osteoblast differentiation) but paradoxically, that cytokine-induced NO is accompanied by increased alkaline phosphatase activity [42]. It is possible that these discrepant results could be explained by differences in the levels of NO achieved or by an interaction with other cytokine-stimulated pathways in osteoblasts as discussed previously in this chapter.

Although osteoblasts express ecNOS and produce low levels of NO constitutively, the role of constitutive NO production on regulation of osteoblast function is unclear. Early work by Riancho and colleagues [43] suggested that basal NO production may play a role in regulating osteoblast-derived IL-6 production and proliferation, but these studies were performed in arginine-free medium and we have failed to find evidence of an autocrine effect of NO on osteoblast growth [42].

Since osteoblasts and osteocytes rapidly produce large amounts of NO in response to fluid flow [11, 44], it could be that the main function of osteoblast-derived NO is to function as an osteoblast-osteoclast signalling molecule, rather than as an autocrine mediator of osteoblast activity. Evidence that this may be the case comes from osteoblast-bone marrow co-cultures, where osteoblast-derived NO provides the main signal for cytokine-induced apoptosis of osteoclast progenitors and for the stimulatory effects of IL-1 on osteoclast formation [32, 45]. Studies *in vivo* also support this concept in showing that increases in bone mass which result from mechanical loading can be blocked by NOS inhibitors [46]. It is currently unclear however, if this effect is due to NO-mediated inhibition of bone resorption, stimulation of bone formation or a combination of both actions. Whatever the underlying mechanisms, these data indicate that NO may act as a transducer for the effects of mechanical strain on the skeleton *in vivo* [44, 47].

Oestrogen provides an important stimulus to production of NO in the vascular system [48] and it has been suggested that this may explain the protective effects of hormone replacement therapy (HRT) on cardiovascular disease in women. Could NO also explain the protective effects of oestrogen on the skeleton? The potential role of NO as a mediator of oestrogen action in bone is supported by experiments in rodents which have shown that the protective effects of oestradiol on bone loss after ovariectomy is abrogated in the presence of NOS inhibitors [35]. This combined with the fact that oestrogen stimulates both ecNOS activity and mRNA levels in human osteoblasts [49] suggest that NO could mediate some actions of sex hormones in bone, although further experiments will be needed to determine the functional consequences of this stimulatory effect on enzyme activity.

Role of NO in regulation of bone turnover in health and disease

The most obvious role for NO in regulation of bone turnover is under conditions of cytokine activation. Inflammatory arthritis is accompanied by activation of the iNOS pathway in both man and experimental animals, as reflected by an elevation in levels of the NO breakdown products nitrate and nitrite in blood, urine and synovial fluid. More recent work has also shown that patients with sepsis have increased production of NO and a dramatic increase in biochemical markers of bone resorption, which are positively correlated with one another [50]. These findings do not of course prove a cause-effect relationship; they do show however, that under conditions of cytokine activation, increases in NO do not appear to suppress bone resorption and indeed raise the possibility that cytokine-induced NO production may enhance bone resorption. Although inhibitors of NO synthesis have been found to reduce joint inflammation in a variety of animal models of arthritis, the effects on periarticular bone have not been investigated and this is an important area for further study. Related studies in animal models of inflammation-induced osteopaenia have confirmed that there is a positive association between NO production and bone loss and more importantly that treatment with NOS inhibitors abrogates systemic bone loss associated with the inflammatory process (K.E. Armour and S.H. Ralston, unpublished data). Taken together, these observations *in vivo*, along with *in vitro* studies support the concept that NO-cytokine interactions may be important in determining whether NO stimulates or inhibits bone loss.

Another potential regulatory role for NO would be in the pathogenesis of post-menopausal osteoporosis. Oestrogen deficiency in rodents is associated with activation of pro-inflammatory cytokine production [51] and there is some evidence to suggest that the same may occur in man [52]. Although cytokine activation might be expected to increase NO production in bone by stimulating the iNOS pathway, studies of urinary NO breakdown products in post-menopausal women have shown that NO production is inhibited [53]. Much of this may derive from down-regulation of ecNOS in the vascular system, but data from *in vitro* work suggest that ecNOS may also be down regulated in bone [49]. Since oestrogen deficiency therefore has the potential to cause opposing effects on activity of the ecNOS and iNOS pathways, the role of NO in the pathogenesis of post-menopausal bone loss is unclear.

The most likely physiological role of NO is in mediating the effects of mechanical stress on the skeleton. The *in vivo* studies with NOS inhibitors and with NO donors in animal models support a role for the L-arginine/NO pathway in this situation, but confirmation that this is indeed the case must await further studies of bone metabolism in knockout mice where various NOS isoforms have inactivated by gene targeting. This is because many of the studies so far have relied on observing effects which result from administration of arginine analogues which could themselves exert non-specific actions on other metabolic pathways.

From the clinical viewpoint it is important to extend the animal studies on the *in vivo* effects of NO donors to humans. Many NO donors are available for clinical use in the treatment of hypertension and angina and it would be relatively simple to study the effects of these agents on bone turnover in man. Studies on the effects of NOS inhibitors on bone metabolism in inflammatory disease states are less easily performed since none of the agents so far available have the required specificity for the iNOS isoform. Although L-NMMA has been used clinically in the treatment of septic shock [54] it is likely that administration of this compound to patients with inflammatory disease or bone disease would cause adverse effects such as hypertension, although this situation may change as more selective inhibitors are developed in the future.

References

1   Palmer RM, Ferrige AG, Moncada S (1987) Nitric oxide release accounts for the biological activity of endothelium-derived relaxing factor. *Nature* 327: 524–526

2   Moncada S, Palmer RMJ, Higgs EA (1991) Nitric oxide: physiology, pathophysiology and pharmacology. *Pharmacol Rev* 43: 109–142

3   Nathan C (1992) Nitric oxide as a secretory product of mammalian cells. *FASEB J* 6: 3051–3064

4   MacIntyre I, Zaid M, Towhidul Alam ASM, Datta HK, Moonga BS, Lidbury PS, Hecker M, Vane JM (1991) Osteoclast inhibition: An action of nitric oxide not mediated by cyclic GMP. *Proc Natl Acad Sci USA* 88: 2936–2940

5   Benjamin N, O'Driscoll F, Dougall H, Duncan C, Smith L, Golden M, McKenzie H (1994) Stomach NO synthesis. *Nature* 368: 502

6   Palmer RMJ (1993) The L-arginine nitric oxide pathway. *Curr Opin Nephrol Hyperten* 2: 122–128

7   Green LC, Wagner DA, Glogowski J, Skipper PL, Wishnock JS, Tannenbaum SR (1982) Analysis of nitrate, nitrite and (15N) nitrate in biological fluids. *Anal Biochem* 126: 131–138

8   Bredt DS, Hwang PM, Glatt CE, Lowenstein C, Reed RR, Snyder SH (1991) Cloned and expressed nitric oxide synthase structurally resembles cytochrome P-450 reductase. *Nature* 351: 714–718

9   Robinson LJ, Weremowicz S, Morton CC, Michel T (1994) Isolation and chromosomal localization of the human endothelial nitric oxide synthase (nos3) gene. *Genomics* 19: 350–357

10   Lowenstein CJ, Glatt CS, Bredt DS, Snyder SH (1992) Cloned and expressed macrophage nitric oxide synthase contrasts with the brain enzyme. *Proc Natl Acad Sci USA* 89: 6711–6715

11   Klein-Nulend J, Semeins CM, Ajubi NE, Nijweide PJ, Burger EH (1995) Pulsating fluid flow increases nitric oxide (NO) synthesis by osteocytes but not periosteal fibroblasts – correlation with prostaglandin upregulation. *Biochem Biophys Res Comm* 217: 640–648

12   Di Rosa M, Radomski M, Carnuccio R, Moncada S (1990) Glucocorticoids inhibit the induction of nitric oxide synthase in macrophages. *Biochem Biophys Res Comm* 172: 1246–1252

13   O'Connor KJ, Moncada S (1991) Glucocorticoids inhibit the induction of nitric oxide synthase and the related cell damage in adenocarcinoma cells. *Biochim Biophys Acta* 1097: 227–231

14   Ding A, Nathan CF, Graycar J, Derynck R, Stuehr DJ, Srimal S (1990) Macrophage deactivating factor and transforming growth factors -beta 1, -beta 2, and beta -3, inhibit induction of macrophage nitrogen oxide synthesis by IFN-gamma. *J Immunol* 145: 904–944

15   Bogdan C, Vodovotz Y, Paik J, Xie Q, Nathan C (1994) Mechanism of suppression of nitric oxide synthase expression by interleukin-4 in primary mouse macrophages. *J Leukocyte Biol* 55: 227–233

16   Cunha FQ, Moncada S, Liew FY (1992) Interleukin-10 (IL-10) inhibits the induction of nitric oxide synthase by interferon-gamma in murine macrophages. *Biochem Biophys Res Comm* 182: 1155–1159

17   Assreuy J, Cunha FQ, Liew FY, Moncada S (1993) Feedback inhibition of nitric oxide synthase activity by nitric oxide. *Br J Pharmacol* 108: 833–837

18   Park SK, Lin HL, Murphy S (1997) Nitric oxide regulates nitric oxide synthase-2 gene expression by inhibiting NF-kappaB binding to DNA. *Biochem J* 322: 609–613

19   Taylor-Robinson AW, Liew FY, Severn A, Xu D, McSorley SJ, Garside P, Padron J, Phillips RS (1994) Regulation of the immune response by nitric oxide differentially produced by T helper type 1 and T helper type 2 cells. *Eur J Immunol* 24: 980–984

20   Blachier F, Selamnia M, Robert V, M'Rabet-Touil H, Duee PH (1995) Metabolism of L-

arginine through polyamine and nitric oxide synthase pathways in proliferative or differentiated human colon carcinoma cells. *Biochim Biophys Acta* 1268: 255–262

21 Stuehr DJ, Olufunmilayo A, Fasehun A, Kwon NS, Gross SS, Gonzalez JA, Levi R, Nathan CF (1991) Inhibition of macrophage and endothelial cell nitric oxide synthase by diphenyleneiodonium and its analogs. *FASEB J* 5: 98–103

22 Mittal CK, Jadhav AL (1994) Calcium-dependent inhibition of constitutive nitric oxide synthase. *Biochem Biophys Res Comm* 203: 8–15

23 Kashiba-Iwatsuki M, Miyamoto M, Inoue M (1997) Effect of nitric oxide on the ligand-binding activity of albumin. *Arch Biochem Biophys* 345: 237–242

24 Ignarro LJ, Kadowitz PJ (1985) The pharmacological and physiological role of cyclic GMP in vascular smooth muscle relaxation. *Ann Rev Pharmacol Toxicol* 25: 171–191

25 Ralston SH, Grabowski PS (1996) Mechanisms of cytokine induced bone resorption: Role of nitric oxide, cyclic guanosine monophosphate and prostaglandins. *Bone* 19: 29–33

26 Lepoivre M, Flaman J, Henry Y (1992) Early loss of the tyrosyl radical in ribonucleotide reductase of adenocarcinoma cells producing nitric oxide. *J Biol Chem* 267: 22994–23000

27 Lipton SA, Choi Y, Pan Z, Lei SZ, Chen HV, Sucher NJ, Loscalzo J, Singel NJ, Stamler JS (1993) A redox based mechanism for the neuroprotective and neurodestructive effects of nitric oxide and related nitroso compounds. *Nature* 364: 626–632

28 Drapier JC, Hibbs JB (1986) Murine cytotoxic activated macrophages inhibit aconitase in tumor cells. Inhibition involves the iron-sulfur prosthetic group and is reversible. *J Clin Invest* 78: 790–797

29 Beckman JS, Beckman TW, Chen J, Marshall PA, Freeman BA (1990) Apparent hydroxyl radical production by peroxynitrite: implications for endothelial injury from nitric oxide and superoxide. *Proc Natl Acad Sci USA* 17: 1620–1624

30 Helfrich MH, Evans DE, Grabowski PS, Pollock JS, Ohshima H, Ralston SH (1997) Expression of nitric oxide synthase isoforms in bone and bone cell cultures. *J Bone Miner Res* 12: 1108–1115

31 Schmidt HHW, Gagne GD, Nakane M, Pollock JS, Miller MF, Murad F (1992) Mapping of neural nitric oxide synthase in the rat suggests frequent co-localisation with NADPH diaphorase but not with soluble guanylate cyclase and novel paraneural functions for signal transduction. *J Histochem Cytochem* 40: 1439–1456

32 van't Hof RJ, Ralston SH (1997) Cytokine induced Nitric Oxide inhibits bone resorption by inducing apoptosis of osteoclast progenitors and suppressing osteoclast activity. *J Bone Miner Res* 12: 1797–1804

33 Ralston SH, Ho LP, Helfrich MH, Grabowski PS, Johnston PW, Benjamin N (1995) Nitric oxide: a cytokine-induced regulator of bone resorption. *J Bone Miner Res* 10: 1040–1049

34 Lowik CWGM, Nibbering PH, Van der Ruit M, Papapoulos SE (1994) Inducible production of nitric oxide in osteoblast-like cells and in fetal bone explants is associated with supression of osteoclastic bone resorption. *J Clin Invest* 93: 1465–1472

35   Wimalawansa SJ, DeMarco G, Gangula P, Yallampalli C, De Marco G (1996) Nitric oxide donor alleviates ovariectomy induced bone loss. *Bone* 18: 301–304

36   Jamal S, Milani G, Lipschutz R, Stone K, Browner WS, Bauer DC, Cummings SR (1997) The therapeutic use of nitrates does not influence post-menopausal osteoporosis. *J Bone Miner Res* 12: S229

37   Brandi ML, Hukkanen M, Umeda T, Moradi-Bidhendi N, Bianchi S, Gross SS, Polak JM, MacIntyre I (1995) Bidirectional regulation of osteoclast function by nitric oxide synthase isoforms. *Proc Natl Acad Sci USA* 92: 2954–2958

38   Kasten TP, Collin-Osdoby P, Patel N, Osdoby P, Krukowski M, Misko TP, Settle SL, Currie MG, Nickols GA (1994) Potentiation of osteoclast bone resorbing activity by inhibition of nitric oxide synthase. *Proc Natl Acad Sci USA* 91: 3569–3573

39   Tsukahara H, Miura M, Tsuchida S, Hata I, Hata K, Yamamoto K, Ishii Y, Muramatsu I, Sudo M (1996) Effect of nitric oxide synthase inhibitors on bone metabolism in growing rats. *Am J Physiol* 270: E840–E845

40   Bender DA (1985) *Amino acid metabolism*, 2nd ed. Wiley, Interscience, London

41   Damoulis PD, Hauschka PV (1997) Nitric oxide acts in conjunction with pro-inflammatory cytokines to promote cell death in osteoblasts. *J Bone Miner Res* 12: 412–423

42   MacPherson H, Noble BS, Ralston SH (1999) Expression and functional role of nitric oxide synthase isoforms in human osteoblast-like cells. *Bone* 24: 179–185

43   Riancho JA, Salas E, Zarrabeitia MT, Olmos JM, Amado JA, Fernandez-Luna JL, Gonzalez-Macias J (1995) Expression and functional role of nitric oxide synthase in osteoblast-like cells. *J Bone Miner Res* 10: 439–446

44   Pitsillides AA, Rawlinson SC, Suswillo RF, Bourrin S, Zaman G, Lanyon LE (1995) Mechanical strain-induced NO production by bone cells: a possible role in adaptive bone (re)modeling? *FASEB J* 9: 1614–1622

45   van't Hof RJ, Ralston SH (1997) Cytokine-induced nitric oxide inhibits bone resorption by inducing apoptosis of osteoclast progenitors and suppressing osteoclast activity. *J Bone Miner Res* 12: 1797–1804

46   Fox SW, Chambers TJ, Chow JW (1996) Nitric oxide is an early mediator of the increase in bone formation by mechanical stimulation. *Am J Physiol* 270: E955–E960

47   Rawlinson SC, Mosley JR, Suswillo RF, Pitsillides AA, Lanyon LE (1995) Calvarial and limb bone cells in organ and monolayer culture do not show the same early responses to dynamic mechanical strain. *J Bone Miner Res* 10: 1225–1232

48   Weiner CP, Lizasoain I, Baylis SA, Knowles RG, Charles IG, Moncada S (1994) Induction of calcium-dependent nitric oxide synthases by sex hormones. *Proc Natl Acad Sci USA* 91: 5212–5216

49   Armour KE, Ralston SH (1998) Estrogen upregulates endothelial constitutive nitric oxide synthase expression in human osteoblast-like cells. *Endocrinology* 139: 799–802

50   Smith LM, Cuthbertson B, Galley H, Webster N, Robins SP, Ralston SH (1998) Bone resorption is increased in critically ill patients, in association with sepsis and increased nitric oxide production. *Bone* 22: 34S

51   Horowitz M (1993) Cytokines and estrogen in bone: anti-osteoporotic effects. *Science* 260: 626–628

52   Ralston SH (1994) Analysis of gene expression in human bone biopsies by polymerase chain reaction: evidence for enhanced cytokine expression in postmenopausal osteoporosis. *J Bone Miner Res* 9: 883–890

53   Rosselli M, Imthurn B, Keller PJ, Jackson EK, Dubey RK (1995) Circulating nitric oxide (nitrite/nitrate) levels in postmenopausal women substituted with 17 beta-estradiol and norethisterone acetate. A two-year follow-up study. *Hypertension* 25: 848–853

54   Petros A, Bennett D, Vallance P (1991) Effect of nitric oxide synthase inhibitors on hypotension in patients with septic shock. *Lancet* 338: 1557–1558

55   Ralston SH (1997) Nitric oxide and bone: what a gas! *Br J Rheumatol* 36: 831–838

56   Grabowski PS, England AJ, Dykhuizen R, Copland M, Benjamin N, Reid DM, Ralston SH (1996) Elevated nitric oxide production in rheumatoid arthritis. Detection using the fasting urinary nitrate: creatinine ratio. *Arthritis Rheum* 39: 643–647

57   van't Hof RJ, Ralston SH (1997) Nitric oxide's function in bone cells. *Curr Op Orthopaed* 8: 19–24

Why does chronic inflammation persist? A radical autoimmune perspective

Joseph Lunec and Helen R. Griffiths

University of Leicester, Division of Chemical Pathology, Hodgkin Building, MRC Centre for Mechanisms in Human Toxicity, Lancaster Road, Leicester LE1 9HN, UK

Introduction

The probability exists that there are as many types of "inflammation" as there are agents which provoke it. To the clinician inflammation, particularly chronic inflammation, represents inter- and intracellular chaos, brought about by the unruly gymnastics of chemicals in the body – a molecular delinquency if you like. It is the clinicians aim to tame, and control this delinquent behaviour. To the cell biologist/biochemist, chronic inflammation and its persistence is an intellectual conundrum, a little like trying to identify the murderer in an Agatha Christie novel. Who or what signalled death for the T cell and where did it happen? What "weapon" was used, cytokines and/or reactive oxygen species (ROS)?

This chapter is an attempt to set the evidence before you, with the help of some of the possible witnesses to the event.

The neutrophilic polymorphonuclear leukocyte (PMN)

Of the cells that infiltrate the tissues in the early stages of the typical acute inflammatory response the predominant cell is the PMN. The PMNs enter the inflammatory focus for the purpose of ingesting and digesting particulate matter such as bacteria, damaged cells or immune complexes. If a foreign substance resists destruction (as does for example, the mycobacterium tuberculosis), a typical focus is established. The major cell types found at such a focus are macrophages, lymphocytes, plasma cells and fibroblasts. These cell types persist long after the initial injury and long after the diminution of PMN. Is it logical to assume then that the former cells mediate the persistent inflammatory response? This may not be the case because chronic inflammation may often have superimposed upon it periods of transient acute inflammation. The clinical observation that classical rheumatoid inflammation is characterised by periods of acute exacerbation and tissue destruction suggests that PMNs may have a role in this exacerbation possibly because of the generation

Free Radicals and Inflammation, edited by P. G. Winyard, D. R. Blake and C. H. Evans

of a new injurious agent quite different from the initial insult. In order to understand how PMNs may do this we must investigate the signals and chemical mediators that PMNs generate, and the consequences of their over-production.

Protein damage during inflammation

The role of phagocytosis in host defence has been recognised since 1882. More recent research implicates oxidative metabolism and proteolytic degradation in the inflammatory killing process [1, 2]. The mediators involve oxygen radicals, hydrogen peroxide, hypochlorous acid (collectively termed ROS), proteases and many others. Under conditions of "frustrated phagocytosis", ROS will be released into the extracellular space targeting to large macromolecules such as IgG, caeruloplasmin and lipoproteins. In an inflammatory focus, for instance the inflamed joint in rheumatoid arthritis, the damage to these macromolecules may elicit a further inflammatory response. The susceptibility of proteins to oxidative damage is well documented [3]. In the inflamed joint, IgG is the major secreted protein and up to 90 mg per day has been calculated to be produced by an active synovium [4]. Studies using monoclonal antibodies, to defined changes in epitope expression on IgG3, have demonstrated the hinge region is chemically altered [5]. If higher order structure is lost the protein assumes the shape of a linear poly-peptide. This alteration of structure may facilitate antibody binding. Complexes of IgG and anti-IgG are a common feature of rheumatoid arthritis particularly localised in the rheumatoid joint [6]. These complexes are considered to play an important role in the pathology. Raised levels of fluorescent IgG, a marker of free radical attack on IgG, are found in synovial fluids suggesting a possible role for the denatured protein promoting a chronic inflammatory response in the synovium [7].

The importance of the deficiencies in N-linked oligosaccharide moieties attached to ASN 297 of the Fc portion in the antigenicity of IgG remains equivocal, although ROS may play a role here also, particularly in relation to loss of galactose [8]. Observations by Murray and Brown [9] in hyperimmunised mice have demonstrated that monoclonal antibodies could be produced which discriminate between IgG generated as part of the immune response and native autologous IgG. These markers suggest that it is possible that following an attenuated immune response to a pathogenic organism an autoantigenic form of IgG could be generated. One of the most compelling pieces of evidence for modified IgG structure occurring in RA is the detection in large quantities of circulating anti IgG antibodies. The generation of such a heterogenous group of antibodies suggests an IgG-antigen driven response. However, the nature of the antigen has always remained elusive. We and others have proposed that modification of IgG by ROS makes human IgG antigenic and facilitates rheumatoid factor binding particularly in synovial fluid [10]. This neutrophil mediated modification of IgG through ROS and subsequent proteolytic modification may be the stimulus for perpetuation of the immune response in RA. The pathophysiological sequelae of RF-IgG immune-complex formation represents a clear mechanism whereby the products of the inflammatory response serve to perpetuate the process by producing autoantigens [11]. We have previously demonstrated this in a model of synovitis, where the introduction of a ROS-modified autologous IgG was shown to result in a worsening of the gross indices of inflammation, increases in lipid peroxidation and further enhancement of IgG autofluorescence [12].

Protease anti-protease imbalance

An important component of the aetiology of certain chronic inflammatory diseases is a genetically determined, or acquired, functional deficiency in the S or Z alleles of alpha-1-protease inhibitor (α1PI, also known as α1-antitrypsin). Studies suggest that circulating levels of α1PI are within the normal range, but that the trypsin inhibitor capacity of serum from asthmatics may be depressed, for reasons that are uncertain [13]. The ability of neutrophils and eosinophils to degranulate and produce ROS is enhanced in asthmatics and their recruitment may effect the structural integrity of a critical methionyl residue associated with α1PI activity; oxidation of this residue markedly impairs anti-elastase function [14]. Similarly studies in synovial fluids aspirated from the inflamed joints of RA patients, suggest that chronic inflammation with recruitment of macrophages and T lymphocytes may be propagated by increased local oxidative stress reactions of this type giving rise to the mediators LTB_4, C_4, D_4 and E_4 and release of IL-8 [15]. Collective evidence suggests an important role for protease-antiprotease balance in the inflammatory events and subsequent appearance and severity of pathological symptoms in both inflammatory joint disease and chronic respiratory disease.

DNA damage during inflammation

Nuclear DNA damage occurs under normal cellular metabolic conditions and is regulated by the cell cycle allowing lesions to be repaired prior to mitosis. Elevated rates of DNA damage, or ineffective repair, appears to occur in autoimmune diseases like RA, insulin dependent diabetes and, in particular, SLE [16, 17]. In SLE, this DNA damage may initiate/or propagate the disease process. Oxidative DNA damage and its repair appears to be a direct effect of the autoimmune process. The immune dysfunction common to chronic inflammatory autoimmune disorders, including RA, SLE and systemic sclerosis, may arise through DNA damage and inadequate or inappropriate repair. Small circulating fragments of DNA (~ 20 Kbases) are a characteristic feature of SLE, as is the generation of antibodies to double-stranded DNA [18, 19]. Nuclear DNA damage occurs during normal cell metabolism. Increased rates of DNA damage, resulting from either high pro-oxidant stress or ineffective repair, or a combination of both are characteristic of the autoimmune diseases SLE and IDDM (insulin-dependent diabetes) [20]. In SLE, DNA damage may initiate and or propagate the disease process and in IDDM, DNA damage appears to be an effect of the autoimmune process.

Antigen driven immune response to DNA damage

The production of autoantibodies in autoimmune disease may arise from either the generation of a specific autoimmune response against selected autoantigens or, as a result of polyclonal B cell activation. The two processes are not necessarily mutually exclusive and there is substantial evidence for an antigen driven response in SLE [21]. We have established, as have others, that oxidative damage to DNA makes the molecule more antigenic with respect to autoantibodies present in SLE sera, and also more immunogenic [22]. More importantly, however, we have shown that not only does modification by oxidative stress to DNA produce specific antibodies against highly specific modifications of bases and sugar moieties, but coincidentally, as part of the polyclonal response, antibodies are generated which have specificity against native double-stranded (ds) and single-stranded (ss) DNA [23]. In studies from our own group, which involved characterisation of epitopes following oxidative modification of DNA using a panel of mouse monoclonals with defined specificity for native regions of DNA, base residues in the DNA backbone and minor regions of (ss) DNA were exposed by oxidative stress, the pattern of epitope modification being characteristic of the denaturing system employed [24]. Similar experiments have been carried out by Ara and Ali [25] where a combination of hydrogen peroxide and UV light was used to generate hydroxyl radical ($\cdot$OH) and denature DNA. SLE patients' sera were found to have a 20–50-fold preference for this oxidatively modified DNA compared to the native molecule. The fact that this antigen was produced by UV light may also be of some significance. UV sensitivity is prevalent in approximately 60–70% of patients with SLE [26]. Furthermore, immunosuppression can be mediated by DNA damage as has been shown recently by Hurks et al. [27].

The Ku antigen and DNA repair

Ku is an antigen with a heterodimer structure composed of 70 and 80 KD proteins. These proteins have an affinity for DNA double-strand ends. It is believed to function in both replication and repair of DNA [28]. In SLE and related disorders autoantibodies develop to the Ku antigen and general studies have been directed to mapping the epitope involved [29]. There is increasing evidence that autoantibody generation in SLE is an antigen driven response and this may arise from neoantigens derived from the interaction between Ku and (ds) DNA ends, which are observed following exposure to oxidative stress [30].

Although DNA strand breaks and base products of oxidative stress are independent processes in terms of free-radical damage they are inextricably linked through the DNA repair process. DNA damage appears to be a common feature of inflammatory autoimmune disease. Autoantibodies to (ss) DNA, (ds) DNA base lesions and so components of the repair system such as PARS (poly-ADP-ribose synthetase), are often found in SLE [31, 32]. In fact compelling evidence exists which suggests that the DNA repair process is dysfunctional in both rheumatoid arthritis and SLE [16, 33]. Peripheral blood lymphocytes from both types of diseases have a greater susceptibility to cytotoxicity caused by oxidative stress compared to age-matched control cells. Patients with SLE show a deficiency in urinary excretion of 8-oxodG, an oxidative lesion of dG which is not observed in RA patients [34]. Many human genes involved in repair of UV induced lesions have now been cloned and positional cloning of the XRCC5 gene (radiation damage repair) has focused on a small region of chromosome 2q [35]. The XRCC5 gene encodes the 80 KD sub-unit of the Ku DNA binding protein, supporting a role for Ku in repair [35]. SCID (sub-combined immune deficiency) murine cells may also provide a useful model for studying the intimate relationship between DNA repair, immunosuppression and autoimmunity; these cells are defective in both repair of ds breaks and VDJ recombination. They also exhibit a deficiency in DNA-dependent protein kinase (DNA-Pk) a protein which forms an activated complex with the DNA and binding proteins Ku p80 and p70 upon association with damaged DNA [36]. Aberration in the repair of oxidatively damaged DNA will result in its persistence and potential for misreading and mispairing. Oxidant strand-breakage above a certain threshold stimulates PARS activity which plays a role in strand-break repair and G2 check-point control. Excessive oxidative damage to DNA especially from an insult such as H_2O_2 may compromise the DNA repair to such an extent that the threshold for signalling apoptosis is exceeded [37].

Apoptosis in autoimmune disease

Programmed cell death or apoptosis of autoreactive T cells is believed to be a control mechanism to guarantee self-tolerance. Many genes are involved in the control of this process, although Fas/apo 1 (CD95) and bcl-2 have received most attention as far as diseases of the immune system are concerned. Cross-linking of the transmembrane receptor Fas expressed on the surface of activated T and B cells by agonistic antibodies or the natural ligand, a novel member of the TNF family, is a powerful stimulus for apoptosis. In contrast, bcl-2 is regarded as having a protective role.

It has recently been reported that the nitric oxide radical (NO·), induced by cytokines, stimulates p53, the tumour suppressor gene, prior to apoptosis, particularly in pancreatic islet cells [38]. Inhibitors of nitric oxide synthase have been shown to be effective at inhibiting p53 expression and apoptosis, and it has been suggested that NO· induced apoptosis in these cells is a result of DNA damage and subsequent p53 expression. Kaneto et al. [39] used isolated pancreatic islet cells to confirm IL-1 induced NO· mediated internucleosomal fragmentation. Streptozotocin has also been shown to be active in inducing islet-cell damage in a similar manner. Genetic studies using apoptosis and non-apoptosis resistant mice have identified chromosome 6 as the region where both type 1 diabetes and control of dexamethazone induced apoptosis are mapped, implicating apoptosis resistance as a pathogenetic mechanism in IDDM [40]. The proto oncogene bcl-2 may inhibit apoptosis by influencing the redox status of the cells although this has been disputed [41]. Increased bcl-2 expression has been identified in a significant proportion of naïve and memory T cells, but not B cells from SLE patients and hence dysregulation of apoptosis has been implicated in pathogenesis of SLE. Furthermore, it has been shown that SLE lymphocytes have a greater than two-fold faster rate of apoptosis compared with normal lymphocytes [42].

A characteristic sequel to active apoptosis is the extracellular release of internucleosomal fragments of DNA. Indeed, this can happen without the necessity for apoptosis taking place. Interaction of these DNA fragments, which are undoubtedly present in normal sera and elevated in SLE sera, with cell surface molecules which may activate production of IL-6. There is evidence that internucleosomal DNA is the major component of plasma DNA in SLE, where apoptosis may represent a mechanism by which antigen is presented to B and T cells [43]. DNA fragments containing oxidised DNA, detected in SLE sera may reflect accelerated apoptosis resulting from increased DNA damage and aberrant repair. The rate of clearance of these ROS damaged fragments, via antibody interaction and particularly complement, may determine increased half-life and pathogenicity of these products [44].

Selective cytotoxicity

Allan et al. have demonstrated the selective depletion of CD^{3+} CD^{8+} T cells by levels of H_2O_2 which can be readily found during the inflammatory response irrespective of the source of the inflammatory foci [45]. The selective lymphocyte depletion may allow uncontrolled help of the B cell response to autoantigen. Subsequent studies by the same authors identified strand breaks to be important in the process of selective lymphocyte depletion by hydrogen peroxide which may ultimately be due to PARS activity [21]. Studies on the phenotype of peripheral blood lymphocytes from SLE patients with active renal disease have shown a decreased percentage of cells which are critical for the activation of CD^{8+} cells. This observation combined with the potential for selective CD^{8+} cell loss during oxidative stress, may promote B cell responsiveness to circulating antigens.

In addition, to a direct role in potentiating the inflammatory response via tissue damage, oxygen radicals also have detrimental effects on the functions of the leukocytes themselves. It has also been suggested that at chronic inflammation foci, where the free radical flux is high and sustained, the levels may exceed those required to abolish lymphocyte function and directly cause cell death. Such events may modify or even modulate lymphocyte function [21, 45]. The rheumatoid synovial membrane has a lymphoid cell infiltrate characteristic of intense immunological activity. Its most striking characteristic is the abnormally high CD^{4+}/CD^{8+} ratio: At least two explanations can be put forward to explain this abnormally high ratio. It may result from poorly suppressed activation and proliferation resulting in an excess of CD^{4+} lymphocytes, or a selective loss or failure to recruit CD^{8+} lymphocytes. Experiments conducted by Allan et al. suggest that CD^{8+} bearing cells may, at least in part predominate as a result of oxidant induced death. We have proposed that oxidant induced lymphocyte killing may favour T cell help by significantly reducing the function of immunoregulator T cells mediating suppression. T suppressor-cell activity has been shown to be significantly depressed in the synovial fluid of RA patients, but normal in the peripheral blood. This supports the proposal that CD^{8+} lymphocytes entering the focus of inflammatory activity and undergoing sustained oxidative activity may be selectively depleted [46].

Cell proliferation during inflammation

ROS, whether they are produced via phagocytic cell activation or through hypoxic cell injury during inflammatory joint disease, may enhance and propagate inflammation through dysregulation of mammalian cell proliferation. Peroxidation of lipids has potential consequences for normal cell proliferation and their effects may be potentiated at foci of inflammation. A characteristic feature of chronic inflammatory disease and particularly RA is an aggressive proliferation of fibroblasts [47]. In RA this may result in an equally aggressive destruction of bone cartilage. *In vivo* it can be expected that during an immune response multiple cytokines are produced simultaneously and interact in complex ways. ROS and lipid peroxides can stimulate fibroblast proliferation *in vitro*, probably through the production of IL-1, TNFα and FGF (fibroblast growth factor). Equally TNFα can stimulate production of ROS and NO˙ *in vivo* [48]. One important and relevant characteristic of proliferating cells is the increased phosphorylation of proteins which can potentially be mediated by ROS.

NF-κB is a protein which activates genes encoding IL-1, IL-6, and TNFα amongst other cytokines, probably via its own activation intracellularly by ROS [49]. Hence here is a potential self-perpetuating cycle of events that once triggered could promote

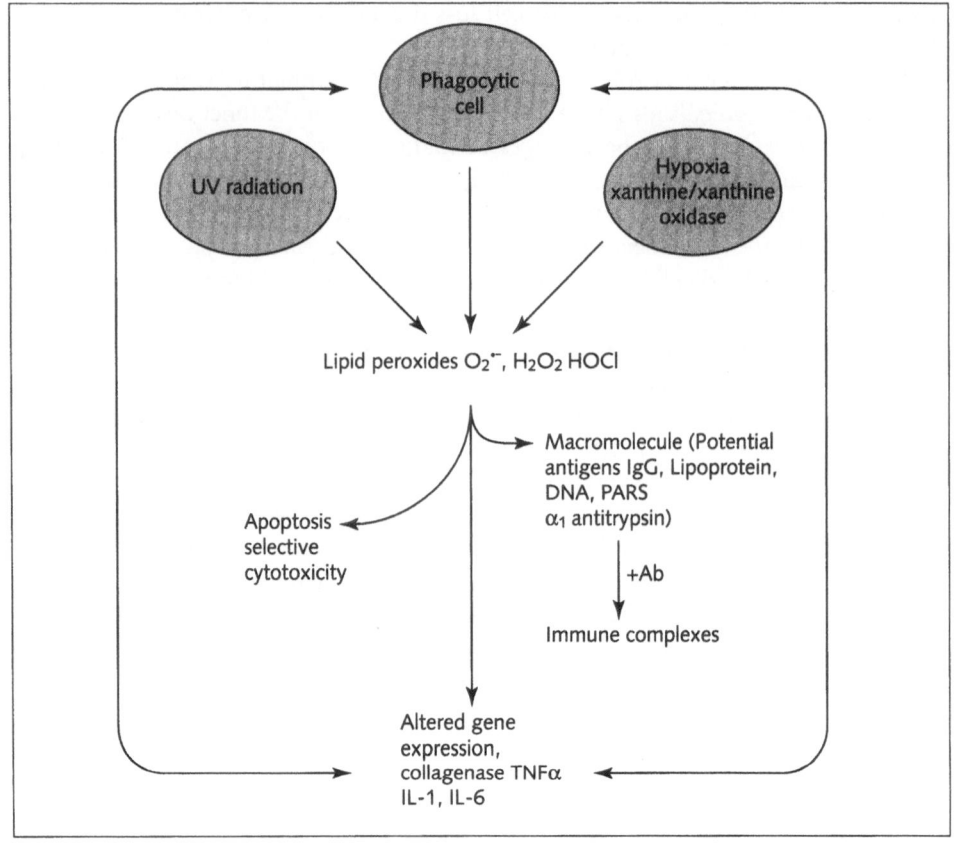

Figure 1
Schematic representation illustrating pivotal role for ROS in perpetuating inflammation.

the chronic inflammatory process including within it the proliferation of cells at the foci of the inflammation. NO˙ has been identified as an important proinflammatory mediator. The high amounts produced by inflamed synovium can lead to bone resorption and diminished bone proliferation, decreased proteoglycan synthesis, activation of metalloproteases and induction of chondrocyte apoptosis. All of these effects contribute to joint damage and could perpetuate inflammation [48].

Conclusions

Herein we have compared several chronic inflammatory autoimmune pathologies in which oxidative stress may influence both initiating and perpetuating stages of the disease process. Not only are oxidative reactions self-perpetuating within the chemistry of their production, they are also clearly important in the perpetuation of inflammatory/autoimmune processes. In RA they may not be the trigger for the disease, but they undoubtedly influence its course and chronicity through cytokine production leading to autoantigenic changes to the pivotal IgG molecule (see Fig. 1). Atherosclerosis represents another chronic inflammatory process with an autoimmune component, where the damage to the lipoprotein macromolecule creates neoantigenic determinants. Increased antigenicity predisposes to immune complex formation. This may be local in the case of the lung or joint, or it may be systemic as in the case of SLE. In SLE the radical reactions may not only be responsible for propagation, but also important in initiation through dysfunction of DNA repair mechanisms in this condition. The evidence, therefore, appears more than circumstantial for ROS being, if not the major rogue in promoting chronic inflammatory disease, then at least an equal "conspirator".

References

1   Lunec J, Griffiths HR, Blake DR (1987) Oxygen radicals in inflammation. *Atlas of Sci* 1: 45–48

2   Krinsky NI (1974) Singlet excited oxygen as a mediator of the antibacterial action of leukocytes. *Science* 186: 363–365

3   Fu S, Davies MJ, Dean RT (1998) Molecular aspects of free radical damage to proteins. In: OI Aruoma, B Halliwell (eds): *Molecular biology of free radicals in human diseases.* OICA International, Saint Lucia, 29–56

4   Smiley JD, Sachs C, Ziff M (1968) *In vitro* synthesis of immunoglobulins by rheumatoid synovial membranes. *J Clin Invest* 47: 624–632

5   Jose SA, Griffiths H, Mageed RA, Jefferis R (1987) Immunogenic and antigenic epitopes of immunoglobulin-XX. Denaturation of human IgG3 by free radicals. *Mol Immunol* 24: 1145–1150

6   Jasin HE (1988) Oxidative crosslinking of immune complexes by human polymorphonuclear leukocytes. *J Clin Invest* 81: 6–15

7   Lunec J, Griffiths HR (1988) Effect of polymorph derived oxidants on IgG in relation to rheumatoid factor binding. *Scand J Rheum Suppl* 75: 148–156

8   Griffiths HR, Lunec J (1991) Effects of reactive oxygen species on immunoglobulin G function. *Mol Asp Med* 12: 107–119

9   Murray JS, Brown JC (1988) Hyperimmunisation alters Fc Gamma antigenicity. Linkage to glycosylation. *J Immunol* 141: 2668–2673

10 Lunec J, Griffiths HR, Brailsford S (1988) Oxygen free radicals denature human IgG and increase its reactivity with rheumatoid factor antibody. *Scand J Rheum Suppl* 75: 140–147

11 Lunec J, Blake DR, McCleary SJ, Brailsford S, Bacon PA (1985) Self perpetuating mech-

anisms of immunoglobulin G aggregation in rheumatoid inflammation. *J Clin Invest* 76: 284–2090

12 Hewitt SD, Lunec J, Morris CJ, Blake DR (1987) Effect of free radical altered IgG on allergic inflammation. *Ann Rheum Dis* 46: 866–874

13 Colp C, Pappas J, Moran D, Lieberman J (1993) Variants of α1-antitrypsin in Puerto Rico children with asthma. *Chest* 103: 812–815

14 Chidwick K, Winyard PG, Zhang Z, Farrell AJ, Blake DR (1991) Inactivation of the elastase inhibility activity of a, antitrypsin in fresh samples of synovial fluid from patients with rheumatoid arthritis. *Ann Rheum Dis* 50: 915–916

15 Fahey JV, Kim KW, Liu J, Boushey HA (1995) Prominent neutrophilic inflammation in sputum from subjects with asthma exacerbation. *J Allergy Clin Immunol* 95: 843–852

16 Bashir S, Harris G, Denman MA, Blake DR, Winyard PG (1993) Oxidative DNA damage and cellular sensitivity to oxidative stress in human autoimmune diseases. *Ann Rheum Dis* 52: 659–666

17 Dandona P, Thusu K, Cook S, Snyder B, Makowski J, Armstrong D, Nicolera T (1996) Oxidative damage to DNA in diabetes mellitus. *Lancet* 347: 444–445

18 Lunec J, Herbert K, Blount S, Griffiths HR, Emery P (1994) A marker of oxidative DNA damage in systemic lupus erythematosus. *FEBS Lett* 348: 131–138

19 Swaak AJG, Groenwold J, Aarden LA, Feltkamp (1981) Detection of anti-ds DNA as a diagnostic tool. *Ann Rheum Dis* 40: 45–49

20 Compton LJ, Steinberg AD, Sano H (1984) Nuclear DNA degradation in lymphocytes of patients with systemic lupus erythematosus. *J Immunol* 133: 213–216

21 Carson DA, Seto S, Wasson DB (1986) Lymphocyte function after DNA damage by toxic oxygen species. *J Exp Med* 163: 74–75

22 Blount S, Griffiths HR, Lunec J (1989) Reactive oxygen species induce antigenic changes in DNA. *FEBS Lett* 245: 100–103

23 Blount S, Griffiths HR, Emery P, Lunec J (1990) Reactive oxygen species modify human DNA eliciting a more descriminating antigen for the diagnosis of Systemic Lupus erythematosus. *Clin Exp Immunol* 81: 384–389

24 Blount S, Griffiths HR, Staines NA, Lunec J (1992) Probing molecular changes induced in DNA by reactive oxygen species with monoclonal antibodies. *Immunol Lett* 34: 115–126

25 Ara J, Ali R (1993) Polynucleotide specificity of anti-reactive oxygen species (ROS) DNA antibodies. *Clin Exp Immunol* 94: 134–139

26 Sontheimer RD (1996) Photoimmunology of lupus erythematosus and dermatomyositis. A speculative review. *Photochem Photobiol* 63 (5): 583–594

27 Hurks HMH, Out-Luiting C, Vermeer BJ, Class FHJ, Mommaas AM (1995) The action spectra for UV-induced suppression of MLR and MECLR show that immuno suppression is mediated by DNA damage. *Photochem Photobiol* 62: 449–453

28 Blier PR, Griffith AJ, Craft J, Hardin JA (1993) Binding of ku protein to DNA. Measurement of affinity for ends and demonstration of binding to nicks. *J Biol Chem* 268: 7594–7601

29   Wen J, Yaneva M (1990) Mapping of epitopes on the 86 kDa subunit of the Ku autoantigen. *Mol Immunol* 27: 973–990

30   Chou CH, Wang J, Knuth MW, Reeves WH (1992) Role of major autoepitope in forming the DNA binding site of the p70 (Ku) antigen. *J Exp Med* 175: 1677–1684

31   Blount S, Griffiths HR, Lunec J (1991) ROS damage to DNA and its role in systemic lupus erythematosus. *Molec Asp Med* 12: 93–105

32   Muller S, Briand JP, Barakat S, Lageux J, Poirrier GG, De Murcia G, Isenberg DA (1994) Autoantibodies reacting with poly-ADP-ribose and with a zinc-finger DNA. *Clin Immunol Immunopathol* 73: 187–196

33   Bhusate LL, Herbert KE, Scott DL, Perret D (1992) Increased DNA strand breaks in mononuclear cells from patients with rheumatoid arthritis and some other diseases. *Ann Rheum Dis* 51: 8–12

34   Blount S, Lunec J, Griffiths HR (1990) Urinary 8-hydroxydeoxyguanosine, a normal repair product is absent in patients with systemic lupus erythematosus. *Int J Rad Biol* 57: 1267–1268

35   Jeggo PA, Carr AM, Lehman AR (1994) Cloning human DNA repair genes. *Int J Rad Biol* 66: 573–577

36   Evans JW, Liu XF, Kirchgessner CU, Brown JM (1996) Induction and repair of chromosome abberrations in scid cells measured in premature chromosome condensation. *Rad Res* 145: 39–46

37   Hu JJ, Dubin N, Kurland D, Ma BL, Roush GC (1995) The effects of hydrogen peroxide on DNA repair activities. *Mut Res – DNA Repair* 336: 193–201

38   Messmer UK, Ankacrona M, Nicotera P, Brune B (1994) p53 expression in nitric oxide induced apoptosis. *FEBS Lett* 355: 23–26

39   Kaneto H, Fujii J, Seo HG, Suzuki K, Matsuoka T, Nakamura M, Tatsumi H, Yamasaki Y, Kamada T, Tanaguchi N (1995) Apoptotic cell death triggered by nitric oxide in pancreatic beta cells. *Diabet* 44: 733–738

40   Penha-Goncalves C, Leijon K, Persson L, Holmberg D (1995) Type 1 diabetes and the control of dexamethasone-induced apoptosis in mice maps to the same region of chromosome 6. *Genomics* 28: 398–404

41   Buttke TM, Sandstrom PA (1994) Oxidative stress as a mediator of apoptosis. *Immunol Today* 15: 7–10

42   Ohsaka S, Hara S, Harigai M, Fukasawa C, Kashiwazaki S (1994) Expression and function of Fas antigen and Bcl-2 in human systemic lupus erythematosus. *Clin Immunol Immunopathol* 73: 109–114

43   Rumore PM, Steinman CR (1990) Endogenous circulating DNA in systemic lupus erythematosus. *J Clin Invest* 86: 69–74

44   Sequi J, Leigh I, Isenberg DA (1991) Relation between antinuclear antibodies and the autoimmune rheumatic diseases and disease type and activity in SLE using a variety of cultured cells. *Ann Rheum Dis* 50: 167–172

45   Allan IM, Lunec J, Salmon M, Bacon PA (1987) Reactive oxygen species selectively

deplete normal T-lymphocytes via a hydroxyl radical mechanism. *Scand J Immunol* 26: 47–53

46 Allan IM, Lunec J, Salmon M, Bacon PA (1986) Selective lymphocyte killing by reactive oxygen species. *Agents and Actions* 19: 351–352

47 Burdon RH (1994) Free radicals in cell proliferation. In: CA Rice-Evans CA, RH Burdon (eds): *Free radical damage and its control*. Elsevier Science, 115–185

48 Jang D, Murrell GAC (1998) Nitric oxide in arthritis. *Free Rad Biol Med* 24: 1511–1519

49 Schrek R, Albermann K, Baeuerle PA (1992) Nuclear factor κB: an oxidative stress response transcription factor of eukaryotic cells (a review). *Free Rad Res Commun* 17: 221–237

Radicals, granuloma formation and fibrosis

George A.C. Murrell

Orthopaedic Research Institute, St George Hospital Campus, University of New South Wales, Kogarah, Sydney 2217, Australia

Introduction

Granulomas and fibrosis

A granuloma is a chronic inflammatory lesion characterized by large numbers of cells of various types (macrophages, lymphocytes, giant cells, fibroblasts) some degrading and some repairing the tissues. Fibrosis is an excessive and persistent accumulation of collagen producing cells – fibroblasts, and their matrix – predominantly Type I collagen. Fibrosis can affect nearly every organ of the body, including the skin. Examples include adhesive capsulitis of the shoulder, Dupuytren's contracture of the hand and foot, cystic fibrosis of the lung and cirrhosis of the liver. Important components of normal wound healing include an infiltration and proliferation of fibroblasts and synthesis of matrix by these cells. Thus the biochemical and histological features of normal wound healing and fibrosis are analogous, with the somewhat arbitrary distinction that in fibrosis there is a persistence of these features – particularly collagen accumulation, and there is no return to "normal" or "baseline" biochemistry and morphology.

Free radicals

A free radical is an atom or molecule with one or more unpaired electrons. These unpaired electrons make these atoms and molecules highly reactive. Free radicals often react with other atoms or molecules to produce more radical species in a chain reaction type effect. With respect to fibrosis and granuloma formation, free radicals may be (1) generated exogenously, for instance inhaled fluorocarbons, (2) initiated by an exogenous source, for instance inhaled silica stimulating production of reactive oxygen species from macrophages, or (3) generated endogenously. A list of endogenous sources of free radicals that may be involved in granuloma formation and fibrosis is illustrated in Table 1. The three major cellular sources of free radicals

Free Radicals and Inflammation, edited by P. G. Winyard, D. R. Blake and C. H. Evans
© 2000 Birkhäuser Verlag Basel/Switzerland

Table 1 - Potential sources of free radicals in fibrosis

Cell type	Initiating event	Enzyme	Free radical
Endothelial cells	ischaemia ethanol	xanthene dehydrogenase xanthene oxidase	$O_2^{\cdot-}$
Endothelial cells	shear stress	endothelial nitric oxide synthase (eNOS)	$NO^{\cdot}$
Macrophage	foreign body zymogen Ca^{2+}	NADPH oxidase	$O_2^{\cdot-}$
Macrophage	pro-inflammatory cytokines (e.g. TNFα, IL-1β)	inducible nitric oxide synthase (iNOS)	$NO^{\cdot}$
Fibroblast	Ca^{2+} shear stress	NADPH oxidase	$O_2^{\cdot-}$
Fibroblast	pro-inflammatory cytokines (e.g. TNFα, IL-1β, IFNα)	iNOS	$NO^{\cdot}$

are likely to be endothelial cells, phagocytic cells and fibroblasts. The two major groups of free radical species are $O_2^{\cdot-}$ (and associated oxygen free radicals) and nitric oxide ($NO^{\cdot}$). $O_2^{\cdot-}$ and $NO^{\cdot}$ may react together to produce a potent oxidant, peroxynitrite. In endothelial cells the normally "benign" xanthine dehydrogenase can be converted to xanthine oxidase (see Harrison, this volume) when exposed to ischaemia or to ethanol with subsequent $O_2^{\cdot-}$ production. Endothelial cells also have a membrane-bound nitric oxide synthase (eNOS or cNOS) which releases small amounts of $NO^{\cdot}$ in a constitutive manner (see Benjamin, this volume). This $NO^{\cdot}$ mediates a number of local effects including vasodilation and decreased platelet aggregation. Macrophages and other phagocytic cells when exposed to foreign bodies activate cytosolic NADPH oxidase to release $O_2^{\cdot-}$ in a "respiratory burst" – a mechanism important in host defense. Macrophages also synthesize inducible nitric oxide synthase (iNOS) when exposed to pro-inflammatory cytokines. Fibroblasts can also release $NO^{\cdot}$ and $O_2^{\cdot-}$ (Tab. 1).

Fibroblasts and free radicals

Oxygen free radicals may act as an intercellular messenger system in fibroblasts. We [1, 2] and others [3, 4] have shown that human fibroblasts in culture release oxygen free radicals via an NADPH oxidase (see Jones and Hancock, this volume) and that when these free radicals were inhibited fibroblast proliferation was inhib-

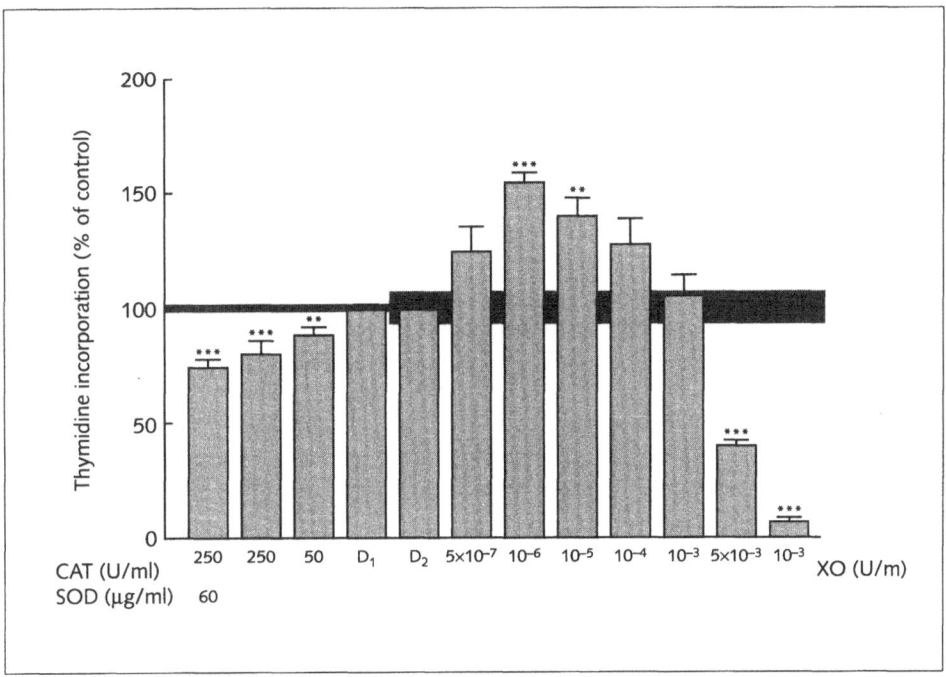

Figure 1
Modulation of fibroblast proliferation by oxygen free radicals.
*The results of two separate experiments are drawn on the same axes for comparison. On the right, exogenous free radicals have been introduced by the addition of increasing concentrations of xanthine oxidase (XO) to media containing 10^{-3} M hypoxanthine. Control (D_2) = 10^{-2} U/ml xanthine oxidase heat denatured at 100°C for 15 min. Mean thymidine incorporated in control group = 13 pmol/10^6 cells. On the left, no exogenous free radicals have been added and endogenous O_2^{-} or H_2O_2 have been scavenged by superoxide dismutase (SOD) and catalase (CAT) respectively. Control (D_1) = 250 U/ml heat denatured CAT and 60 μg/ml heat denatured SOD. Mean thymidine incorporated in control group = 53 pmol/10° cells. Expressed mean ± SEM % of control, n = 6. *Significantly different from control (* = p < 0.05, ** = p < 0.01, *** = p < 0.001 by two-tailed Student's t-test). From [1] with permission.*

ited [1]. Human fibroblasts in culture when exposed to high concentration of free radicals were damaged. However, lower, more physiological exogenous concentrations of free radicals were associated with a stimulation of fibroblast proliferation (Fig. 1) [1, 5]. This "hormetic" effect of low concentrations of oxygen free radicals on fibroblast proliferation was strikingly similar to the "hormetic" effects of low doses of radiation noted by Luckey in a number of animal and cellular systems [6].

Human keratinocytes in culture express eNOS [7] and when stimulated by interferon can express iNOS [7, 8]. The roles of nitric oxide released by these enzymes in keratinocyte physiology have yet to be explored.

Granulomas and free radicals

There is good evidence that both oxygen free radicals and nitric oxide are involved in granuloma formation. Gossart et al. [9] demonstrated that intratracheal installation of silica in rats lead to an increase in alveolar macrophage oxygen free radical production at days 3–28 and a rise in tumor necrosis factor-α (TNFα) production. Free radical scavenger pre treatment reversed granuloma formation, TNFα production and free radical release.

iNOS has been identified in the inflammatory lesions of pulmonary granulomatosis induced in rats by intratracheal installation of zymosan or silica [10]. The iNOS was expressed in neutrophils, monocyte-derived macrophages, and bronchiolar epithelial cells in the pulmonary lesions and was accompanied by electron spin resonance spectroscopy evidence of nitric oxide release and immunochemical evidence for the generation of peroxynitrite anion. Administration of nitric oxide synthase inhibitors suppressed NO$^{\cdot}$ production, reduced monocyte/macrophage infiltration and inhibited the induction of the monocyte chemoattractant protein-1 in the lesions [10]. Tsuji et al. [11] induced pulmonary granulomas by the intratracheal injection of dextran beads in two strains of mice – a genetically high granuloma responder and a genetically low responder. Interleukin-1α (IL-1α) and iNOS were induced in the cells accumulated around the beads during the early phase (1 to 3 days) of granuloma formation, whereas TNFα was induced in the cells around the beads at the later resolution phase (3 to 7 days). In low responder mice, IL-1α and TNFα was not detected throughout the period. The authors concluded that IL-1 and NO$^{\cdot}$ produced by recruited macrophages may take part in the early, macrophage-dependent phase of granuloma formation whereas TNFα may be responsible for the difference in innate resistance or susceptibility to granuloma formation.

Iuvone et al. [12] evaluated the role of NO$^{\cdot}$ in another model of granuloma formation – subcutaneous implantation of carrageenin-soaked polyether sponges in rats. They found that granulomatous tissue formation, cell infiltration and NO$_2^{\cdot-}$ (a stable end product of NO$^{\cdot}$) production were reduced, in a dose-dependent manner, by a nitric oxide synthase inhibitor and increased by its substrate L-arginine, suggesting that endogenous NO$^{\cdot}$ also plays a modulating role in this model of granuloma formation.

Matrix synthesis and free radicals

There is little data on the effects of oxygen free radicals on matrix synthesis, however Schaffer et al. [13] have shown in a rat model that nitric oxide may modulate matrix synthesis. Wound fibroblasts isolated from polyvinyl alcohol sponges implanted in rats synthesized and released NO and expressed iNOS. Inhibition of endogenous NO synthesis had no effect on fibroblast proliferation. However, fibroblast-mediated collagen contraction was enhanced and collagen synthesis was significantly decreased by inhibiting nitric oxide synthase. Schaffer et al. [13–15] have also shown that systemic inhibition of wound nitric oxide synthesis decreased wound mechanical strength. We have shown that nitric oxide synthase was expressed from day 1–15 in healing rat Achilles tendons and that inhibition of nitric oxide synthase reduced the cross-sectional area and load to failure properties of healing rat Achilles tendons by 30% [16, 17]. These data imply that wound fibroblasts are phenotypically altered during the healing process to synthesize NO, which, in turn, regulates their collagen synthetic and contractile activities. This regulation of matrix synthesis in wound healing is in contradistinction to the modulation of matrix synthesis by NO˙ in articular cartilage where NO˙ decreases collagen and protoglycan synthesis [18–22].

Animal models of fibrosis

Lung

21-Aminosteroids, potent inhibitors of iron-dependent lipid peroxidation protected rats from bleomycin-induced pulmonary fibrosis [23].

Liver

In a rat model for secondary biliary fibrosis the main pathway for the hepatic oxidation of ethanol to acetaldehyde has been shown to be associated with the reduction of NAD to NADH. NADH inhibited xanthine dehydrogenase activity, resulting in a shift of purine oxidation to xanthine oxidase, thereby promoting the generation of oxygen-free radical species. In addition, induction of the microsomal system resulted in enhanced acetaldehyde production, which in turn impaired defense systems against oxidative stress (for a review see [24]). Restoration or supplementation of oxidative defense systems has been achieved by the administration of a mixture of polyunsaturated phospholipids (polyenylphosphatidylcholine). This approach provided total protection against alcohol-induced septal fibrosis and cirrhosis in the baboon and it abolished an associated twofold rise in hepatic F2-isoprostanes, a product of lipid peroxidation. A similar effect was observed in rats given CCl_4.

Human model of fibrosis

There is little information regarding the potential role of nitric oxide in fibrosis in human models of fibrosis. There is however, good circumstantial evidence regarding the roles of oxygen free radicals in several forms of fibrosis in humans.

Thyroid

Free radical damage and fibrosis caused by selenium deficiency are thought to be involved in the pathogenesis of myxoedematous cretinism. Work by Contempre et al. [25] indicates that in selenium deficiency, an active fibrotic process occurs in the thyroid, in which the inflammatory reaction and an excess of TGFβ play a key role.

Lung

In idiopathic pulmonary fibrosis Jack et al. [26] have found evidence of increased lipid peroxidation in the serum and that these levels correlated with disease activity. Saleh et al. [27] have also shown strong expression of nitrotyrosine (a byproduct of protein nitration by peroxynitrite) and nitric oxide synthase in macrophages, neutrophils and alveoli epithelium in patients with early to intermediate idiopathic pulmonary fibrosis.

Patients with cystic fibrosis are thought to be more susceptible to oxidative cell injury than normal healthy children due to both the impaired absorption of antioxidant nutrients and the increased oxidative stress caused by chronic pulmonary infections [28] due to the lack of surfactant. As a consequence, free radical attack on unsaturated fatty acids of lipid structures leading to lipid peroxidation and damaging effects on proteins may occur. Furthermore, in the lung there is evidence that antiproteases are inactivated by oxygen free radicals released from inflammatory cells [29]. Supplementation with beta-carotene has corrected the increased lipid peroxidation in children with cystic fibrosis [30].

Hand

Dupuytren's contracture is a fibrotic condition of the palmar fascia of the hand associated with microvascular ischaemia [31, 32]. The condition occurs more frequently in elderly, white males and has associations with diabetes, cigarette smoking and AIDS. We explored a potential role for free radicals in this condition and found a six-fold increase in the substrates for xanthine oxidase in the fascia of Dupuytren's contracture compared with control fascia [33]. Allopurinol, an inhibitor of xanthene oxidase reversed the contracture in a series of patients with this condition [34]. We hypothesized that age, genetic and environmental factors may contribute to microvessel narrowing with consequent localized ischaemia and free radical generation. Endothelial xanthine oxidase-derived free radicals may both damage the surrounding stroma and stimulate fibroblasts to proliferate. Proliferating fibroblasts lay down and contract collagen (with their myofibrillar bundles) in lines of stress. Progressive pericyte damage, fibroblast proliferation and deposition of collagen is likely to encourage further microvessel ischaemia, narrowing and basal lamina laminating with a positive feedback effect consistent with the progressive nature of the condition (Fig. 2) [32, 35, 36].

Liver

Liver cirrhosis following persistent ethanol consumption is associated with nutritional deficiencies and direct toxic effects of the metabolism of ethanol [37]. As in animal models, in humans the main pathway of ethanol metabolism involves liver alcohol dehydrogenase which catalyzes the oxidation of ethanol to acetaldehyde, with a shift to a more reduced state, and results in metabolic disturbances, such as hyperlactacidemia, acidosis, hyperglycemic, hyperuricemia and fatty liver. More toxic manifestations of ethanol metabolism are produced by an accessory pathway, the microsomal ethanol oxidizing system involving an ethanol-inducible cytochrome P450 (2E1). After chronic ethanol consumption a 4- to 10-fold induction of 2E1 has been found associated not only with increased acetaldehyde generation but also with production of oxygen radicals that promote lipid peroxidation [24, 37].

Summary

In summary free radicals are likely to play an important, but by no means an exclusive role in wound healing and fibrosis. Following an initial surgical or traumatic incident including the inhalation or implantation of foreign material there is a "granulomatous" reaction which includes an accumulation of macrophages and phagocytic cells. These cells produce a milieu of cytokines, release oxygen free radicals, induce nitric oxide synthase, nitric oxide, and peroxynitrite. This early inflammatory series of events and the inflammatory cells are replaced over 7–21 days with fibroblasts. The fibroblasts synthesize and are usually replaced by a collagenous matrix. In fibrotic conditions such as Dupuytren's contracture and alcoholic cirrhosis, the initiating – oxygen free radical driven – events for fibroblast proliferation may persist and the "fibrotic" process continues (Fig. 3). The roles of nitric oxide

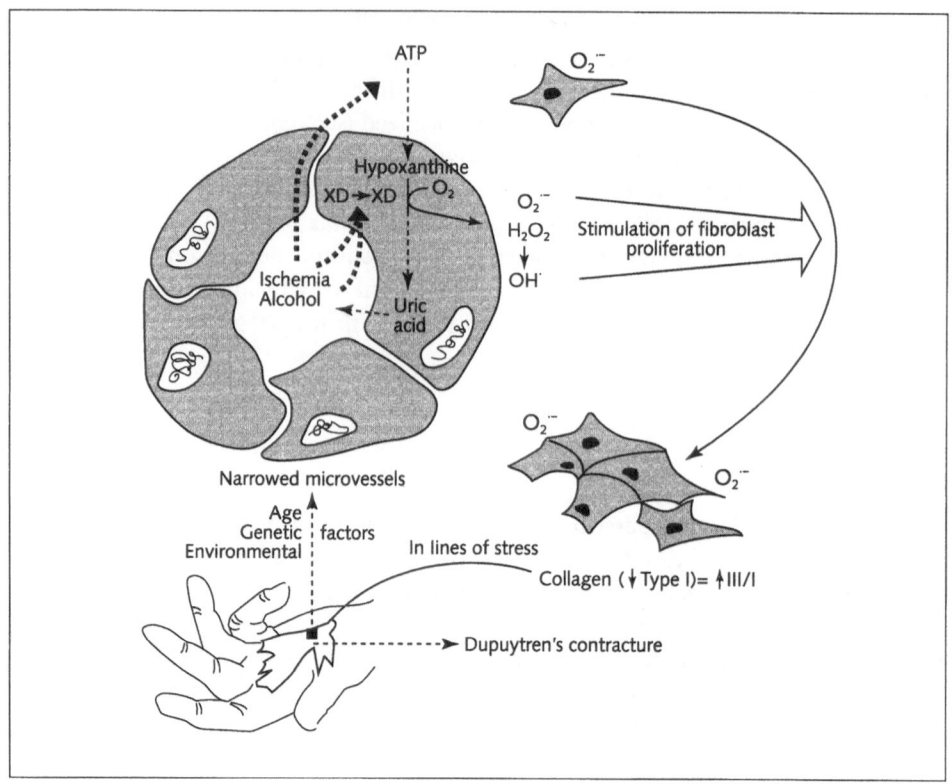

Figure 2

Hypothesis for the pathogenesis of Dupuytren's contracture.

A number of factors (genetic, age, sex, race) may lead to the characteristic thickening of endothelial cells, basal lamina lamination and narrowing of the lumen of microvessels in the palmar fascia. Localized ischemia and alcohol cause adenosine triphosphate (ATP) break-down to the purine bases, hypoxanthine and xanthine, and the conversion of xanthine dehy-drogenase (XD) to xanthine oxidase (XO) with resultant oxygen free radical (O_2^{-}, $OH^{\cdot}$) and H_2O_2 release. HIV infection and cigarette smoking are also associated with increased free radical generation. Oxygen free radicals may damage pericytes and lead to pericyte regen-eration with consequent further layering of basal laminae, and fibroblast proliferation. Oxy-gen free radicals released by the fibroblasts themselves may also further stimulate fibroblast proliferation. The collagen produced by fibroblasts in areas of high cell density (nodules) is initially highly disorganized and relatively depleted of type I collagen, but gradually becomes aligned in lines of stress resulting in the characteristic fibrous "cords" that are pal-pated beneath palmar skin and extend into the fingers of patients with Dupuytren's con-tracture. Progressive fibroblast proliferation and collagen deposition may further compro-mise microvessels with a positive feedback effect consistent with the progressive nature of the condition. Adapted from [32] with permission.

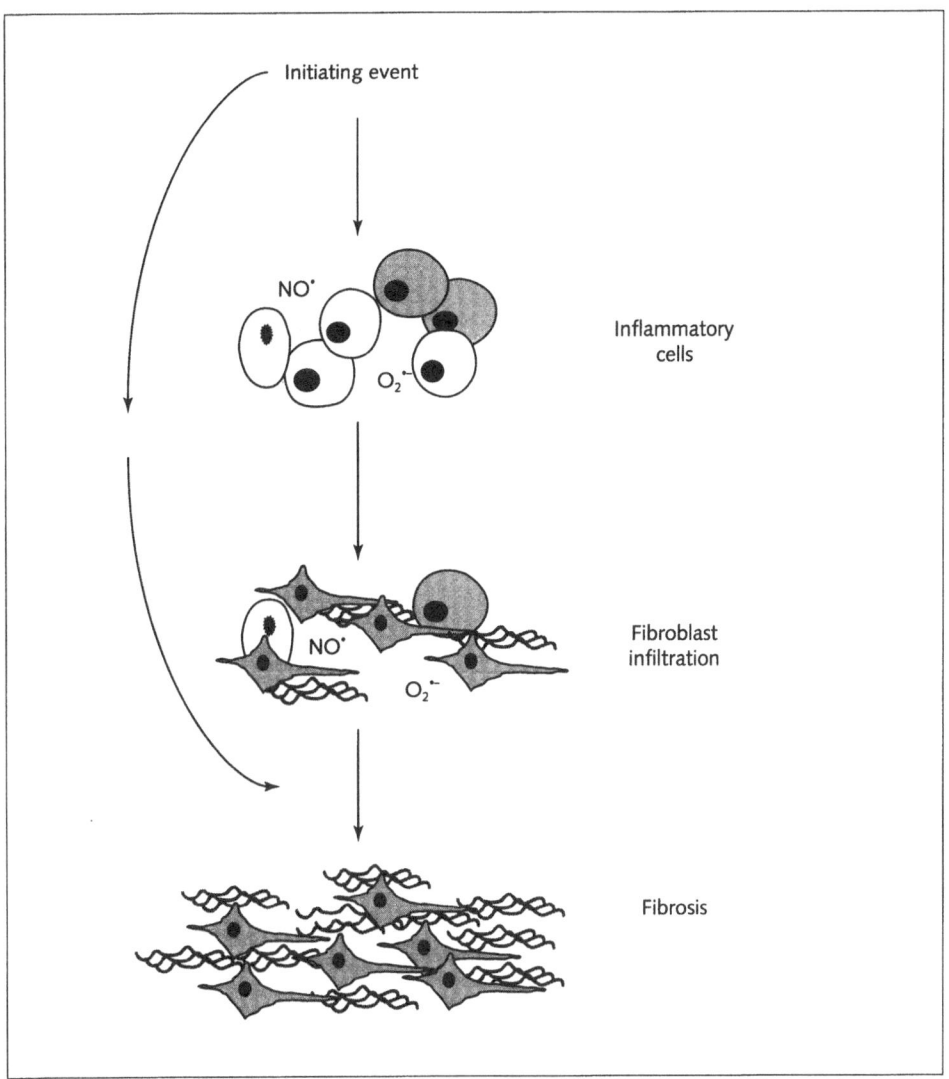

Figure 3
Schematic illustration of granuloma formation and fibrosis.
Inflammatory cells are recruited following an initiating event (e.g. trauma, foreign body). These cells release a milieau of cytokines, free radicals and nitric oxide. These cytokines and radicals attract and recruit fibroblasts. Fibroblasts proliferate and lay down a collagenous matrix. In the event that the initiating event persists and/or the inflammatory cells persist with releasing NO˙ and $O_2^{˙-}$, fibroblast proliferation, matrix synthesis and hence fibrosis persist. Agents which inhibit nitric oxide synthesis and/or oxygen free radical production have the potential therapeutic application as an "anti-fibrotic agent".

and oxygen free radicals in this process appear to be of enough significance that pharmacological manipulation of their production and promulgation may prove to be a fruitful clinical strategy for limiting granuloma formation and fibrosis.

References

1   Murrell GAC, Francis MJO, Bromley L (1990) Modulation of fibroblast proliferation by oxygen free radicals. *Biochem J* 265: 659–665
2   Murrell GAC, Francis MJO, Bromley L (1989) Fibroblasts release superoxide free radicals. *Biochem Soc Trans* 17: 483–484
3   Meier B, Cross AR, Hancock JT, Kaup FJ, Jones TG (1991) Identification of a super-oxide-generating NADPH oxidase system in human fibroblasts. *Biochem J* 275: 241–245
4   Meier B, Jesaitis AJ, Emmendörffer A, Roesler J, Quinn MT (1993) The cytochrome b-5558 molecules involved in the fibroblast and polymorphonuclear leucocyte superoxide-generating NADPH oxidase systems are structurally and genetically distinct. *Biochem J* 289: 481–486
5   Murrell GAC, Francis MJO, Bromley L (1989) Oxygen free radicals stimulate fibroblast proliferation. *Biochem Soc Trans* 17: 484
6   Luckey TD (1991) *Radiation hormesis.* CRC Press, Boca Raton
7   Wang R, Ghahary A, Shen YJ, Scott PG, Tredget EE (1996) Human dermal fibroblasts produce nitric oxide and express both constitutive and inducible nitric oxide synthase isoforms. *J Invest Dermatol* 106: 419–427
8   Arany I, Brysk MM, Brysk H, Tyring SK (1996) Regulation of inducible nitric oxide synthase mRNA levels by differentiation and cytokines in human keratinocytes. *Biochem Biophys Res Comm* 220: 618–622
9   Gossart S, Cambon C, Orfila C, Seguelas MH, Lepert JC, Rami J, Carre P, Pipy B (1996) Reactive oxygen intermediates as regulators of TNF-alpha production in rat lung inflammation induced by silica. *J Immunol* 156: 1540–1548
10 Setoguchi K, Takeya M, Akaike T, Suga M, Hattori R, Maeda H, Ando M, Takahashi K (1996) Expression of inducible nitric oxide synthase and its involvement in pulmonary granulomatous inflammation in rats. *Am J Pathol* 149: 2005–2022
11 Tsuji M, Dimov VB, Yoshida T (1995) *In vivo* expression of monokine and inducible nitric oxide synthase in experimentally induced pulmonary granulomatous inflammation. Evidence for sequential production of interleukin-1, inducible nitric oxide synthase, and tumor necrosis factor. *Am J Pathol* 147: 1001–1015
12 Iuvone T, Carnuccio R, Di Rosa M (1994) Modulation of granuloma formation by endogenous nitric oxide. *Eur J Pharmacol* 265: 89–92
13 Schaffer MR, Efron PA, Thornton FJ, Klingel K, Gross SS, Barbul A (1997) Nitric oxide, an autocrine regulator of wound fibroblast synthetic function. *J Immunol* 158: 2375–2381

14   Schaffer MR, Tantry U, Ahrendt GM, Wasserkrug HL, Barbul A (1997) Acute protein-calorie malnutrition impairs wound healing: a possible role of decreased wound nitric oxide synthesis. *J Am Coll Surg* 184: 37–43

15   Schaffer MR, Tantry U, Efron PA, Ahrendt GM, Thornton FJ, Barbul A (1997) Diabetes-impaired healing and reduced wound nitric oxide synthesis: a possible pathophysiologic correlation. *Surgery* 121: 513–519

16   Murrell GAC, Szabo C, Hannafin JA, Jang D, Dolan MM, Deng X-H, Doty SB, Warren RF (1995) Modulation of tendon healing by nitric oxide. In: *41st Annual Meeting of the Orthopaedic Research Society*. Orlando, Florida, 219

17   Murrell GAC, Szabo C, Hannafin JA, Jang D, Dolan MM, Deng X, Murrell DF, Warren RF (1997) Modulation of tendon healing by nitric oxide. *Inflamm Res* 46: 19–27

18   Taskiran D, Stafanovic-Racic M, Georgescu H, Evans C (1994) Nitric oxide mediates suppression of cartilage proteoglycan synthesis by interleukin-1. *Biochem Biophys Res Comm* 200: 142–8

19   Hauselmann HJ, Oppliger L, Michel BA, Stefanovic-Racic M, Evans CH (1994) Nitric oxide and proteoglycan synthesis by human articular chondrocytes in alginate culture. *FEBS Letts* 352: 361–364

20   Stafonovic-Racic M, Taskiran D, Georgescu HI, Evans CH (1995) Modulation of chondrocyte proteoglycan synthesis by endogenously produced nitric oxide. *Inflamm Res* 44: S217–S227

21   Stefanovic-Racic M, Morales TI, Taskiran D, McIntyre LA, Evans CH (1996) The role of nitric oxide in proteoglycan turnover by bovine articular cartilage organ cultures. *J Immunol* 156: 1213–1220

22   Stefanovic-Racic M, Mollers MO, Miller LA, Evans CH (1997) Nitric oxide and proteoglycan turnover in rabbit articular cartilage. *J Orthop Res* 15: 442–449

23   McLaughlin GE, Frank L (1994) Effects of the 21-aminosteroid, U74389F, on bleomycin-induced pulmonary fibrosis in rats. *Crit Care Med* 22: 313–319

24   Lieber CS (1997) Role of oxidative stress and antioxidant therapy in alcoholic and non-alcoholic liver diseases. *Adv Pharmacol* 38: 601–628

25   Contempre B, Le Moine O, Dumont JE, Denef JF, Many MC (1996) Selenium deficiency and thyroid fibrosis. A key role for macrophages and transforming growth factor beta (TGF-beta). *Mol Cell Endo* 124: 7–15

26   Jack CI, Jackson MJ, Johnston ID, Hind CR (1996) Serum indicators of free radical activity in idiopathic pulmonary fibrosis [see comments]. *Am J Resp Crit Care Med* 153: 1918–1923

27   Saleh D, Barnes PJ, Giaid A (1997) Increased production of the potent oxidant peroxynitrite in the lungs of patients with idiopathic pulmonary fibrosis. *Am J Resp Crit Care Med* 155: 1763–1769

28   Brown RK, Kelly FJ (1994) Evidence for increased oxidative damage in patients with cystic fibrosis. *Ped Res* 36: 487–493

29   Winklhofer-Roob BM (1994) Oxygen free radicals and antioxidants in cystic fibrosis: the concept of an oxidant-antioxidant imbalance. *Acta Paed* (Suppl) 83: 49–57

30 Lepage G, Champagne J, Ronco N, Lamarre A, Osberg I, Sokol RJ, Roy CC (1996) Supplementation with carotenoids corrects increased lipid peroxidation in children with cystic fibrosis [published erratum appears in *Am J Clin Nutr* 1997 Feb; 65(2): 578] [see comments]. *Am J Clin Nutr* 64: 87–93

31 Kischer CW, Speer DP (1984) Microvascular changes in Dupuytren's contracture. *J Hand Surg* 58–62

32 Murrell GAC, Francis MJO, Howlett CR (1989) Dupuytren's contracture: fine structure in relation to aetiology. *J Bone Joint Surg* 71B: 367–373

33 Murrell GAC, Francis MJO, Bromley L (1987) Free radicals and Dupuytren's contracture. *Br Med J* 295: 1373–1375

34 Murrell GAC, Pilowsky E, Murrell TGC (1987) A hypothesis on the resolution of Dupuytren's contracture with allopurinol. *Spec Sci Techn* 10: 107–112

35 Murrell GAC (1988) *Studies on Dupuytren's contracture.* D Phil Thesis, Oxford University

36 Murrell GAC (1991) The role of the fibroblast in Dupuytren's contracture. *Hand Clinics* 7: 1–12

37 Lieber CS (1997) Ethanol metabolism, cirrhosis and alcoholism. *Clin Chim Acta* 257: 59–84

Reactive oxygen species, nitric oxide and apoptosis

Christopher A. Bombeck, Jianrong Li and Timothy R. Billiar

Department of Surgery, University of Pittsburgh, A1010 Presbyterian University Hospital, 200 Lothrop Street, Pittsburgh, PA 15261, USA

The emergence of apoptosis

For multicellular organisms, control of individual cell death is essential to the main-tenance of homeostasis throughout the various conditions that influence life. Devel-opment requires the coordinated growth of cells, as well as the elimination of non-functioning or neoplastic cells [1]. This control was initially observed in the mor-phologic development of insects, where it was termed programmed cell death. However in 1972, Wyllie and Kerr recognized a similar phenomenon with associat-ed nuclear changes in ischemic hepatocytes and called it apoptosis [2]. This is a Greek word, which refers to the life cycle of a tree, whose leaves fall away, eventu-ally allowing the emergence of new leaves to sustain the whole. The morphological characteristics of apoptosis include nuclear fragmentation (which programmed cell death does not), chromatin condensation, plasma membrane blebbing, relative pre-servation of organellar structure, and preservation of plasma membrane continuity [3]. Phosphatidylserine (PS) is rearranged to the outer leaflet of the cellular mem-brane, allowing identification of the apoptotic cell by macrophages which then engulf the cell without the initiation of an inflammatory response, as is the case in necrotic cell death [4]. In this way, apoptosis allows the tidy disposal of cells rather than the littered result of necrosis.

In the late 1980s the investigation into the genetic control of apoptosis was large-ly conducted in the nematode, *Caenorhabditis elegans* [5–7]. This work identified several genes such as *ced-3* and *ced-9* which, when hyperexpressed, would respec-tively induce or inhibit apoptosis. Interest in this field exploded in the early 1990s when a high degree of conservation was demonstrated between the *C. elegans* cell death gene *ced-3*, and the mammalian gene for the interleukin-1β-converting enzyme (ICE, caspase-1) [8–11]. Sequence similarity between the *C. elegans* gene *ced-9* and the mammalian gene *bcl-2* soon followed [12, 13]. This discovery further suggested significance for the apoptotic machinery, which has been conserved across several phyla [14].

Free Radicals and Inflammation, edited by P. G. Winyard, D. R. Blake and C. H. Evans

Table 1 - Reactive oxygen species and reactive nitrogen species

O_2^-	Superoxide anion (radical)
H_2O_2	Hydrogen Peroxide
$^{\cdot}OH$	Hydroxyl (radical)
$^1O_2$	Singlet molecular oxygen
$RO^{\cdot}$	Alkoxyl (radical)
$ROO^{\cdot}$	Peroxyl (radical)
ROOH	Organic hydroperoxide
HOCl	Hypochlorous acid
$Fe^{2+}O$	Ferryl ion
$NO^{\cdot}$	Nitric oxide (radical)
$NO_2^{\cdot}$	Nitrogen dioxide (radical)
$OONO^-$	Peroxynitirite anion

The process of apoptotic cell death can be divided into three distinguishable phases: initiation, effector and degradation [15]. There are many different stimuli that can induce the initiation phase of apoptosis. These include physiologic activators (i.e. TNF, Fas ligand, calcium), damage-related inducers (i.e. heat shock, p53, free radicals, cytolytic T cells), therapy-associated agents (i.e. chemotherapeutic drugs, gamma and UV radiation) and toxins (i.e. ethanol, β-amyloid peptide) [16–18]. It is in the effector phase that common pathways toward cell death can be identified. Since the 1970s it has been known that mitochondrial Ca^{2+} overload leads to a non-specific permeabilization of the inner mitochondrial membrane. While it is controversially discussed in the literature, the events of mitochondrial membrane permeability transition (MMPT, MPT or PT) represent a dedicated step towards apoptosis. Most authors agree that this is the result of the opening of an inner membrane channel or pore, which allows the equilibration of solutes up to 1500 Da in mass, and is inhibited by cyclosporin A [19–23]. PT leads to the disruption of the mitochondrial transmembrane potential ($\Delta\psi$), cytochrome c redistribution into the cytosol, calcium flux and caspase-3 activation [24–28]. These changes induce the characteristics of the degradation phase of apoptosis: (1) changes in the cytoplasmic redox state, including decreased levels of reduced glutathione (GSH) and enhanced generation of free radicals; (2) membrane flipping of phosphatidylserine residues; (3) nuclear fragmentation and chromatin condensation [2, 4, 29, 30]. The large body of data characterizing the *ced-9* homologue, Bcl-2, as an inhibitor of mitochondrial membrane pore formation as well as the development of apoptosis, further emphasizes the importance of PT in controlled cell death [31–35].

While the molecular ordering of the cell death pathway remains to be fully characterized, advances in this field continue to implicate other compounds in the mechanism of apoptosis. This applies to "oxygen free radicals," which is a term loosely used in reference to several reactive biomolecular compounds containing oxygen. Some of the compounds considered to be free radicals lack an unpaired electron, and therefore are not radicalic at all (i.e. H_2O_2). However, as these nonradicalic and radicalic compounds are often regarded together, they are more appropriately termed reactive oxygen species (ROS) (Tab. 1) [36]. They are usually of low-molecular weight, easily diffuse across cellular membranes and considered to be reactive enough to alter essential biological molecules. With respect to apoptosis, ROS can be involved in all three of its phases. They are facultative inducers of the mitochondrial permeability transition as well as byproducts thereof. Conversely, they can also inhibit apoptosis through the modulation of caspases and the induction of other protective factors.

Generation of reactive oxygen species (ROS)

Reactive oxygen species are formed in several different ways: as the byproduct of the catalytic action of oxidases, synthases, irradiation, or as the result of leaked electrons from the respiratory chain. In addition, metals including iron, copper, chromium, and vanadium undergo redox cycling, while cadmium, mercury, nickel and lead, deplete cellular stores of reduced glutathione, resulting in the production of ROS such as superoxide, hydrogen peroxide and the hydroxyl radical [37]. While the reactivity of $O_2^{\cdot-}$ is quite modest, this can be increased by several orders of magnitude through the conversion of $O_2^{\cdot-}$ to the hydroxyl radical ($^{\cdot}OH$), which reacts with organic molecules in a diffusion-limited manner [36]. Both $O_2^{\cdot-}$ and its dismutation product hydrogen peroxide (H_2O_2), can produce the $^{\cdot}OH$ through reactions that are catalyzed by transition metals.

Fenton reaction	$Fe^{2+} + H_2O_2 + H^+ \longrightarrow Fe^{3+} + {}^{\cdot}OH + H_2O$
Haber-Weiss reaction	$O_2^{\cdot-} + H_2O_2 + H^+ \longrightarrow O_2 + {}^{\cdot}OH + H_2O$

The Haber-Weiss reaction can be catalyzed by iron or copper; however these metals must be released from their storage and transport proteins to be catalytically active [37]. It is in this way that some xenobiotics , as well as calcium and aluminum, may indirectly induce ROS-mediated effects by facilitating the release of iron from protein complexes and allowing it to participate in these reactions [38, 39].

The mitochondria are continuously generating ROS as a result of the monoelectronic reduction of oxygen in the electron-transport chain, and as much as 2% of the total mitochondrial oxygen consumption results in the production of superoxide anion ($O_2^{\cdot-}$) [40]. To maintain redox equilibrium, mitochondria possess an efficient antioxidant mechanism in the enzymes: superoxide dismutase (SOD), glutathione peroxidase, glutathione reductase, NAD(P) transhydrogenase as well as in the compounds: glutathione, NADPH, vitamins E and C [30]. Catalase is also an effective antioxidant enzyme. However, it exists mainly in the cytosol and has rarely been identified within the mitochondria. When these checks are overwhelmed, the intracellular stores of GSH and NADPH decrease favoring the accumulation of H_2O_2 and an oxidative stress. *In vitro*, both endogenous and exogenous sources of oxidative stress have been shown to induce PT in the presence of Ca^{2+} [41]. The induction of PT is inhibited when mitochondria are incubated in anaerobic medium or in the presence of o-phenanthroline, an intracellular iron-chelator that inhibits the production of ROS through the Fenton reaction [42]. It has been further demonstrated that the formation of ROS goes on to induce apoptosis in thymocytes and human umbilical vein endothelial cells (HUVECs), and this effect is inhibited by iron-chelation and enzymatic detoxification of ROS [43]. Recent studies suggest that there are at least two distinct sites in the mitochondrial inner membrane, which affect the probability of the mitochondrial transition pore being open or closed, as a function of oxidative state. The first site seems to be in redox equilibrium with the pyridine nucleotide (PN) pool and the second site appears to involve two cysteinyl residues, whose oxidation results in the formation of a disulfide bridge leading to pore formation [28, 41, 44]. Taking these findings together Vercesi et al. [30], present a coherent scheme for the molecular processes involved in ROS-induced PT. Intramitochondrial Ca^{2+} interacts with the inner mitochondrial membrane components (i.e. cardiolipin) thus altering the substructure of this lipid membrane as well as the functionality of the resident enzymes. This alteration may lead to increased mitochondrial production of ROS, which has been seen in the presence of elevated levels of Ca^{2+} [42, 44]. Second, the increased electron-leakage from the electron-transport chain augments matrix levels of $O_2^{\cdot-}$. The Ca^{2+} may also contribute to Fe^{2+} mobilization further increasing the production of H_2O_2 and $^{\cdot}OH$ through the Fenton reaction. These changes induce an oxidative stress in the matrix, which as described above, induces PT and leads to the cytosolic migration of ROS and other mitochondrial components. In the cytosol, cytochrome c, dATP, and the *ced-4* homologue APAF-1, activate caspase-9, which goes on to cleave caspase-3. Once activated, caspase-3 migrates to the nucleus where it cleaves death substrates (i.e. poly ADP-ribose polymerase, caspase-activated deoxyribonuclease) contributing to the degradative changes seen in apoptotic death [27, 45]. These ideas are strengthened by reports that demonstrate the inhibition of apoptosis in settings where the removal of ROS is facilitated. Hockenbery et al. [31] demonstrated that a murine B-cell line was protected from apoptotic death by pretreatment with N-acetylcysteine, an antioxidant that is capable of the direct reduction of ROS, as well as increasing intracellular levels of reduced glutathione. GSH is an effective antioxidant, which is capable of reacting with H_2O_2 to produce water. It also has the ability to scavenge the hydroxyl radical. Hockenbery and coworkers also found protection from apoptosis in a B cell line that was engineered to hyperexpress glutathione peroxidase, an enzyme that inactivates H_2O_2 by facilitating its conversion to water.

Exogenous sources of ROS have been shown to induce apoptosis [30, 31]. While apoptosis induced by neutrophils (PMN) infiltrating the murine liver, has been described [46–48], the role of PMN-produced ROS in this toxicity has not been fully characterized. Monocytes, macrophages and polymorphonuclear cells migrate into inflamed tissues in response to chemotactic factors, where they release ROS generated with NADPH oxidase and myeloperoxidase [49, 50]. These ROS readily diffuse through the membranes of resident cells allowing them to react with the essential cell and tissue molecules therein. One of the best-studied reactions to follow is lipid peroxidation [36], in which polyunsaturated fatty acids are oxidized to produce fatty acid peroxyradicals which may decompose to low molecular weight ketones and aldehydes, thus contributing to membrane destabilization. The products of lipid peroxidation may inactivate membrane transport proteins and enzymes as well (i.e. Ca^{2+}-ATPase) which has been shown to increase intracellular levels of Ca^{2+} [51]. In this way, ROS released by infiltrating inflammatory cells may potentially contribute to resident cell damage and apoptotic destruction.

The role of NO in apoptosis

Nitric oxide (NO), nitrogen dioxide (NO_2) and peroxynitrite ($ONOO^-$) are reactive nitrogen species. They are either the direct products of, or the byproducts of the nitric oxide synthases (NOS). Over the past ten years, NO has been the subject of intense investigation and three distinct isoforms of NOS have been identified: neuronal NOS (nNOS or NOS1), inducible NOS (iNOS or NOS2) and endothelial NOS (eNOS or NOS3) [52–54]. nNOS and eNOS are calcium/calmodulin-dependent enzymes that are constitutively expressed, whereas iNOS is typically expressed in response to specific stimuli, and its activation is independent of elevations in intracellular Ca^{2+} [55–58]. While eNOS constitutively produces NO in picomolar amounts under physiologic conditions, iNOS can be induced to produce nanomolar amounts of NO.

Nitric oxide has been shown to exert both protective and damaging actions in various cell types. Several reports suggest that NO and its metabolites induce tissue injury [59–63], and inhibit enzymes such as aconitase and cytochrome c oxidase [64, 65]. NO has also been shown to directly induce apoptosis in various cell lines, including macrophages, neurons, pancreatic β-cells, and thymocytes [60, 66–68]. The mechanism of the proapoptotic signal of NO is not clear. However the accumulation of the tumor suppressor protein p53 has been linked to apoptosis in some cells exposed to DNA damaging agents, thus suggesting that the accumulation of p53 seen in NO-induced apoptosis is the result of a direct DNA damaging effect of nitric oxide [66]. This is consistent with other reports suggesting the proapoptotic effect of NO is most likely related to deamination of DNA [69, 70]. Still others have suggested that the proapoptotic effect of NO is mediated through the potentiation of the mitochondrial permeability transition. Hortelano et al. [61] cultured murine thymocytes in the presence of the NO donor, GSNO (1 mM). They noted apoptotic changes that were inhibited by cyclosporin A and bongkrekic acid, both known inhibitors of PT. This finding is consistent with previous reports that demonstrate the colloidosmotic swelling of isolated mitochondria in response to various NO donors [41, 71].

However, other studies have shown that there is a protective role for NO as well [72–77]. NO has been characterized as a neurotransmitter [78]. It has been shown to preserve microvascular perfusion through its inhibition of platelet aggregation, erythrocyte agglutination and intravascular thrombosis [79, 80]. NO also limits smooth muscle cell proliferation and thereby inhibits the progression of atherosclerotic lesions [81, 82]. While it is speculative at present, the antiatherosclerotic effect of NO may be potentiated by its antiapoptotic effect on endothelial cells. Increased endothelial cell turnover, as well as an increased number of cells undergoing apoptosis, characterizes regions where atherosclerotic lesions develop [83, 84]. Reduced shear stress and unsteady blood flow are also present, which correlates with decreased concentrations of NO [85]. Indeed, recent investigation suggests that the increased apoptotic turnover of vascular smooth muscle cells involved in coronary atherosclerotic lesions may contribute to plaque rupture and subsequent myocardial infarction [86].

A great deal of the investigation into the toxic potential of NO has been conducted in hepatic models, and many of these studies have yielded conflicting results. Several of these differences may be secondary to experimental design. First, most studies have solely utilized nonselective NOS inhibitors, denigrating the potential differences among the NOS isoforms. Second, all have administered these inhibitors as a bolus, without organ-specific direction. To address these issues, we devised experiments in which various NOS inhibitors were delivered continuously to the portal vein of rats, using Alzet osmotic pumps, thus blocking NOS activity for up to 7 days [87, 88]. Rats received a bolus of LPS during the constant infusion of either saline, selective inhibitors of iNOS or non-selective inhibitors of both eNOS and iNOS. After 24 h of nonselective inhibition with NMA and L-NAME, there was a significant rise in serum transaminases compared to controls, indicative of hepatocellular necrosis. ICAM-1 expression was also increased, and there was a significant increase in the number of infiltrating neutrophils on histologic examination of the liver. NIL and AG, the iNOS selective inhibitors [89, 90], both blocked elevations in serum nitrite and induced the same development of hepatocellular necrosis as the nonselective inhibitors. However with NIL, neutrophil accumulation was not significantly increased from controls, as it was with L-NAME. Even though, the NIL treated animals showed no increase in necrosis, they did manifest evidence of increased apoptotic cell death. All of these effects were attenuated by the simultaneous administration of V-PYRRO/NO, a donor that concentrates release of NO in the liver. These findings suggest that differences exist between selective and nonselective inhibition of the NOS isoforms in the liver, and reveal an important anti-apoptotic function for NO.

We have also investigated the protective effect of NO on cultured hepatocytes when it is added with an exogenous donor [91]. Pre-exposure of hepatocytes to S-nitoso-N-acetyl-penicillamine (SNAP), an NO donor, rendered them resistant to TNF/ActD induced toxicity. Further study showed that this effect was related to the induction of heat shock protein 70 (HSP70) and it was blocked by the addition of a specific anti-sense oligonucleotide to HSP70. However this type of bolus administration of SNAP probably does not mimic the more sustained release of NO that follows from iNOS expression. To test this idea, we used a human liver cell line that has been designed to stably express human iNOS. Sustained production of NO in these cells did not decrease viability and it offered a protective effect against the toxicity of TNF/ActD. Interestingly, HSP70 was not induced in this model, but the cells had to be producing NO to enjoy protection. Genaro et al. [92], found that murine B-cells had a delayed onset of apoptosis when cultured in the presence of NO or cGMP. They also noted that NO induced a sustained expression of the protooncogene bcl-2, at both the protein and mRNA levels. Dimmeler et al. [69], similarly found in human endothelial cells, that the TNFα induced cleavage of Bcl-2 was also inhibited by NO. This sustained expression of Bcl-2, as induced by NO, might further confer a survival advantage to these cells.

More recent studies into the mechanism by which lower concentrations of NO prevent apoptosis have shown multiple sites for its action. One of the first molecular targets for NO to be discovered was the heme protein, guanylate cyclase [93]. NO stimulates elevations in cGMP, which inhibits the activation of caspase-3-like activity in hepatocytes [94]. NO also directly inhibits the activity of activated caspases by s-nitrosylating the sulfhydryl group in the active site of the enzyme [69, 95]. To investigate whether this reaction was specific for caspase-3, our group utilized seven purified human recombinant caspases, and examined the effect of NO on their enzymatic activities. We found that NO reversibly inhibited them all[96]. Dithiothreitol was able to reverse the NO inhibition, indicating the direct S-nitrosylation of the caspase catalytic cysteine residue by NO. Furthermore, NO produced by donors, iNOS induction or iNOS gene transfer, are all effective at blocking hepatocyte death in vitro. To demonstrate the same protection in vivo, we used a liver-specific NO donor, V-PYRRO/NO [97]. When administered continuously following TNF/GalN in rats it inhibited apoptosis and reduced plasma AST/ALT levels by > 90%. In addition, NO treatment prevented the increases in caspase-3-like activity seen in the TNF/GalN controls. Taken together these data support an anti-apoptotic role for NO in hepatocytes. Low rates of production may be adequate to signal via certain pathways such as cGMP, or caspase-3, whereas increasing rates lead to the induction of protective effects of HSP70. At some point, however, threshold for its own toxicity is reached and NO may no longer have cytoprotective effect.

While our understanding of the molecular mechanism of apoptosis is in evolution, it seems clear that reactive oxygen species and reactive nitrogen species are intimately involved therein. Further studies into the roles of nitric oxide and the redox modulation of mitochondrial permeability transition offer great potential for gaining control of apoptotic cell death.

References

1   Sarafian T, Bredesen D (1994) Invited commentary: Is apoptosis mediated by reactive oxygen species? *Free Rad Res* 21: 1–8

2   Kerr JF, Wyllie AH, Currie AR (1972) Apoptosis: a basic biological phenomenon with wide-ranging implications in tissue kinetics. *Br J Cancer* 26: 239–257

3   Wyllie AH, Kerr JF, Currie AR (1980) Cell death: the significance of apoptosis. *Internat Rev Cytology* 68: 251–306

4   Castedo M, Hirsch T, Susin SA et al (1996) Sequential acquisition of mitochondrial and plasma membrane alterations during early lymphocyte apoptosis. *J Immunol* 157: 512–521

5   Ellis HM, Horvitz HR (1986) Genetic control of programmed cell death in the nematode C. elegans. *Cell* 44: 817–829

6   Fixsen W, Sternberg P, Ellis H et al (1985) Genes that affect cell fates during the development of *Caenorhabditis elegans*. *Cold Spring Harb Symp Quant Biol* 50: 99–104

7   Hengartner MO, Ellis RE, Horvitz HR (1992) *Caenorhabditis elegans* gene ced-9 protects cells from programmed cell death. *Nature* 356: 494–499

8   Kumar S, Kinoshita M, Noda M et al (1994) Induction of apoptosis by the mouse Nedd2 gene, which encodes a protein similar to the product of the *Caenorhabditis elegans* cell death gene ced-3 and the mammalian IL-1 beta-converting enzyme. *Genes Dev* 8: 1613– 1626

9   Yuan J, Shaham S, Ledoux S et al (1993) The C. elegans cell death gene ced-3 encodes a protein similar to mammalian interleukin-1 beta-converting enzyme. *Cell* 75: 641–652

10 Miura M, Zhu H, Rotello R et al (1993) Induction of apoptosis in fibroblasts by IL-1 beta-converting enzyme, a mammalian homolog of the C. *elegans* cell death gene ced-3. *Cell* 75: 653–660

11 Vaux DL, Weissman IL, Kim SK (1992) Prevention of programmed cell death in *Caenorhabditis elegans* by human bcl-2. *Science* 258: 1955–1957

12 Fernandes-Alnemri T, Litwack G, Alnemri ES (1994) CPP32, a novel human apoptotic protein with homology to Caenorhabditis elegans cell death protein Ced-3 and mammalian interleukin-1 beta- converting enzyme. *J Biol Chem* 269: 30761–30764

13 Hengartner MO, Horvitz HR (1994) C. elegans cell survival gene ced-9 encodes a functional homolog of the mammalian proto-oncogene bcl-2. *Cell* 76: 665–676

14 Steller H (1995) Mechanisms and genes of cellular suicide. *Science* 267: 1445–1449

15 Kroemer G, Petit P, Zamzami N et al (1995) The biochemistry of programmed cell death. *FASEB J* 9: 1277–1287

16 Thompson C (1995) Apoptosis in the pathogenesis and treatment of disease. *Science* 267: 1456–1462

17 Leist M, Gantner F, Naumann H et al (1997) Tumor necrosis factor-induced apoptosis during the poisoning of mice with hepatotoxins. *Gastroenterology* 112: 923–934

18 Nagata S (1997) Apoptosis by death factor. *Cell* 88: 355–365

19 Hunter DR, Haworth RA (1979) The Ca^{2+}-induced membrane transition in mitochondria. I. The protective mechanisms. *Arch Biochem Biophys* 195: 453–459

20 Hunter DR, Haworth RA (1979) The Ca^{2+}-induced membrane transition in mitochondria. III. Transitional Ca^{2+} release. *Arch Biochem Biophys* 195: 468–477

21 Haworth RA, Hunter DR (1979) The Ca^{2+}-induced membrane transition in mitochondria. II. Nature of the Ca^{2+} trigger site. *Arch Biochem Biophys* 195: 460–467

22 Fournier N, Ducet G, Crevat A (1987) Action of cyclosporine on mitochondrial calcium fluxes. *J Bioenerg Biomembr* 19: 297–303

23 Halestrap AP, Davidson AM (1990) Inhibition of Ca^{2+}-induced large-amplitude swelling of liver and heart mitochondria by cyclosporin is probably caused by the inhibitor binding to mitochondrial-matrix peptidyl-prolyl cis-trans isomerase and preventing it interacting with the adenine nucleotide translocase. *Biochem J* 268: 153–160

24 Zamzami N, Marchetti P, Castedo M et al (1995) Reduction in mitochondrial potential constitutes an early irreversible step of programmed lymphocyte death *in vivo*. *J Exp Med* 181: 1661–1672

25 Vander HM, Chandel NS, Williamson EK et al (1997) Bcl-xL regulates the membrane potential and volume homeostasis of mitochondria. *Cell* 91: 627–637

26 Marchetti P, Castedo M, Susin SA et al (1996) Mitochondrial permeability transition is a central coordinating event of apoptosis. *J Exp Med* 184: 1155–1160

27 Li P, Nijhawan D, Budihardjo I et al (1997) Cytochrome c and dATP-dependent formation of Apaf-1/caspase-9 complex initiates an apoptotic protease cascade. *Cell* 91: 479–489

28 Costantini P, Chernyak BV, Petronilli V et al (1996) Modulation of the mitochondrial permeability transition pore by pyridine nucleotides and dithiol oxidation at two separate sites. *J Biol Chem* 271: 6746–6751

29 Kroemer G, Zamzami N, Susin SA (1997) Mitochondrial control of apoptosis. *Immunol Today* 18: 44–51

30 Vercesi AE, Kowaltowski AJ, Grijalba MT et al (1997) The role of reactive oxygen species in mitochondrial permeability transition. *Biosci Rep* 17: 43–52

31 Hockenbery DM, Oltvai ZN, Yin XM et al (1993) Bcl-2 functions in an antioxidant pathway to prevent apoptosis. *Cell* 75: 241–251

32 Kane DJ, Sarafian TA, Anton R et al (1993) Bcl-2 inhibition of neural death: decreased generation of reactive oxygen species. *Science* 262: 1274–1277

33 Reed J (1997) Double identity for proteins of the bcl2 family. *Nature* 387: 773

34 Susin SA, Zamzami N, Castedo M et al (1996) Bcl-2 inhibits the mitochondrial release of an apoptogenic protease. *J Exp Med* 184: 1331–1341

35 Yang J, Liu X, Bhalla K et al (1997) Prevention of apoptosis by Bcl-2: release of cytochrome c from mitochondria blocked. *Science* 275: 1129–1132

36 de Groot H (1994) Reactive oxygen species in tissue injury. *Hepatogastroenterology* 41: 328–332

37 Stohs SJ, Bagchi D (1995) Oxidative mechanisms in the toxicity of metal ions. *Free Rad Biol Med* 18: 321–336

38 Ryan TP, Aust SD (1992) The role of iron in oxygen-mediated toxicities. *Crit Rev Toxicol* 22: 119–141

39 Merryfield ML, Lardy HA (1982) Ca^{2+}-mediated activation of phosphoenolpyruvate carboxykinase occurs via release of Fe^{2+} from rat liver mitochondria. *J Biol Chem* 257: 3628–3635

40 Cadenas E, Boveris A, Ragan CI et al (1977) Production of superoxide radicals and hydrogen peroxide by NADH-ubiquinone reductase and ubiquinol-cytochrome c reductase from beef-heart mitochondria. *Arch Biochem Biophys* 180: 248–257

41 Zoratti M, Szabo I (1995) The mitochondrial permeability transition. *Biochim Biophys Acta* 1241: 139–176

42 Castilho RF, Kowaltowski AJ, Meinicke AR et al (1995) Permeabilization of the inner mitochondrial membrane by Ca^{2+} ions is stimulated by t-butyl hydroperoxide and mediated by reactive oxygen species generated by mitochondria. *Free Rad Biol Med* 18: 479–486

43 Jacob AK, Hotchkiss RS, DeMeester SL et al (1997) Endothelial cell apoptosis is accelerated by inorganic iron and heat via an oxygen radical dependent mechanism. *Surgery* 122: 243–253

44 Castilho RF, Kowaltowski AJ, Vercesi AE (1996) The irreversibility of inner mitochondrial membrane permeabilization by Ca^{2+} plus prooxidants is determined by the extent of membrane protein thiol cross-linking. *J Bioenerg Biomembr* 28: 523–529

45 Sakahira H, Enari M, Nagata S (1998) Cleavage of CAD inhibitor in CAD activation and DNA degradation during apoptosis. *Nature* 391: 96–99

46 Kondo T, Suda T, Fukuyama H et al (1997) Essential roles of the Fas ligand in the development of hepatitis. *Nature Medicine* 3: 409–413

47 Chisari FV, Ferrari C (1995) Hepatitis B virus immunopathogenesis. *Ann Rev Immunol* 13: 29–60

48 Ando K, Moriyama T, Guidotti LG et al (1993) Mechanisms of class I restricted immunopathology. A transgenic mouse model of fulminant hepatitis. *J Exp Med* 178: 1541–1554

49 Anonymous (1992) *Basic science review for surgeons*. W.B. Saunders, Philadelphia, 45–49

50 Jaeschke H (1995) Mechanisms of oxidant stress-induced acute tissue injury. *Proc Soc Exp Biol Med* 209: 104–111

51 Comporti M (1985) Lipid peroxidation and cellular damage in toxic liver injury. *Lab Invest* 53: 599–623

52 Morris SMJ, Billiar TR (1994) New insights into the regulation of inducible nitric oxide synthesis. *Am J Physiol* 266: E829–E839

53 Nathan C (1992) Nitric oxide as a secretory product of mammalian cells. *FASEB J* 6: 3051–3064

54 Billiar TR (1995) Nitric oxide. Novel biology with clinical relevance. *Annals Surg* 221: 339–349

55 Geller DA, Nussler AK, Di SM et al (1993) Cytokines, endotoxin, and glucocorticoids regulate the expression of inducible nitric oxide synthase in hepatocytes. *Proc Natl Acad Sci USA* 90: 522–526

56 Geller DA, de VM, Russell DA et al (1995) A central role for IL-1 beta in the *in vitro* and *in vivo* regulation of hepatic inducible nitric oxide synthase. IL-1 beta induces hepatic nitric oxide synthesis. *J Immunol* 155: 4890–4898

57 Geller DA, Freeswick PD, Nguyen D et al (1994) Differential induction of nitric oxide synthase in hepatocytes during endotoxemia and the acute-phase response. *Archives Surg* 129: 165–171

58 Geller DA, Di SM, Nussler AK et al (1993) Nitric oxide synthase expression is induced in hepatocytes in vivo during hepatic inflammation. *J Surg Res* 55: 427–432

59 Billiar TR, Curran RD, West MA et al (1989) Kupffer cell cytotoxicity to hepatocytes in coculture requires L-arginine. *Archives Surg* 124: 1416–1420

60 Brune B, Sandau K (1995) The role of NO in cell injury. *Toxicol Lett* 82/83: 233–237

61 Hortelano S, Dallaporta B, Zamzami N et al (1997) Nitric oxide induces apoptosis via triggering mitochondrial permeability transition. *FEBS Lett* 410: 373–377

62 Thomae KR, Joshi PC, Davies P et al (1996) Nitric oxide produced by cytokine-activated pulmonary artery smooth muscle cells is cytotoxic to cocultured endothelium. *Surgery* 119: 61–66

63 Szabo C, Southan GJ, Thiemermann C (1994) Beneficial effects and improved survival in rodent models of septic shock with S-methylisothiourea sulfate, a potent and selective inhibitor of inducible nitric oxide synthase. *Proc Natl Acad Sci USA* 91: 12472–12476

64 Stadler J, Billiar TR, Curran RD et al (1991) Effect of exogenous and endogenous nitric oxide on mitochondrial respiration of rat hepatocytes. *Am J Physiol* 260: C910–C916

65 Cleeter MW, Cooper JM, Darley-Usmar VM et al (1994) Reversible inhibition of cytochrome c oxidase, the terminal enzyme of the mitochondrial respiratory chain, by nitric oxide. Implications for neurodegenerative diseases. *FEBS Lett* 345: 50–54

66 Messmer UK, Ankarcrona M, Nicotera P et al (1994) p53 expression in nitric oxide-induced apoptosis. *FEBS Lett* 355: 23–26

67 Fehsel K, Kroncke KD, Meyer KL et al (1995) Nitric oxide induces apoptosis in mouse thymocytes. *J Immunol* 155: 2858–2865

68 Albina JE, Cui S, Mateo RB et al (1993) Nitric oxide-mediated apoptosis in murine peritoneal macrophages. *J Immunol* 150: 5080–5085

69 Dimmeler S, Zeiher A (1997) Nitric oxide and apoptosis: another paradigm for the double-edged role of nitric oxide. *Nitric Oxide: Biology and Chemistry* 1: 275–281

70 Nguyen T, Brunson D, Crespi CL et al (1992) DNA damage and mutation in human cells exposed to nitric oxide *in vitro*. *Proc Natl Acad Sci USA* 89: 3030–3034

71 Bernardi P (1996) The permeability transition pore. Control points of a cyclosporin A-sensitive mitochondrial channel involved in cell death. *Biochim Biophys Acta* 1275: 5–9

72 Wink DA, Hanbauer I, Krishna MC et al (1993) Nitric oxide protects against cellular damage and cytotoxicity from reactive oxygen species. *Proc Natl Acad Sci USA* 90: 9813–9817

73 Wink DA, Cook JA, Pacelli R et al (1995) Nitric oxide (NO) protects against cellular damage by reactive oxygen species. *Toxicol Lett* 82–83: 221–226

74 Tenneti L, D'Emilia DM, Lipton SA (1997) Suppression of neuronal apoptosis by S-nitrosylation of caspases. *Neurosci Lett* 236: 139–142

75 Nishida J, McCuskey RS, McDonnell D et al (1994) Protective role of NO in hepatic microcirculatory dysfunction during endotoxemia. *Am J Physiol* 267: G1135–G1141

76 Mueller AR, Platz KP, Langrehr JM et al (1994) The effects of administration of nitric oxide inhibitors during small bowel preservation and reperfusion. *Transplantation* 58: 1309–1316

77 Mannick JB, Asano K, Izumi K et al (1994) Nitric oxide produced by human B lymphocytes inhibits apoptosis and Epstein-Barr virus reactivation. *Cell* 79: 1137–1146

78 Anonymous (1995) Behavioral abnormalities in male mice lacking neuronal nitric oxide synthase. *Nature* 378: 383–386

79 Harbrecht BG, Billiar TR, Stadler J et al (1992) Inhibition of nitric oxide synthesis during endotoxemia promotes intrahepatic thrombosis and an oxygen radical-mediated hepatic injury. *J Leukocyte Biol* 52: 390–394

80 Harbrecht BG, Billiar TR, Stadler J et al (1992) Nitric oxide synthesis serves to reduce hepatic damage during acute murine endotoxemia. *Crit Care Med* 20: 1568–1574

81 Cooke JP, Dzau VJ (1997) Nitric oxide synthase: role in the genesis of vascular disease. *Annu Rev Med* 48: 489–509: 489–509

82 Yu S, Hung L, Lin C (1997) cGMP-elevating agents suppress proliferation of vascular smooth muscle cells by inhibiting the activation of epidermal growth factor singaling pathway. *Circulation* 95: 1269–1277

83 Caplan B, Schwartz C (1973) Increased endothelial cell turnover in areas of *in vivo* Evans Blue uptake in the pig aorta. *Atherosclerosis* 17: 401–417

84 Isner J, Kearney M, Bortman S et al (1995) Apoptosis in human atherosclerosis and restenosis. *Circulation* 91: 2703–2711

85 Morigi N, Donadelli R, Aiello S et al (1995) Nitric oxide synthesis by cultured endothelial cells is modulated by flow conditions. *Circ Res* 76: 536–543

86 Bennett M, Littlewood T, Schwartz S et al (1997) Increased sensitivity of human vascular smooth muscle cells from atherosclerotic plaques to p53-mediated apoptosis. *Circ Res* 81: 591–599

87 Luss H, DiSilvio M, Litton AL et al (1994) Inhibition of nitric oxide synthesis enhances

the expression of inducible nitric oxide synthase mRNA and protein in a model of chronic liver inflammation. *Biochem Biophys Res Comm* 204: 635–640

88   Ou J, Carlos T, Watkins S et al (1997) Differential effects of nonselective nitric oxide synthase (NOS) and selective inducible NOS inhibition on hepatic necrosis, apoptosis, ICAM-1 expression, and neutrophil accumulation during endotoxemia. *Nitric Oxide: Biology and Chemistry* 1: 404–416

89   Moore WM, Webber RK, Jerome GM et al (1994) L-N6-(1-iminoethyl)lysine: a selective inhibitor of inducible nitric oxide synthase. *J Med Chem* 37: 3886–3888

90   Ruetten H, Thiemermann C (1996) Prevention of the expression of inducible nitric oxide synthase by aminoguanidine or aminoethyl-isothiourea in macrophages and in the rat. *Biochem Biophys Res Comm* 225: 525–530

91   Kim YM, deVera ME, Watkins SC et al (1997) Nitric oxide protects cultured rat hepatocytes from tumor necrosis factor-alpha-induced apoptosis by inducing heat shock protein 70 expression. *J Biol Chem* 272: 1402–1411

92   Genaro AM, Hortelano S, Alvarez A et al (1995) Splenic B lymphocyte programmed cell death is prevented by nitric oxide release through mechanisms involving sustained Bcl-2 levels. *J Clin Invest* 95: 1884–1890

93   Moncada S, Higgs A (1993) The L-arginine-nitric oxide pathway. *N Engl J Med* 329: 2002–2012

94   Kim YM, Talanian RV, Billiar TR (1997) Nitric oxide inhibits apoptosis by preventing increases in caspase-3-like activity via two distinct mechanisms. *J Biol Chem* 272: 31138–31148

95   Haendeler J, Weiland U, Zeiher A et al (1997) Effects of redox-related congeners of NO on apoptosis and caspase-3 activity. *Nitric Oxide: Biology and Chemistry* 1: 282–293

96   Li J, Billiar TR, Talanian RV et al (1997) Nitric oxide reversibly inhibits seven members of the caspase family via S-nitrosylation. *Biochem Biophys Res Commun* 240: 419–424

97   Saavedra JE, Billiar TR, Williams DL et al (1997) Targeting nitric oxide (NO) delivery *in vivo*. Design of a liver-selective NO donor prodrug that blocks tumor necrosis factor-alpha-induced apoptosis and toxicity in the liver. *J Med Chem* 40: 1947–1954

Evolving measurements of radical products – how much do they tell us about inflammation?

Harparkash Kaur[1] and Barry Halliwell[2]

[1]Northwick Park Institute of Medical Research, Department of Surgical Research, Watford Road, Harrow, Middlesex HA1 3UJ, UK; [2]Department of Biochemistry, National University of Singapore, 10 Kent Ridge Crescent, Singapore 119260

Introduction

It is now widely accepted that reactive oxygen species (ROS) such as superoxide radical ($O_2^{\cdot-}$), hydrogen peroxide (H_2O_2) and hydroxyl radical ($^{\cdot}OH$) reactive chlorine species (RCS) such as hypochlorous acid (HOCl) and reactive nitrogen species (RNS) such as nitrogen monoxide (nitric oxide, $NO^{\cdot}$) and oxoperoxonitrate (peroxynitrite, $ONOO^-$) contribute to considerable tissue injury during chronic inflammation (reviewed in [1]).

Some of these species may arise as a result of normal metabolism, i.e. $NO^{\cdot}$ is synthesised from the amino acid L-arginine by vascular endothelial cells, phagocytes and many other cell types. It serves many useful functions, such as regulation of blood pressure and platelet function, but it is toxic when produced in excess i.e. in conditions such as chronic inflammation, stroke and septic shock [1–4]. Tissue injury will recruit and activate phagocytes (neutrophils, monocytes, macrophages and eosinophils) which produce $O_2^{\cdot-}$ and H_2O_2 as a defence mechanism [5]. Additionally neutrophils (but not macrophages) produce the enzyme myeloperoxidase which uses H_2O_2 to oxidise chloride ions into HOCl as a killing mechanism against foreign organisms [6]. This essential defence mechanism can go wrong in several diseases such as rheumatoid arthritis (RA) and inflammatory bowel disease (IBD) where excessive phagocytic activation results in tissue damage mediated by ROS, RNS and RCS [1, 3].

The rest of this chapter will outline methodology used to study the role of free radicals with reference to RA where damage to important biomolecules such as lipids [7, 8], proteins [9, 10], DNA [11, 12], uric acid [13], polysaccharides [14] and ascorbic acid [15, 16] has been shown to be increased.

It is however important to point out here that all ROS and RNS are not necessarily free radicals as these are collective terms used to include radical and non-radical agents. A free radical is defined as "any species capable of independent existence

Free Radicals and Inflammation, edited by P. G. Winyard, D. R. Blake and C. H. Evans

that contains one or more unpaired electrons" and a superscript dot is used to denote this species [1, 17]. Species such as H_2O_2, HOCl and $ONOO^-$ are non-radicals. H_2O_2 cannot damage most biological macromolecules directly but exerts most of its deleterious effect by becoming converted into the highly reactive $^\bullet OH$ [1], which reacts at diffusion controlled rates with almost all molecules in living cells. By contrast, HOCl can chlorinate many molecules directly (e.g. lipids [18]). $ONOO^-$ is poorly reactive but products of isomerisation and decomposition of its protonated form ONOOH can oxidise and nitrate many biomolecules [19–21].

Production of hydroxyl radicals

Hydroxyl radical is produced in living organisms by several mechanisms and its properties have been well documented by radiation chemists [22]. It can be produced *in vivo* by the following processes:

(1) We are continuously exposed to low-wavelength electromagnetic radiation which causes homolytic fission of O–H bonds in water to give $H^\bullet$ and $^\bullet OH$

$$H_2O \longrightarrow H^\bullet + {}^\bullet OH$$

(2) The Fenton reaction is the classic reaction between iron (II) salts and H_2O_2 generating $^\bullet OH$

$$H_2O_2 + Fe^{2+} \longrightarrow {}^\bullet OH + OH^- + Fe^{3+}$$

Copper ions also produce $^\bullet OH$ from H_2O_2 and tissue injury releases both Fe^{2+} and Cu^+ from their protein bound state [23–25]. "Catalytic" bleomycin detectable iron is found in some synovial fluids aspirated from inflamed knee joints [26] and the iron within such synovial fluid samples has been demonstrated to be directly capable of stimulating lipid peroxidation [27]. Furthermore, infusion of iron complexes into RA patients was found to exacerbate preexisting synovitis and the effect appeared to be mediated by iron-promoted lipid peroxidation [28]. There is a correlation between iron status and disease pathology for RA patients [29] and a relationship between disordered iron metabolism and chronic inflammation has been established [30]. "Catalytic" phenanthroline detectable copper ions on the other hand have not been detected in synovial fluid from RA patients [31]. H_2O_2 is produced *in vivo* by dismutation of $O_2^{\bullet-}$ and by several oxidase enzymes, including xanthine oxidase (XO) [1, 17]. The latter enzyme is found in the endothelium of the synovium of RA patients [32]. H_2O_2 itself inhibits proteoglycan synthesis in cartilage [33], thus contributing to cartilage destruction in RA by interfering with the repair of proteolytic and oxidative damage.

(3) Oxoperoxonitrite (ONOO⁻) is produced by the rapid reaction of $O_2^{\cdot-}$ with $NO^{\cdot}$ [34] and the synthesis of both $O_2^{\cdot-}$ and $NO^{\cdot}$ appears to be increased in RA [35]. ONOO⁻ can be directly damaging to a few biological molecules, e.g. it can oxidise protein thiol groups and methionine residues [20]. In addition, at physiological pH, ONOO⁻ protonates to peroxynitrous acid (ONOOH) which decays to give a wide range of cytotoxic products whose chemical identity is not well established. Simple homolytic fission of ONOOH would produce nitrogen dioxide radical ($NO_2^{\cdot}$) and $^{\cdot}OH$; but there is considerable debate about the production of "free $^{\cdot}OH$" [36, 37]. Other products include nitrate (NO_3^-) and the nitronium ion (NO_2^+). Some of these species will nitrate aromatic amino acids, hence the formation of nitroaromatics (especially 3-nitrotyrosine) is taken to be a marker of ONOO⁻ generation [19] (discussed later). ONOO⁻ also reacts rapidly with carbon dioxide (CO_2) to form a strongly oxidising intermediate, nitrosoperoxycarbonate, $ONOOC(O)O^-$, which is predicted to consist of an equimolar mixture of $CO_3^{\cdot-}$- and $NO_2^{\cdot}$ free radicals [36]. Indeed, both the toxicity of ONOO⁻ towards bacteria and its ability to nitrate tyrosine were found to increase in the presence of CO_2 [38]. Formation of $ONOOC(O)O^-$ is feasible at sites of inflammation, such as in the inflamed rheumatoid joint which is hypoxic and will have a substantially higher level of CO_2.

(4) In a pathway apparently independent of metal ions HOCl reacts with $O_2^{\cdot-}$ to generate $^{\cdot}OH$ [39].

$$HOCl + O_2^{\cdot-} \longrightarrow O_2 + {}^{\cdot}OH + Cl^-$$

Detection of reactive species

Elucidation of the precise role of ROS/RNS/RCS in inflammation has been hampered because it is difficult to measure them *in vivo* [40]. The only technique that can detect free radicals directly is electron spin resonance (ESR) spectroscopy and the only persistent radicals that can be detected *in vivo* by direct ESR are the ascorbate radical and the ubiquinol radical (reduced coenzyme Q radical – $COQH^{\cdot}$). Most radicals are highly reactive with very short half-lives and two approaches have been adopted to study them. The first is trapping (spin trapping and aromatic hydroxylation) and the second involves the measurement of the end products of free radical attack on the biomolecules (discussed later).

In the trapping methods, the radical reacts with a trap molecule to produce a molecule of greater stability that can then be measured. The Spin trapping method is the most utilised trapping method, in which the radical reacts with a trap molecule (the so called spin trap) to give a more persistent radical which is then detected by ESR.

The spin trap 3,5-dibromo-4-nitrosobenzenesulphonic acid (DBNBS) was tailored for use in aqueous or hydrophilic environments (reviewed in [41]). Blake et al. have used this trap to demonstrate the presence of ROS in synovial tissue samples taken from patients undergoing knee joint replacement [42]. The samples were subjected to hypoxia-reoxygenation cycles *in vitro* and were found to generate ROS measured as the radical cation DBNBS$^{\cdot+}$. The amount of ROS measured correlated with the degree of inflammation i.e. the more inflamed the tissue, the greater the amount of ROS (and the larger the signal due to DBNBS$^{\cdot+}$). Other spin traps such as α-phenyl-*tert*-butyl nitrone and 5,5-dimethylpyrroline-N-oxide have been useful in detecting certain free radicals *in vitro* and in whole animals, but the shortfall of all currently available spin traps is that they have not been successful in detecting $O_2^{\cdot-}$ or $\cdot OH$ *in vivo*. Indeed, it is not clear if they are safe for administration to humans.

Aromatic hydroxylation and nitration

Aromatic hydroxylation is an alternative trapping method which relies on the reaction of $\cdot OH$ under physiological conditions with aromatic compounds at diffusion controlled rates, giving rise to hydroxylated products. The products are then measured using high performance liquid chromatography (HPLC) (reviewed in [43]). Salicylic acid (SA) was the first aromatic compound to be used to trap $\cdot OH$ in whole animals. Attack of $\cdot OH$ upon SA produces two major products of hydroxylation: 2,3-dihydroxybenzoate (2,3-DHB) and 2,5-dihydroxybenzoate (2,5-DHB). 2,5-DHB can also be generated by the action of cytochromes P-450 on salicylate, whereas 2,3-DHB appears to be produced only as a result of $\cdot OH$ participation and thereby serves as an index of $\cdot OH$ production *in vivo* [44]. Fairly high doses of salicylate are sometimes given to RA patients whereby it accumulates in concentration that would be sufficient to trap some $\cdot OH$ *in vivo*. Indeed elevated concentrations of 2,3-DHB have been detected in body fluids of rheumatoid patients taking aspirin, providing evidence consistent with the view that these subjects are generating $\cdot OH$ *in vivo* [45]. Elevated levels of 2,3-DHB have also been found in carefully controlled diabetic patients following the administration of 1 g aspirin [46]. We have developed an HPLC method that measures both the hydroxylated and nitrated products of SA (Fig. 1). The product of nitration, 5-nitrosalicylic acid, is a potential marker of RNS formation [37]. Salicylate does have some disadvantages for its use *in vivo* as it has a high affinity for Fe^{3+}, which might disturb iron-dependent $\cdot OH$ generation. It also suppresses glycosaminoglycan synthesis by cartilage, inhibits cyclooxygenase and causes microbleeding in the stomach.

An alternative detector molecule is the amino acid phenylalanine (Phe) which is about five times slower to react with $\cdot OH$ than SA but it has no known inhibitory affects on biochemical functions and little or no acute toxicity at millimolar con-

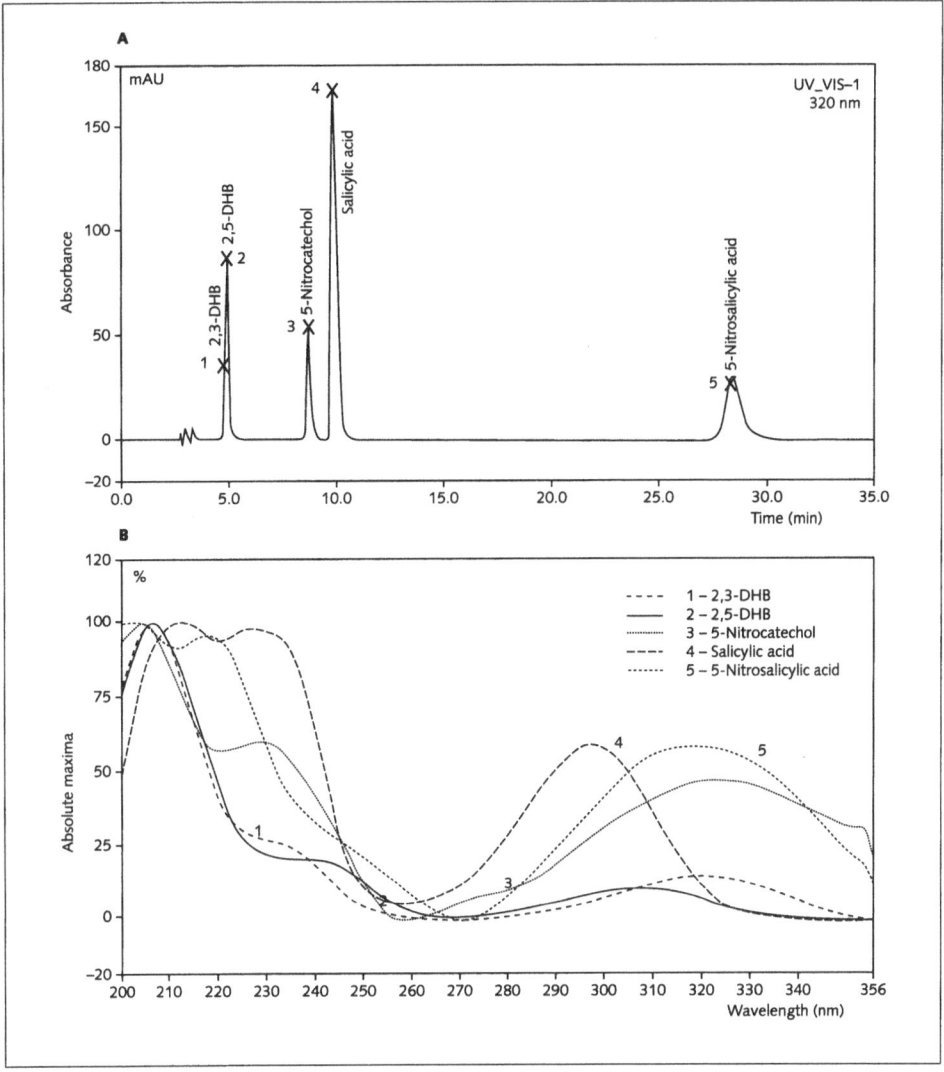

Figure 1

(A) HPLC separation of a standard mixture of salicylate and its hydroxylation and nitration products following our published procedure [37] (2,3-DHB each at 25 μM, 5-nitrocatechol at 25 μM, 5-nitrosalicylic acid at 25 μM and salicylic acid at 1.25 μM). Essentially 100 μl of the standard mixture was injected onto a nucleocil C_{18} column 5 micron (30 × 406 mm) with a Hibar guard column and 500 mM KH_2PO_4-KOH (pH 6.6) plus methanol (80:20, v/v) as the eluent at a flow rate of 1 ml min^{-1}. Detection was on a photo-diode array detector (Gynkotek-UVD 340, Dionex, UK, Ltd) set at 320 nm. Peaks eluting before 4 min are due to the solvent front. (B) UV absorbance spectrum of each peak on the photo-diode array detector.

centrations. Trapping of ˙OH by Phe yields p-, m- and o-tyrosines; only p-tyrosine is produced by the enzyme phenylalanine hydroxylase. We have shown that aspirated synovial fluid and blood from some RA patients collected directly into Phe and SA does give products of hydroxylation (measured on HPLC) suggesting that ˙OH does contribute to injury at sites of chronic inflammation and may also contribute to systemic damage [47].

Attack of various RNS ($ONOO^-$, $NO_2^˙$ etc.) upon tyrosine (both free and protein bound) leads to production of 3-nitrotyrosine (3-NT), which can be measured immunologically or by HPLC or gas chromatography-mass spectroscopy (GC/MS) techniques (reviewed in [48]). In order to improve sensitivity 3-NT can be reduced to aminotyrosine which is easily detected by e.c.d., but the peak appears very close to the injection front, hence it is difficult to determine (personal observation). Production of not only $O_2^{˙-}$ but also NO˙ appears to be increased in RA patients measured in terms of increased nitrite (NO_2^-) levels in serum and synovial fluid from these patients [35]. There is also an increase in the levels of 3-NT, consistent with $ONOO^-$ formation in vivo [49]. Figure 2 shows the separation and absorbance spectra of tyrosines (p-, m-, and o-), Phe, p-nitrophenylalanine and 3-NT using our improved HPLC conditions (use of a photo-diode array detector helps to authenticate the peaks). 3-chlorotyrosine (3-ClT, results not shown) a product from the reaction of HOCl with tyrosine is also separated on the same chromatogram with a retention time greater by 1 min than Phe but well resolved from 3-NT. 3-ClT is another potential bio-marker indicating the presence of reactive chlorine species (RCS), e.g. HOCl and NO_2Cl in inflammatory conditions [50, 51].

Assays for measuring end products of lipid damage

Cellular membranes are composed of a variety of polyunsaturated fatty acid esters (PUFA). Disruption of these membranes results in cellular dysfunction and subsequent death, often involving lipid peroxidation.

Diene conjugation and the TBA test

PUFA have a characteristic methylene interupted double bond arrangement or the "skipped diene" unit ($-CH=CH-CH_2-CH=CH-$). This unit is particularly susceptible to abstraction of hydrogen from the central CH_2 by a reactive free radical, marking the first stage in the peroxidation process. In fact other molecules with this arrangement in their structure (such as vitamin A and carotenoids) also undergo peroxidation. The resultant carbon radical tends to undergo molecular rearrangement and reaction with oxygen that lead to the formation of conjugated dienes which can be detected by their characteristic UV absorbance (230–235 nm) [52].

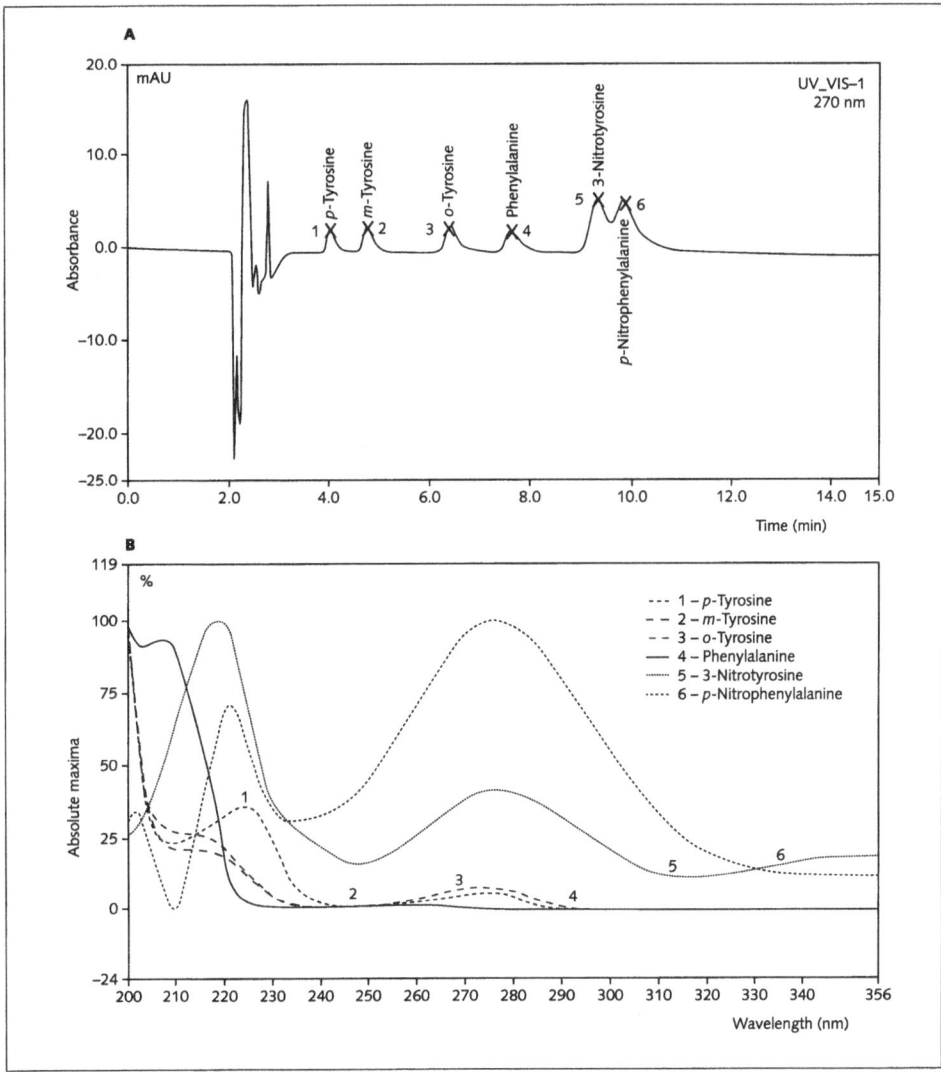

Figure 2

(A) HPLC separation of a standard mixture of phenylalanine and its hydroxylation and nitration products (p-, m-, o-, and 3-nitro-tyrosines, p-nitrophenylalanine, 5 µM each; and phenylalanine, 200 µM following our published procedure [33]). Essentially 100 µl of the standard mixture was injected onto a nucleocil C_{18} column 5 micron (25 × 406 mm) with a Hibar guard column and 500 mM KH_2PO_4-KOH (pH 3.01) plus methanol (90:10, v/v) as the eluent at a flow rate of 1 ml min^{-1}. Detection was on a photo-diode array detector (Gynkotek-UVD340, Dionex, UK, Ltd) set at 270 nm. Peaks eluting before 4 min are due to the solvent front. (B) UV absorbance spectrum of each peak on the photo-diode array detector.

Measuring this UV absorbance should be a useful index of the early stage in lipid damage but application of simple diene conjugate methods to human body fluids has measured products from bacterial fatty acid metabolism and not due to radical mediation as anticipated [53].

The peroxyl radical formed by reaction with oxygen can react with a second molecule containing a skipped diene unit, i.e. an adjacent fatty-acid side chain or with a protein. This is the propagation stage and the repetitive radical chain process is otherwise known as lipid peroxidation. There is no simple method for accessing lipid peroxidation but decomposition or degradation of peroxides results in end products such as the cytotoxic aldehydes-malondialdehyde (MDA) and 4-hydroxy-nonenal (HNE); both cause damage to proteins and to DNA [54, 55]. Detection of these end products of lipid peroxidation continues to be one of the criteria used to implicate free radicals in pathophysiological processes, but they do not give a measure of the degree of inflammation. Increased levels of both free MDA [56] and HNE [57] have been measured in plasma of rheumatoid patients, extending the findings of several earlier researchers who measured lipid peroxidation in serum and synovial fluid of RA patients by the "classical" spectrophotometric thiobarbituric acid (TBA) test which relies on reaction of MDA with TBA to generate a chromogen (TBA-MDA-TBA). The chromogen is measured by absorbance at 532 nm or fluorescence at 553 nm after extraction into an organic solvent (butan-1-ol) [7, 58]. This method measures all TBA reactive material, some of which is not necessarily lipid derived, i.e. material arising from amino acids, carbohydrates and aldehydes other than MDA. An HPLC–based TBA test has been developed which offers greater specificity provided that butylated hydroxytoluene is added with the TBA reagents [53].

Isoprostanes

A more chemically-robust method evolved recently measures a series of prostaglandin (PG) F_2-like compounds, termed F_2-isoprostanes, that are produced *in vivo* by the free radical-catalysed peroxidation of arachidonic acid independent of the cyclooxygenase enzyme [59]. The isoprostanes produced in humans circulate in plasma and are excreted in urine. The majority of plasma isoprostanes are esterified to phospholipids rather than free and sensitive assays to measure them have been described [59, 60]. Plasma levels of 35 ± 6 pg/mL and urinary levels of 1600 ± 600 pg/mg creatinine have been measured in healthy volunteers indicating ongoing lipid peroxidation even in non-disease states [40]. Measurement of F_2-isoprostanes may offer a sensitive, specific, and noninvasive method for measuring oxidative stress in inflammatory conditions. Recent evidence suggests that isoprostanes derived from eicosapentaenoic acid (EPA) and decosahexaenoic acid (DHA) could conceivably be useful biomarkers of peroxidation of these fatty acids *in vivo* [61, 62].

Oxidation products of linoleic acid

Oxidation of linoleic acid leads to pro-inflammatory products that induce the release of interleukin-1β from macrophages. Linoleic acid hydroperoxides are transformed to a very small extent to MDA, thereby escaping determination with the TBA-test. The amounts of 9-hydroxy-10,12-octadecadienoic acid (9-HODE) and 13-hydroxy-9,11-octadecadienoic acid (13-HODE) are increased by a factor of 20–50 in the low density lipoproteins of patients suffering from RA compared to healthy age matched controls [63]. Additionally 9-HODE has been found to stimulate inflammation [64]. Base line levels of these compounds need to be established as they might be directly involved in the pathology and joint destruction in RA.

The hydrocarbon breath test

Ethane and pentane are the hydrocarbons representing the very end of the free-radical-induced PUFA degradation cascade. They are proposed as objective, non-specific and noninvasive markers of lipid peroxidation. The method relies on collecting exhaled air through a mouthpiece into a pentane or ethane impermeable collection bag and analysed against ambient air by GC/MS. Increases in pentane levels have been found in patients suffering acute asthma [65], IBD [66] and in RA [8]. Increased ethane levels have also been reported in IBD [67]. This method does have drawbacks in that the yield of hydrocarbons is very low in comparison to other degradation products. Additionally pentane is not the best marker as it is lipid soluble to a greater extent than ethane and will partition into body fat stores from atmospheric contamination by these gases. Pentane is also metabolised by cytochromes P-450 and is often inseparable (on GC) from isoprene which is also excreted in exhaled air. Therefore, ethane could be a better marker. Application of this technique does require care to be taken to confine subjects to controlled environments breathing air of known hydrocarbon content – a difficult feat but not impossible to accomplish [68]. The validation of hydrocarbons as markers needs to be carried out in conjunction with other markers of lipid peroxidation but such studies are rare. While this test does offer a noninvasive screening procedure, rendering insight into the role of oxidative stress in a given patients disease process and the effects of intervention strategies; it will not provide the clinician with a specific diagnosis.

Protein damage

Oxidative damage to proteins may be particularly informative regarding the role of free radicals *in vivo*. For example, it affects the function of receptors, enzymes, transport proteins and it can contribute towards secondary damage to other biomolecules e.g. inactivation of DNA repair enzymes and loss of fidelity of DNA polymerases in replicating DNA [69].

Evidence to support the view that protein damage occurs in inflammatory synovitis comes from the observation that methionine[358] residues on α_1-antiproteinase (α_1-AP) are oxidised to methionine sulphoxide, rendering the molecule less active [70]. α_1-AP is the main serine proteinase inhibitor in human plasma, and one of its main roles is to protect connective tissue from degradation by elastase. Oxidised α_1-AP is found in synovial fluid aspirated from inflamed rheumatoid joints [71] and from the lung fluid of patients with acute respiratory distress syndrome (ARDS) and emphysema [72]. Experiments carried out *in vitro* indicate that oxidants such as HOCl and ONOO$^-$ are capable of inactivating α_1-AP [73, 74] and it is therefore likely that these species may inactivate α_1-AP *in vivo*. In order to ascertain which species is involved *in vivo*, Western blotting could be used to compare the α_1-AP isolated from the inflamed joint with a commercial sample of α_1-AP cleaved specifically by known oxidants.

Peroxides of proteins are formed from carbon radicals [75] in a similar manner to lipid peroxides and they can generate peroxyl radicals. Protein peroxides may contribute to measurements of peroxide levels in human tissues and body fluids by assay determinations such as the xylenol orange [76] or iodometric methods [77]. This could explain why lipid peroxides measured by these methods tend to be higher (often in the µM range) than those achieved by more-specific techniques for measuring lipid peroxides [53].

Damage to specific amino acid residues in proteins can be accessed using several assays: such as measuring L-DOPA (produced by tyrosine hydroxylation) [78], valine hydroxides (produced from valine hydroperoxide) [79], tryptophan hydroxylation and ring opened products [80], 2-oxohistidine [81], dityrosine [48] and hydroxylated products of phenylalanine; *ortho-* and *meta*-tyrosines [82]. The levels of any one, or preferably more than one, of these products could indicate the amount of protein damage but to date only the hydroxylated products of phenylalanine have been determined in RA fluids (discussed earlier [47]).

The end products of oxidative attack on proteins (particularly histidine, arginine, lysine and proline) leads to the formation of "protein carbonyls" that can be measured after reaction with 2,4-dinitrophenylhydrazine (DNPH) [83]. Increased levels of protein carbonyls have been detected in RA synovial fluid [84]. The assay does not give information regarding the amino acid residue damaged or the protein involved, hence Western-blotting assays based on the use of anti-DNPH antibodies have also been developed [85, 86]. Amounts measured may be higher due to binding of proteins with end products of lipid peroxidation (cytotoxic aldehydes) generating "carbonyls" which need to be distinguished from carbonyls caused by protein oxidation especially as levels of HNE are reported to be elevated in RA [57].

DNA damage

The chemistry of DNA damage by several ROS/RNS/RCS has been well characterised *in vitro* [21, 22, 87–90]. Attack of $^{\cdot}OH$ upon DNA generates a multiplicity of products from all four DNA bases [87] whereas $O_2^{\cdot-}$ and H_2O_2 do not appear to react with DNA bases. The pattern of damage to the purine and pyrimidine bases conveys the fingerprint of $^{\cdot}OH$ attack, suggesting that $^{\cdot}OH$ formation occurs within the nucleus *in vivo* [91, 92]. By contrast, singlet oxygen ($^1O_2$) appears to selectively attack guanine [88].

The most common procedure employed to assay oxidative DNA damage is the measurement of 8-hydroxydeoxyguanosine (8-OHdG) by HPLC with electrochemical detection (HPLC-e.c.d) after enzymic hydrolysis of DNA [93]. Increases in urinary excretion of 8-OHdG in RA patients [11] and significantly higher 8-OHdG than healthy controls have also been reported in lymphocyte DNA from patients with RA, systemic lupus erythematosus, vasculitis and Behcets' disease [12]. HPLC-e.c.d. may not be a quantitative assay of 8-OHdG because of incomplete enzymic hydrolysis (e.g. oxidised bases can interfere with the action of nucleases [94] and possible deglycosylation of 8-OHdG during sample handling (discussed in [91])). An alternative procedure is acidic hydrolysis of DNA, followed by derivatisation of modified bases and analysis by GC-MS with selected ion monitoring (SIM) [94]. This method measures multiple base-damage products and the chemical pattern of base modification can give information about the species causing the damage. However, the derivatisation procedures required for GC/MS can lead to "artefactual" generation of some base damage during the derivatisation if O_2 is not completely excluded [40]. This can be minimised by performing derivatisation at low temperature in the presence of a reducing agent [95]. The levels of 8-hydroxylated guanine (8-OHG) in cell DNA determined by GC/MS are usually higher than those obtained using HPLC-e.c.d, although it is not clear as yet which result is correct (discussed in [91]).

We have developed an HPLC-e.c.d. method (not requiring derivatisation) that allows measurement of 8-OHG, three of the other oxidised bases, and three methylated bases [96]. Ultimately liquid chromatography-mass spectroscopy will be the answer to overcoming problems associated with derivatisation [40] provided sensitivity of a satisfactory level can be achieved.

Polysaccharide damage – Oxidation of hyaluronate

Hyaluronic acid (HA) is a glycosaminoglycan consisting of polymerised units of glucuronic acid and N-acetyl glucosamine. It maintains the high viscosity of synovial fluid. Interest in the role of free radicals in inflammation has its origins in the pioneering work of McCord, who observed a decrease in viscosity of synovial fluid of RA patients which could be reproduced *in vitro* by exposing purified HA to a $O_2^{\cdot-}$-

231

Table 1 - Markers and potential markers of oxidative damage studied in rheumatoid disease.

Biomolecule	Current markers	Comment and potential marker/s
Lipid	(TBA)$_2$-MDA [7, 53] 4-hydroxy-2-nonenal [57] Exalation of pentane [8]	Increase in lipid peroxidation is consistent with decreased α-tocopherol (per unit lipid) in synovial fluid [100] and detection of "Foam cells" containing oxidised low density lipoprotein in rheumatoid synovium [101]. Isoprostanes may offer a highly specific *in vivo* method to ascertain the precise role played by lipid peroxidation in tissue injury [59].
Protein	Fluorescent proteins [80] α_1-Antiproteinase [71] *o*- and *m*-tyrosines [47, 82] 3-Nitrotyrosine [49] Protein carbonyls [83]	Fluorescence maybe due to oxidative damage to proteins. Tyrosines (*o*-, *m*-, NO_2- and Cl-) are specific products but they are metabolised to other products [43] in the body. The protein carbonyl assay measures the end product of oxidative damage to proteins but the identity of the molecular nature of the carbonyls is unknown. 3-Chlorotyrosine is detected by HPLC and GC/MS and is a marker of HOCl mediation [50]. 2-Oxohistidine is a new marker but tedious to synthesise [81]. Dityrosine can be measured by fluorescence [48].
DNA	8-Hydroxydeoxy-guanosine [11, 12]	A spectrum of base damage products can be measured using GC/MS-SIM (see text and [88] provided damage during the extraction procedure can be minimised [40]. 8-Nitroguanine may be useful marker of RNS such as $ONOO^-$ [102] and 5-chlorocytosine a marker of HOCl [90] damage to DNA.
Hyaluronic acid	See text.	
Uric acid	Allantoin [13]	Uric acid is an *in vivo* marker of damage by several ROS (including $^{\cdot}OH$, but not $O_2^{\cdot-}$ or H_2O_2) resulting in allantoin as the major prodct. Concentration of allantoin is higher in serum and synovial fluid of RA patiets compared to controls [13]. Other products formed are oxonic acid, parabanic acid, oxaluric acid and cyanuric acid [103].
Ascorbate	Depletion and oxidation of ascorbic acid in serum and synovial fluid [15, 16]	Ascorbate is depleted during its action as an antioxidant. Activated neutrophils are known to oxidise ascorbate rapidly [104].

generating system, rendering it less viscous [97]. The active species was demonstrated to be the iron dependent formation of $^{\cdot}$OH involving $O_2^{\cdot-}$ and H_2O_2 [98]. Hydroxyl radical causes random fragmentation of hyaluronate, eventually producing oligosaccharides that have been recognised from the chemical pattern of damage recorded in synovial fluid using nuclear magnetic resonance spectroscopy [14]. Other oxidants such as HOCl also react with the glycosaminoglycan chain of hyaluronic acid to cause depolymerisation and recently $ONOO^-$ has been observed to degrade HA [99].

Conclusion

There is ongoing production of ROS/RNS/RCS in the body that is not completely combated by antioxidant defences. Hence there is a level of steady-state damage in humans that rises in most disease states, showing an increase in measured indices of damage to biomolecules (Tab. 1). All markers studied indicate the involvement of reactive species in the inflammatory process, but the measured parameters cannot as yet provide the clinician with a specific diagnosis. The precise role played by oxidants is uncertain because until recently the methodology employed was not as rigorous. There is a rapid development of new and improved assays (i.e. isoprostanes for lipid damage; m-, o-, Cl-, NO_2-tyrosines and 2-oxohistidine for protein damage; plus methodology for measuring oxidised, chlorinated and nitrated DNA bases) applicable to humans that need to be fully evaluated and validated. Application of a number of markers should allow specific evaluation of the role of reactive species in the pathology of a given disease.

Acknowledgement
The authors are very grateful to the Arthritis and Rheumatism Council for research support. Harparkash Kaur dedicates this chapter to the memory of the late Mr. Richard Aldridge.

References

1   Halliwell B, Gutteridge JMC (1999) *Free radicals in biology and medicine*, 3rd ed. Oxford University Press, UK
2   Moncada S, Higgs (1993) The L-arginine-nitric oxide pathway. *N Engl J Med* 329: 2002–2011
3   Grisham MB (1994) Oxidants and free radicals in inflammatory bowl disease. *Lancet* 344: 859–861

4   Anggard E (1994) Nitric oxide: Mediator, murderer and medicine. *Lancet* 343: 1199–1206

5   Babior BM, Woodman RC (1990) Chronic granulomatous disease. *Sem Hematol* 27: 247–259

6   Weiss SJ (1989) Tissue destruction by neutrophils. *N Engl J Med* 320: 365–376

7   Rowley DA, Gutteridge JMC, Blake DR, Farr M, Halliwell B (1984) Lipid peroxidation in rheumatoid arthritis: thiobarbituric-reactive material and catalytic iron salts in synovial fluid from rheumatoid patients. *Clin Sci* 66: 691–695

8   Humad S, Zarling E, Clapper M and Skosey JL (1988) Breath pentane excretion as a marker of disease activity in rheumatoid arthritis. *Free Rad Res Commun* 5: 101–106

9   Lunec J, Blake DR, McCleary SJ, Brailford S, Bacon PA (1985) Self-perpetuating mechanisms of immunoglobulin G aggregation in rheumatoid inflammation. *J Clin Invest* 76: 2084–2090

10   Griffiths HR, Lunec J (1991) Effects of reactive oxygen species on immunoglobulinG function. *Mol Aspects Med* 12: 107–119

11   Lunec J, Herbert K, Blount S, Griffiths HR, Emery P (1994) 8-Hydroxydeoxyguanosine: a marker of DNA damage in systemic lupus erythematosus. *FEBS Lett* 348: 131–138

12   Bashir S, Harris G, Denman MA, Blake DR, Winyard PG (1993) Oxidative damage and cellular sensitivity to oxidative stress in human autoimmune diseases. *Ann Rheum Dis* 52: 659–666

13   Grootveld M, Halliwell B (1987) Measurement of allantoin and uric acid in human body fluids. A potential index of free radical reactions *in vivo*. *Biochem J* 243: 803–808.

14   Grootveld M, Henderson EB, Farrell A, Blake DR, Parkes HG, Haycock P (1991) Oxidative damage to hyaluronate and glucose in synovial fluid during exercise of the inflamed rheumatoid joint. *Biochem J* 273: 459–467

15   Lunec J, Blake DR (1985) The determination of dehydroascorbic acid in the serum and synovial fluid of patients with rheumatoid arthritis. *Free Rad Res Commun* 1: 32–39

16   Situnayake RD, Turnham DI, Kootathep S, Chirico S, Lunec J, Davis M, McConkey B (1991) Chain breaking antioxidant status in rheumatoid arthritis: clinical and laboratory correlates. *Ann Rheum Dis* 50: 81–86

17   Halliwell B, Gutteridge JMC (1989) *Free radicals in biology and medicine*. Clarendon Press, Oxford

18   Carr AC, van den Berg JJ, Winterbourn CC (1996) Chlorination of cholesterol in cell membranes by hypochlorous acid. *Arch Biochem Biophys* 332: 63–69

19   Beckman JS, Chen J, Ischiropoulous H, Crow JP (1994) Oxidative chemistry of peroxynitrite. *Methods Enzymol* 233: 229–240

20   Pryor WA, Squadrito GL (1995) The chemistry of peroxinitrite – a product from the reaction of nitric oxide with superoxide. *Am J Phys* 268: L699–L722

21   Spencer JPE, Wong J, Jenner A, Aruoma OI, Cross CE, Halliwell B (1996) Base modification and strand breakage in isolated calf thymus DNA and in DNA from human skin epidermal keratinocytes exposed to peroxynitrite or 3-morpholinosydnonimine. *Chem Res Toxicol* 9: 1152–1158

22 Sonntag von C (1987) *The chemical basis of radiation biology*. Taylor and Francis, London

23 Biemond P, Swaak AJG, Van Eijk HG, Koster JF (1986) Intraarticular ferritin-bound iron in rheumatoid arthritis. *Arthritis Rheum* 29: 1187–1193

24 Halliwell B, Aruoma OI, Mufti G, Bomford A (1988) Bleomycin detectable iron in serum from leukaemic patients before and after chemotherapy. *FEBS Lett* 241: 202–204

25 Puppo A, Halliwell B (1988) Formation of hydroxyl radicals from hydrogen peroxide in the presence of iron. Is haemoglobin a biological Fenton catalyst? *Biochem J* 249: 185–190

26 Gutteridge JMC (1987) Bleomycin-detectable iron in knee-joint synovial fluid from arthritic patients and relationships to the extracellular antioxidant activities of caeroplasmin, transferrin and lactoferrin. *Biochem J* 245: 415–421

27 Gutteridge JMC, Rowley DA, Halliwell B (1982) Superoxide-dependent formation of hydroxyl radicals and lipid peroxidation in the presence of iron salts. Detection of catalytic iron and anti-oxidant activity in extracellular fluids. *Biochem J* 206: 605–609

28 Winyard PG, Blake DR, Chirico S, Gutteridge JMC, Lunec J (1987) Mechanism of exacerbation of rheumatoid synovitis by total-dose iron-dextran infusion: *in vivo* demonstration of iron-promoted oxidative stress. *Lancet* I: 69–72

29 Halliwell B, Hoult JRS, Blake DR (1988) Oxidants, inflammation, and anti-inflammatory drugs. *FASEB J* 2: 2867–2873

30 Means JT, Krantz SB (1992) Progress in understanding the pathogenesis of the anemia of chronic disease. *Blood* 80: 1639–1647

31 Winyard PG, Pall H, Lunec J, Blake DR (1987) Non-caeruloplasmin copper (Phenanthroline-copper) is not present in fresh serum or synovial fluid from patients with rheumatoid arthritis. *Biochem J* 247: 245–247

32 Stevens CR, Benboubetra M, Harrison R, Sahinoglu T, Smith EC, Blake DR (1991) Location of xanthine oxidase to synovial endothelium. *Ann Rheum Dis* 50: 760–762

33 Schalkwijk J, van den Berg WB, Van de putte LBA, Joosten LAB (1986) An experimental model for hydrogen peroxide-induced tissue damage. Effect of a single inflammatory mediator on (peri) articular tissues. *Arthritis Rheum* 29: 532–538

34 Huie RE, Padmaja S (1993) The reaction of NO with superoxide. *Free Rad Res Commun* 18: 195–199

35 Farrell AJ, Blake DR, Palmer RMJ, Moncada S (1992) Increased concentrations of nitrite in synovial fluid and serum samples suggest increased nitric oxide synthesis in rheumatic diseases. *Ann Rheum Dis* 51: 1219–1222

36 Merenyi G, Lind J (1997) Thermodynamics of peroxynitrite and its CO_2 adduct. *Chem Res Toxicol* 10: 1216–1220

37 Kaur H, Whiteman M, Halliwell B (1997) Peroxynitrite-dependent aromatic hydroxylation and nitration of salicylate and phenylalanine. Is hydroxyl radical involved? *Free Rad Res* 26: 71–82

38 Lymar SV, Jiang Q, Hurst JK (1996) Mechanism of carbon dioxide-catalysed oxidation of tyrosine by peroxynitrite. *Biochemistry* 35: 7855–7861

39 Candeias LP, Patel KB, Stratford MRL, Wardman P (1993) Free hydroxyl radicals are formed on reaction between the neutrophil derived species superoxide anion and hypochlorous acid. *FEBS Lett* 333: 151–153

40 Halliwell B (1996) Oxidative stress, nutrition and health. Experimental strategies for optimisation of nutritional antioxidants intake in humans. *Free Rad Res* 25: 57–74

41 Kaur H (1996) A water soluble C-nitroso-aromatic spin-trap-3,5-dibromo-4-nitroso-benzenesulphonic acid. "The Perkins spin-trap". *Free Rad Res* 24: 409–420

42 Singh D, Nazhat NB, Fairburn K, Sahinoglu T, Blake DR, Jones P (1995) Electron spin resonance spectroscopic demonstration of the generation of reactive oxygen species by diseased human synovial tissue following *ex vivo* hypoxia-reoxygenation. *Ann Rheum Dis* 54: 94–99

43 Kaur H, Halliwell B (1994) Detection of hydroxyl radicals by aromatic hydroxylation. *Methods Enzymol* 233: 67–82

44 Ingelman-Sundberg M, Kaur H, Terelius Y, Persson JO, Halliwell B (1991) Hydroxylation of salicylate by microsomal fractions and cytochrome P-450. Lack of production of 2,3-dihydroxybenzoate unless hydroxyl radical formation is permitted. *Biochem J* 276: 757–853

45 Grootveld M, Halliwell B (1986) Aromatic hydroxylation as a potential measure of hydroxyl radical formation *in vivo*. Identification of hydroxylated derivatives of salicylate in human body fluids. Biochem J 237: 499–504Æ

46 Ghiselli A, Laurenti O, Mattia GD, Mariani G, Ferro-Luzzi A (1992) Salicylate hydroxylation as an early marker of *in vivo* oxidative stress in diabetic patients. *Free Rad Biol Med* 13: 621–626

47 Kaur H, Edmonds SE, Blake DR, Halliwell B (1996) Hydroxyl radical generation by rheumatoid blood and knee joint synovial fluid. *Ann Rheum Dis* 55: 1–6

48 Vliet van der A, Eiserich JP, Kaur H, Cross CE, Halliwell B (1996) Nitrotyrosine as biomarker for reactive nitrogen species. *Methods Enzymol* 269: 175–184

49 Kaur H, Halliwell B (1994) Evidence for nitric oxide mediated oxidative damage in chronic inflammation. *FEBS Lett* 350: 9–12

50 Kettle AJ (1996) Neutrophils convert tyrosyl residues in albumin to chlorotyrosine. *FEBS Lett* 379: 103–106

51 Eiserich JP, Cross CE, Jones DA, Halliwell B, van der Vliet A (1996) Formation of nitrating and chlorinating species by reaction of nitrite with hypochlorous acid. *J Biol Chem* 271: 19199–19208

52 Esterbauer H, Gebicki J, Puhl H and Jurgens G (1992) The role of lipid peroxidation and antioxidants in the oxidative modification of LDL. *Free Rad Biol Med* 13: 341–390

53 Halliwell B, Chirico S (1993) Lipid peroxidation: its mechanism, measurement, and significance. *Am J Clin Nutr* 57: 715S–725S

54 Douki T, Ames BN (1994) An HPLC-EC assay for $1,N^2$-propano adducts of 2'-deoxyguanosine with 4-hydroxynonenal and other α,β-unsaturated aldehydes. *Chem Res Toxicol* 7: 511–518

55 Chaudary AK, Nokubo M, Reddy GR, Yeola SN, Morrow JD, Blair IA, Marnett LJ

(1994) Detection of endogenous malondialdehyde-deoxyguanosine adducts in human liver. *Science* 265: 1580–1582

56   Gambhir JK, Lali P, Jain AK (1997) Correlation between blood antioxidant levels and lipid peroxidation in rheumatoid arthritis. *Clin Biochem* 30: 351–355

57   Selley ML, Bourne DJ, Bartlett MR, Tymms KE, Brook AS, Duffield AM, Ardlie NG (1992) Occurrence of (E)-4-hydroxy-2-nonenal in plasma and synovial fluid of patients with rheumatoid arthritis and osteoarthritis. *Ann Rheum Dis* 51: 481–484

58   Merry P, Grootveld M, Lunec J, Blake DR (1991) Oxidative damage to lipids within the inflamed human joint provides evidence of radical-mediated hypoxic-reperfusion injury. *Am J Clin Nutr* 56: 362S–369S

59   Morrow JD, Roberts LJ (1997) The isoprostanes: unique bioactive products of lipid peroxidation. *Prog Lipid Res* 36: 1–21

60   Roberts LJ, Morrow JD (1996) The generation and actions of isoprostanes. *Biochem Pharmacol* 51: 1–9

61   Nourooz-Zadeh J, Halliwell B, Anggard EE (1997) Evidence for the formation of F3-isoprostanes during peroxidation of eicosapentaenoic acid. *Biochem Biophys Res Comm* 236: 467–472

62   Nourooz-Zadeh J, Liu HCE, Anggard EE, Halliwell B (1997) F4-isoprostanes: A novel class of prostenoids formed during peroxidation of decosahexaenoic acid (DHA). *Biochem Biophys Res Comm* 242: 338–344

63   Jira W, Spiteller G, Richter A (1997) Increased levels of lipid oxidation products in low density lipoproteins of patients suffering from rheumatoid arthritis. *Chem Phys Lipids* 87: 81–89

64   Ku G, Thomas CE, Akeson AL, Jackson RL (1992) Induction of interleukin-1β expression from peripheral blood monocyte-derived macrophages by 9-hydroxy-octadeca-dienoic acid. *J Biol Chem* 267: 14183–14188

65   Olopade CO, Zakkar M, Swedler WI, Rubinstein I (1997) Exhaled pentane levels in acute asthma. *Chest* 111: 862–865

66   Kokoszka J, Nelson RL, Swedler WI, Skosey JL, Abcarian H (1993) Determination of inflammatory bowel disease activity by breath pentane analysis. *Dis Colon Rectum* 36: 597–601

67   Sedghi S, Keshavarzian A, Klamut M, Eiznhamer D, Zarling EJ (1994) Elevated breath ethane levels in active ulcerative colitis: Evidence for excessive lipid peroxidation. *Am J Gastroenterol* 89: 2217–2221

68   Kneepkens FCM (1997) Assessment of oxidative stress and antioxidant status in humans: The hydrocarbon breath test. In: Aruoma OI, Cuppett SL (eds): *Antioxidant methodology – in vivo and in vitro concepts*. AOCS Press, Illinois, 23–38

69   Wiseman H, Halliwell B (1996) Damage to DNA by reactive oxygen and nitrogen species: Role in inflammatory disease and progression to cancer. *Biochem J* 313: 17–29

70   Wong PS, Travis J (1980) Isolation and properties of alpha-1-proteinase inhibitor from human rheumatoid synovial fluid. *Biochem Biophys Res Comm* 96: 1449–1454

71   Chidwick K, Winyard PG, Zhang Z, Farrell AJ, Blake DR (1991) Inactivation of the elas-

tase inhibitory activity of α_1-antitrypsin in fresh samples of synovial fluid from patients with rheumatoid arthritis. *Ann Rheum Dis* 50: 915–916

72 Carp H, Miller F, Hoidal JR, Janoff A (1982) Potential mechanism of emphysema: alpha proteinase inhibitor recovered from lungs of cigarette smokers contains oxidised methionine and has decreased elastase inhibitory capacity. *Proc Natl Acad Sci USA* 79: 2041–2045

73 Matheson NR, Wong PS, Travis J (1979) Enzymatic inaction of human alpha-1-proteinase inhibitor by neutrophil myeloperoxidase. *Biochem Biophys Res Comm* 88: 402–409

74 Moreno JJ, Pryor WA (1994) Inactivation of α_1-antiproteinase inhibitor by peroxynitrite. *Chem Res Toxicol* 5: 425–431

75 Fu S, Gebicki S, Jessup W, Gebicki JM, Dean RT (1995) Biological fate of amino acid, peptide and protein hydroperoxides. *Biochem J* 311: 821–827

76 Jiang ZY, Woodland ACS, Wolff SP (1992) Lipid hydroperoxide measurement by oxidation of Fe^{2+} in the presence of xylenol orange: Comparison with the TBA assay and iodometric method. *Lipids* 26: 853–856

77 Thomas SM, Jessup W, Gebicki JM, Dean RT (1989) A continuous-flow automated assay for iodometric estimation of hydroperoxides. *Anal Biochem* 176: 353–359

78 Gieseg SP, Simpson JA, Charlton TS, Duncan MW, Dean RT (1993) Protein bound, 3,4-dihydroxyphenylalanine is a major reductant formed during hydroxyl radical damage to proteins. *Biochem* 32: 4780–4786

79 Maskos Z, Rush JD, Koppenol WH (1992) The hydroxylation of tryptophan. *Arch Biochem Biophys* 296: 514–520

80 Griffiths HR, Lunec J, Blake DR (1992) Oxygen radical induced fluorescence in proteins; identification of the fluorescent tryptophan metabolite, N-formylkynurenine, as a biological index of radical damage. *Amino Acids* 3:183–194

81 Uchida K, Kawakishi S (1994) Identification of oxidised histidine generated at the active site of Cu,Zn-superoxide dismutase exposed to H_2O_2. *J Biol Chem* 269: 2405–2410

82 Kaur H, Halliwell B (1994) Aromatic hydroxylation of phenylalanine as an assay for hydroxyl radicals. Measurement of hydroxyl radical formation from ozone and in blood from premature babies using improved HPLC methodology. *Anal Biochem* 220: 11–15

83 Levine RL, Garland D, Oliver CN, Amici A, Climent I, Lenz AG, Ahn BW, Shaltiel S, Stadman ER (1990) Determination of carbonyl content in oxidatively modified protein. *Methods Enzymol* 186: 464–487

84 Chapman ML, Rubin BR, Gracy RW (1989) Increased carbonyl content of proteins in synovial fluid from patients with rheumatoid arthritis. *J Rheumatol* 16: 15–18

85 Levine RL, Williams JA, Stadman ER, Shacter (1994) Carbonyl assays for determinination of oxidatively modified proteins. *Methods Enzymol* 233: 346–357

86 Keller J, Halmes NC, Hinson JA, Pumford NR (1993) Immuno-chemical detection of oxidised proteins. *Chem Res Toxicol* 6: 430–433

87 Dizdaroglu M (1993) Chemistry of free radical damage to DNA and nucleoproteins.

In: B Halliwell, OI Aruoma (eds): *DNA and free radicals*. Ellis Harwood, Chichester, UK, 19–39

88 Cadet J, Ravant JL, Buchko GW, Yeo HC, Ames BN (1994) Singlet oxygen DNA damage: chromatographic and mass spectrometric analysis of damage products. *Methods Enzymol* 234: 79–88

89 deRojas-Walker T, Tamir S, Ji H, Wishnock JS, Tennenbaum SR (1995) Nitric oxide induces oxidative damage in addition to deamination in macrophage DNA. *Chem Res Toxicol* 8: 473–477

90 Whiteman M, Jenner A, Halliwell B (1997) Hypochlorous acid-induced base modification in isolated calf thymus DNA. *Chem Res Toxicol* 10: 1240–1246

91 Halliwell B, Dizdaroglu M (1992) The measurement of oxidative damage to DNA by HPLC and GC/MS techniques. *Free Rad Res Comm* 16: 75–87

92 Nackerdien Z, Olinski R, Dizdaroglu M (1992) DNA base damage in chromatin of g-irradiated cultured human cells. *Free Rad Res Comm* 16: 259–273

93 Floyd RA, Watson JJ, Wong PK, Altmiller DH, Rickard RC (1986) Hydroxyl-free radical adduct of deoxyguanosine: sensitive detection and mechanism of formation. *Free Rad Res Comm* 1: 163–172

94 Dizdaroglu M (1994) Chemical determination of oxidative DNA damage by gas chromatography-mass spectrometry. *Methods Enzymol* 234: 3–16

95 Jenner A, England TG, Aruoma OI, Halliwell B (1998) Measurement of oxidative DNA damage by gas chromatography/mass spectroscopy. The use of ethanethiol to prevent artefactual generation of oxidised DNA bases. *Biochem J* 331: 365–369

96 Kaur H, Halliwell B (1996) Measurement of oxidised and methylated DNA bases by HPLC with electrochemical detection. *Biochem J* 318: 21–23

97 McCord JM (1997) Free radicals and inflammation. *Science* 185: 529–531

98 Halliwell B (1978) Superoxide-induced generation of hydroxyl radicals in the presence of iron salts. Its role in degradation of hyaluronic acid by a superoxide-generating system. *FEBS Lett* 96: 238–242

99 Li M, Rosenfield L, vilar RE and Cowman MK (1997) Degradation of hyaluronan by peroxynitrite. *Arch Biochem Biophys* 341: 245–250

100 Fairburn K, Grootveld M, Ward RJ, Abiuka C, Kus M, Williams RB, Winyard PG, Blake DR (1992) α-Tocopherol, lipids and lipoproteins in knee-joint synovial fluid and serum from patients with inflammatory joint disease. *Clin Sci* 83: 657–664

101 Winyard PG, Tatzber F, Esterbauer H, Kus ML, Blake DR, Morris CJ (1993) Presence of foam cells containing oxidised low density lipoprotein in the synovial membrane from patients with rheumatoid arthritis. *Ann Rheum Dis* 52: 677–680

102 Yermilov V, Ribio J, Becci M, Friesen MD, Pignatelli B, Oshima H (1995) Formation of 8-nitroguanine by reaction of guanine with peroxynitrite *in vivo*. *Carcinogenesis* 16: 2045–2050

103 Kaur H, Halliwell B (1990) Action of biologically-relevant oxidising species upon uric acid. Identification of uric acid oxidation products. *Chem Biol Interac* 237: 314–321

104 Wasko P, Rotrosen D, Levine M (1989) Ascorbic acid transport and accumulation in human neutrophils. *J Biol Chem* 264: 18996–19002

Do antioxidants have a role in the therapy of human inflammatory diseases?

Sally E. Edmonds

Oxford Regional Rheumatic Diseases Research Centre, Stoke Mandeville Hospital NHS Trust, Mandeville Road, Aylesbury, Bucks HP21 8AL, UK

Introduction

An antioxidant may be defined as "any compound that protects biological systems against the potentially harmful effects of processes or reactions that can cause excessive oxidations" [1]. Therefore, although the term "antioxidant" is often restricted to the chain-breaking antioxidants such as vitamin E, it should embrace a wide variety of substances that protect against oxidation. The relative importance of an individual antioxidant in a biological system such as plasma or low-density lipoprotein (LDL), depends on both the nature of the oxidant stress imposed upon that system and the type of target molecule to be protected from oxidative damage. Antioxidants can act at different levels in the oxidative sequence and may have multiple mechanisms of action. Oxidative reactions may be inhibited by: removing metal catalysts; removing oxygen; inactivating key intermediates; scavenging initiating radicals or breaking the chain reactions of initiated sequences. Antioxidants therefore include enzymes such as superoxide dismutase (SOD), catalase and glutathione peroxidase; metal-binding proteins such as transferrin, caeruloplasmin and albumin; other water-soluble antioxidants such as ascorbate and uric acid, as well as the lipid-soluble antioxidants, the tocopherols, the carotenoids and the quinones.

Oxidative processes undoubtedly occur in inflammatory diseases, although the aetiopathogensis of the latter is almost certainly multi-factorial. Treating these diseases with antioxidants is therefore a rational approach, but might be expected to have only a small effect. However, even a small benefit, without side-effects, would be welcome in diseases where, at best, disease activity can only be suppressed, and where the drugs currently used have potentially toxic and occasionally fatal side-effects. Oxidants also play a role in signal transduction and the use of antioxidants may therefore offer a "two-pronged attack" in the treatment of inflammation. This will be discussed in more detail below. Before discussing the use of antioxidants in inflammatory diseases such as rheumatoid arthritis (RA), we should examine some of the evidence for the occurrence of oxidative reactions and indeed, what relevance these processes have to the pathogenesis of the individual disease.

Free Radicals and Inflammation, edited by P. G. Winyard, D. R. Blake and C. H. Evans
© 2000 Birkhäuser Verlag Basel/Switzerland

The evidence for oxidation in inflammatory diseases

There is both direct and indirect evidence for the occurrence of oxidative processes in inflammatory diseases. The demonstration of damage to biomolecules, including the presence of certain products of oxidation, and the presence of reactive oxygen species (ROS) in inflammatory states, all lend support to the fact that oxidative reactions occur. It is a lot more difficult to demonstrate the significance of these reactions in terms of disease pathogenesis.

The inflammatory joint disease RA lends itself to the investigation of oxidants and oxidative reactions. Inflammatory synovial fluid (SF) is readily aspirated from joints such as the knee, where ROS, and the products of ROS damage may be measured. Recently, the ability of SF and blood from patients with RA to generate the highly toxic hydroxyl radical ($^{\cdot}$OH) has been demonstrated [2]. If oxidising species such as $^{\cdot}$OH are generated at sites of inflammation, then clearly, oxidative damage can occur and may be an important factor in the perpetuation of a particular disease. In RA, free radical-mediated oxidative modification of proteins, including immunoglobulin G (IgG) [3, 4], and α_1-antitrypsin (AAT) [5, 6] has been demonstrated. Lipid peroxidation can also readily occur as an oxygen radical-mediated process. Thiobarbituric acid reactive substances (TBARS) – products of lipid peroxidation – have been measured in synovial fluid (SF) from patients with RA before and after exercise [7]. Levels of TBARS rose significantly following exercise, indicating a rise in lipid peroxidation, probably mediated by reactive oxygen species (ROS), produced during exercise-induced hypoxia-reperfusion cycles. In addition, the cytotoxic propagation product of lipid peroxidation, (E)-4-hydroxy-2-nonenal, is present in elevated concentrations in the plasma of patients with RA [8]. It is probable that the main constituent of synovial fluid (SF), hyaluronic acid (HA), is subject to oxidative fragmentation in RA [9]. Several intermediates and end products of free-radical attack on HA have been characterised *in vitro* and their elevation in the SF and sera of rheumatoid patients over those of normal controls has been demonstrated [10]. Low molecular weight fragments of HA have interesting biological properties that may perpetuate synovitis and the prevention of oxidative damage to HA may therefore be a useful therapeutic manoeuvre.

Perhaps most important, in terms of the pathogenesis of inflammatory synovitis, is the oxidative modification of lipoproteins. A number of researchers have proposed that the microvasculature has a pathogenetic role in RA and that some of the histopathological changes in rheumatoid synovitis are similar to those noted adjacent to atherosclerotic plaques [11]. Oxidised LDL (o-LDL) is recognised and engulfed by the scavenger receptors of macrophages which then become lipid-laden foam cells. The formation of foam cells is an early event in the genesis of atherosclerotic plaques and o-LDL has been shown to be present in these plaques by immunostaining with antibodies raised against o-LDL. It has been shown that such o-LDL is present in rheumatoid synovium [12]. As o-LDL is a specific chemoattractant for circulating human monocytes and oxidation of LDL at or near endothelial cells results in monocyte binding [13], it is reasonable to propose that the oxidative modification of LDL contributes to inflammatory synovitis. In theory, therefore, if the oxidation of LDL could be prevented or reduced with the use of lipid-soluble antioxidants such as vitamin E, it should be possible to influence the inflammatory process.

Free radical-mediated oxidative damage has been implicated in the pathogenesis of a number of other inflammatory diseases, including adult respiratory distress syndrome [14], and periodontitis [15].

There is good evidence that the major chain-breaking, lipid-soluble antioxidant, vitamin E, is beneficial in preventing atherosclerotic disease. As already discussed, although atherosclerosis is not primarily an inflammatory disease, the pathogenesis, in terms of the oxidative modification of LDL, may be something the two conditions have in common. Two large prospective studies have examined the association between the intakes of vitamin E and the risk of coronary heart disease (CHD) in middle-aged Americans. In the first of these [16], 87 000 healthy female nurses were recruited. It was found that women with the highest intakes of vitamin E had a relative risk of CHD of 0.66, compared to those with the lowest intakes. In the second [17], 40 000 male health care professionals were investigated. Men who had consumed vitamin E supplements for at least 2 years had a relative risk of 0.63 of fatal or non-fatal myocardial infarction (MI), or undergoing bypass graft or angioplasty when compared to men who did not take supplements. More recently, a double-blind, placebo-controlled study of 2002 patients with angiographically proven coronary atherosclerosis was undertaken [18]. The treatment group received either 400 or 800 IU of vitamin E daily and all patients were followed up for a mean of 510 days. The primary end-points were a combination of cardiovascular death and non-fatal MI as well as non-fatal MI alone. The authors conclude that in patients with proven atherosclerosis, vitamin E substantially reduces the rate of non-fatal MI, with beneficial effects apparent after 1 year of treatment.

There is therefore substantial evidence to suggest that oxidative processes occur in inflammatory diseases, as exemplified by RA, and that these processes have some importance in terms of disease pathogenesis. There is also evidence that antioxidants, when used prophylactically in diseases where oxidation of lipoproteins occurs, are beneficial. Cells, of course, have their own "inbuilt" antioxidant defence mechanisms and it is a subject of much debate whether it is worth supplementing these with exogenous antioxidants or not. There are conflicting data about antioxidant activity in patients with RA. One group measured antioxidant enzyme activity in RA SF and found no SOD at all, with only low levels of catalase [19]. This was confirmed in part in another study which showed no increase in SOD in RA SF and a slight elevation of glutathione peroxidase, but found catalase to be markedly elevated [20]. Other studies have demonstrated elevated SOD activity in RA [21, 22]. However, intra-articular SOD has been used therapeutically in RA with some benefit [23], suggesting that these patients may be deficient. The total peroxyl radical trapping antioxidant ability (TRAP) has been found to be significantly lower in 20 patients with RA than in 20 healthy controls [24]. This study demonstrated that the concentration of ascorbic acid was lower in RA plasma, and that the major determinant of TRAP *in vitro* was serum uric acid in RA and serum vitamin E in controls. Other workers have also found patients with RA to be vitamin C deficient [25].

Overt deficiency of vitamin E in humans is extremely rare, and supplementing the diet of patients with chronic inflammatory diseases with vitamin E simply because they may be "deficient" does not seem to be a logical rationale. There have been claims however, that people with chronic inflammatory arthritis have lower levels of vitamin E than healthy subjects [26, 27]. It is possible that patients with inflammatory diseases such as RA may be locally vitamin E deficient. There is indirect evidence that patients with RA may be consuming vitamin E at an increased rate in their joints. It has been demonstrated that SF concentrations of α-tocopherol are significantly lower relative to those of paired serum samples [28], although serum levels in these patients did not differ significantly from those of control serum. Even when other variables, such as LDL concentration, are taken into account, there remained a significant depletion of α-tocopherol, consistent with it being consumed within the inflamed joint via its role in terminating the process of lipid peroxidation.

Another study has looked at antioxidant status and the risk of developing RA [29]. These workers studied 1419 Finnish adults. During a median follow up of 20 years, 14 individuals, initially free of arthritis, developed RA. α-tocopherol, β-carotene and selenium were measured in these individuals and in two sex and age-matched controls per incident case, from stored serum samples. Elevated risks of developing RA were observed at low levels of all three antioxidants, but none of the associations were significant. The index combining the serum levels of the three however, gave a relative risk of 8.3 and presented a significant gradient. A further, more recent study, has also suggested that serum concentrations of α-tocopherol, β-carotene and retinol are lower among people who subsequently develop RA than among the general population [30]. The same may also be true of systemic lupus erythematosus, although these results were less convincing [30].

It may be therefore, that an individual's antioxidant status may be one of many factors which influences whether they develop an inflammatory disease such as RA, or not, as appears to be the case with coronary artery disease. This is, of course, quite a different thing to treating established inflammatory diseases with antioxidants. What then is the evidence that antioxidants are beneficial in the treatment of inflammatory diseases?

Very few randomised, placebo-controlled trials of antioxidants in human inflammatory diseases, including arthritis, have been conducted, and almost none are suitably powered. Early pilot studies of vitamin E in a variety of rheumatic diseases led to further investigation of this antioxidant as a possible useful drug in arthritis [31, 32]. It is far from clear what the rationale for conducting these studies was, given that they were looking at inflammatory and non-inflammatory arthritides alike. Another early study compared the efficacy of mefanamic acid, a non-steroidal anti-inflammatory drug (NSAID), with vitamin E used as a "placebo" [33]. This study was inadequately powered, and not surprisingly, the results showed no difference between vitamin E and mefanamic acid. A further single-blind crossover study with 32 patients followed [34]. A "significant improvement" in symptoms was observed in 51.7% of cases and a minor improvement in 24.2%. Although it is not clear, the authors are presumably attributing the success of vitamin E to its antioxidant and assumed anti-inflammatory effects. In 1986, the first placebo-controlled double-blind study on the efficacy of vitamin E in patients suffering from a variety of arthritides, although not including RA, was published [35]. Patients taking placebo were able to reduce their analgesic drugs by 25%, whereas the reduction in analgesic therapy in the vitamin E group was 50% – a statistically significant difference from the placebo group. However, no benefit of vitamin E over diclofenac sodium (another NSAID) was demonstrated in patients with ankylosing spondylitis by another group of workers [36].

Several studies have suggested that dietary supplementation with fish oils, rich in ω-3 polyunsaturated fatty acids (PUFA), may lead to considerable relief of pain in patients who have RA [37–39]. These oils contain α-tocopherol which is added to prevent peroxidation. However, a later study has shown that the beneficial effects of fish oil supplementation cannot be ascribed to the antioxidant properties of α-tocopherol per se [40].

In a further double-blind, controlled study of vitamin E in RA, patients received 400 mg of d-α-tocopherol acetate three times a day, or 50 mg of diclofenac sodium, also three times a day [41]. Laboratory as well as clinical parameters such as early morning stiffness were monitored. Analysis of the clinical parameters resulted in a significant improvement in both groups, with no significant difference between the vitamin E and diclofenac groups. During the 3-week study, the patients were hospitalised. It is quite possible that the improvements seen in the clinical parameters were simply a result of the patients being in hospital, and it is not possible from this non-placebo controlled study to prove any benefit of vitamin E. More recently, we have conducted a double-blind, placebo-controlled trial of vitamin E in patients with RA [42]. The aim of this study was not only to investigate the anti-inflammatory effects of vitamin E, but also, given that previous studies have suggested an independent analgesic effect of vitamin E, to investigate its analgesic effects, using a wide range of clinical and laboratory parameters. Forty-two patients with RA were recruited and given either α-tocopherol, 600 mg twice a day, or placebo. All laboratory measures of inflammatory activity and oxidative modification were unchanged and clinical indices of inflammation were not influenced by the treatment. However, parameters for pain were significantly decreased after vitamin E when compared with placebo, suggesting that vitamin E may have a small but significant analgesic activity independent of any peripheral anti-inflammatory effect. This study needs confirmation, but there is a potential mechanism by which vitamin E may exert its analgesic activity. Nitric oxide (NO) is one of the free radicals that has been implicated in central pain processing [43, 44] and interacts with vitamin E. This mechanism is still being elucidated, but it is known that there is a loss of α-tocopherol in the presence of the syndnonimine SIN-1, a compound that spontaneously decomposes to yield both NO and superoxide. Addition of NO to α-tocopherol results in the loss of vitamin E and quinone formation, indicating that NO (or one of its products) reacts with α-tocopherol [45]. Depletion of vitamin E by this process could contribute to injury in neuronal tissues. Furthermore, vitamin E partially inhibits the activation of the transcription factor NFκB [46], and the latter influences nitric oxide synthase (NOS) gene expression. Vitamin E may be useful therefore, as an adjunct to standard anti-rheumatic treatment even though it may be acting centrally through its interactions with NO and NFκB rather than as a peripheral antioxidant. Indeed, although this study failed to demonstrate any anti-inflammatory effect of vitamin E, it could, in theory, modulate the inflammatory response also via its interaction with NFκB. It is becoming increasingly apparent that in addition to promoting direct toxicity, ROS may also initiate and/or amplify inflammation via the upregulation of several different genes involved in the inflammatory response. This may occur by the activation of certain transcription factors, such as NFκB. Activation of NFκB produces an amplification of the inflammatory response by upregulating the production of various pro-inflammatory cytokines such as IL-2 [47], IL-6 [48] and TNFα [49]. There is also evidence that NFκB is a dominant regulator in the transcription of genes for leukocyte adhesion molecules such as E-selectin, ICAM-1 and VCAM-1 [50]. The inhibition of NFκB activation by a variety of antioxidants, including vitamin E, is a logical rationale for investigating their effect in human inflammatory diseases, but this theory has yet to be translated into practice.

As already indicated, the number of properly controlled trials of antioxidants in inflammatory diseases are few. One such however is a 20-week, double-blind, placebo-controlled crossover trial of a mixture of antioxidants, including vitamin E, selenium, vitamin C, β-carotene and methionine, in acute and chronic pancreatitis [51]. This combination appeared to have a beneficial effect in both acute and chronic pancreatitis, but it is impossible to tell which of the antioxidants or which combination of these was achieving the desired effects.

Perhaps one of the reasons that so few controlled trials of antioxidants have been conducted in inflammatory diseases is that pilot studies have not been encouraging. For example, a study of eight patients with ulcerative colitis (confined to the rectum) failed to show any benefit of vitamin E supplementation, as measured by the mucosal release of prostaglandin E_2 and leukotriene B_4 [52]. This is perhaps not surprising, as the antioxidant status of patients with inflammatory bowel disease (IBD) –

as with other inflammatory diseases – is not clear cut. In one recent study, children with IBD have been shown to have decreased plasma levels of ascorbic acid, whilst at the same time, having increased levels of glutathione peroxidase, glutathione and vitamin E [53]. Another study has demonstrated decreased total peroxyl radical scavenging capacity in IBD, with decreased levels of urate, glutathione and ubiquinol-10, whilst levels of α-tocopherol were unchanged [54]. A further study used amplified chemiluminescence to measure ROS production by colonic biopsy specimens from rats with acetic acid induced colitis [55]. Chemiluminescence was reduced by the antioxidants dimethyl sulphoxide and ascorbate, and the authors suggest that these compounds merit further assessment in the treatment of IBD –these studies are awaited.

Another recent study has shown that enhanced oxidative stress initiates a fibrogenesis cascade in the liver of patients with chronic hepatitis C, and that that cascade can be prevented by the administration of d-α-tocopherol [56]. In addition, vitamin E significantly decreased the carbonyl modifications of plasma proteins – a sensitive index of oxidative stress. However, 8 weeks of vitamin E treatment did not significantly affect serum alanine aminotransferase levels, hepatitis C virus titres or histological degree of hepatocellular inflammation or fibrosis. It seems therefore, that although oxidative processes may play a part in the pathogenesis of this disease, the administration of antioxidants may not have any effect on disease outcome.

Conclusions

Although there is overwhelming evidence that oxidative stress occurs in human inflammatory diseases, the jury is still out as far as the significance of that stress is concerned, and has not yet been supplied with sufficient evidence to decide whether or not antioxidants have a major role to play in the treatment of these diseases. The synergistic relationships between various antioxidants have also to be fully elucidated. The relationship between vitamin E and vitamin C *in vitro* is well documented [57], although how these two vitamins interact *in vivo* is not so clear [58]. Certainly *in vitro*, the absence of agents such as vitamin C may actually lead to tocopherol-mediated oxidation [59], and lipid peroxidation may be accelerated by an increase in the level of vitamin E within LDL. Indeed, the pro-oxidant capabilities of vitamin E are well documented [60], and it is not hard to imagine that other antioxidants may become pro-oxidants given the right (or wrong!) set of conditions.

It is likely however, that no antioxidant works in isolation and until we have a better understanding of the "working relationships" between various antioxidants, it will be difficult to design clinical trials effectively. In addition, there must exist a balance between antioxidant defence and repair systems and pro-oxidant mechanisms of tissue destruction. It may only be possible to influence that balance with the use of antioxidants before an oxidative insult has occurred. The studies of vitamin E in ischaemic heart disease have certainly suggested that this is true, and other successful animal studies have used a pre-treatment approach, beginning days to weeks before injury. One such looked at the effect of giving vitamin E at the onset of a progressive inflammatory injury and found it to be protective [61]. As far as vitamin E is concerned, it may need to be incorporated into biological membranes before any insult occurs – administering it after the insult may simply be too late.

It is often argued that although administering vitamins and other antioxidants may not do any good, "at least they won't do any harm". It is already clear that large (or even small) doses of one antioxidant may upset the delicate balance of others, and under certain circumstances may actually become pro-oxidant. Indeed, a randomised, double-blind, placebo-controlled primary prevention trial of vitamin E and β-carotene, given alone or together to male smokers, showed an increased incidence of lung cancer in the group given β-carotene alone [62]. Some would go as far as to attribute a whole range of side-effects to even quite small doses of vitamin E [63].

In summary, therefore, oxidative stress plays a role in the pathogenesis of human inflammatory diseases. Preliminary evidence suggests that antioxidant therapy may have a small but significant effect, without the same risk of side-effects as "conventional" treatment. Clearly, many more properly controlled and randomised trials need to be conducted before antioxidants can be routinely used in the management of these conditions.

References

1   Krinsky NI (1992) Mechanism and action of biological antioxidants. *Proc Soc Exp Biol Med* 200: 248–254
2   Kaur H, Edmonds SE, Blake DR, Halliwell B (1996) Hydroxyl radical generation by rheumatoid blood and knee joint synovial fluid. *Ann Rheum Dis* 55: 915–920
3   Lunec J, Blake DR, Brailsford S, Bacon PA (1985) Self-perpetuating mechanisms of IgG aggregation in rheumatoid inflammation. *J Clin Invest* 76: 2084–2090
4   Lunec J, Wakefield A, Brailsford S, Blake DR (1986) Free radical altered IgG and its interaction with rheumatoid factor In: Rice-Evans C (ed): *Free radicals, oxidant stress and drug action,* Vol 2. Richelieu Press, London, 151–167
5   Zhang Z, Winyard PG, Chidwick K, Farrell A, Pemberton P, Carrell RW, Blake DR (1990) Increased proteolytic cleavage of α_1-antitrypsin (α_1-proteinase inhibitor) in knee-joint synovial fluid from patients with rheumatoid arthritis. *Biochem Soc Trans* 18: 898–899
6   Zhang Z, Farrell AJ, Blake DR, Chidwick K, Winyard PG (1993) Inactivation of synovial fluid α_1-antitrypsin by exercise of the inflamed rheumatoid joint. *FEBS Lett* 321: 274–278

7   Blake DR, Merry P, Unsworth J, Kidd BL, Outhwaite J, Ballard R, Morris C, Gray L, Lunec J (1989) Hypoxic-reperfusion injury in the inflamed human joint. *Lancet* i: 289–293

8   Selley ML, Bourne DJ, Bartlett MR, Tymms KE, Brook AS, Duffield AM, Ardlie NG (1992) Occurrence of (E)-4-hydroxy-2-nonenal in plasma and synovial fluid of patients with rheumatoid arthritis and osteoarthritis. *Ann Rheum Dis* 51: 481–484

9   Henderson EB, Grootveld M, Farrell A, Smith EC, Thompson PW, Blake DR (1991) A pathological role for damaged hyaluronan in synovitis. *Ann Rheum Dis* 50: 196-200

10   Grootveld MC, Henderson EB, Farrell A, Blake DR, Parkes HG, Haycock P (1991) Oxidative damage to hyaluronate and glucose in synovial fluid during exercise of the inflamed rheumatoid joint Detection of abnormal low-molecular mass metabolites by proton-nmr spectroscopy. *Biochem J* 273: 459–467

11   Rothschild BM and Masi AT (1982) Pathogenesis of rheumatoid arthritis: a vascular hypothesis. *Semin Arthritis Rheum* 12: 11–31

12   Winyard PG, Tatzber F, Esterbauer H, Kus ML, Blake DR, Morris CJ (1993) Presence of foam cells containing oxidised low density lipoprotein in the synovial membrane from patients with rheumatoid synovitis. *Ann Rheum Dis* 52: 677–680

13   Brown MS and Goldstein JL (1983) Lipoprotein metabolism in the macrophage: implications for cholesterol deposition in atherosclerosis. *Ann Rev Biochem* 52: 223–261

14   Tate RM, Repine JE (1983) Neutrophils and the adult respiratory distress syndrome. *Free Rad Biol Med* 6: 53–60

15   Kimura S, Yonemura T, Kaya H (1993) Increased oxidative product formation by peripheral blood polymorphonuclear leukocytes in human periodontal diseases. *J Periodon Res* 28: 197–203

16   Stampfer MJ, Hennekens CH, Manson JE, Colditz GA, Rosner B, Willett WC (1993) Vitamin E consumption and the risk of coronary disease in women. *N Engl J Med* 328: 1444–1449

17   Rimm EB, Stampfer MJ, Ascherio A, Giovannucci E, Colditz GA, Willett WC (1993) Vitamin E consumption and the risk of coronary heart disease in men. *N Engl J Med* 328: 1450–1456

18   Stephens NG, Parsons A, Schofield PM, Kelly F, Cheeseman K, Mitchinson MJ, Brown MJ (1996) Randomised controlled trial of vitamin E inpatients with coronary disease: Cambridge Heart Antioxidant Study (CHAOS). *Lancet* 347: 781–786

19   Blake DR, Hall ND, Terby DA, Haliwell B, Gutteridge JMC (1981) Protection against superoxide and hydrogen peroxide in synovial fluid from rheumatoid patients. *Clin Sci* 61: 483–486

20   Biedmond P, Swaak AJG, Koster JF (1984) Protective factors against free radicals and hydrogen peroxide in rheumatoid arthritis synovial fluid. *Arthritis Rheum* 27:760–765

21   Igari T, Kaneda H, Horiuchi S, Ono S (1982) A remarkable increase of superoxide dismutase activity in synovial fluid of patients with rheumatoid arthritis. *Clin Orthop* 162: 282–287

22   Sato H, Takahashi T, Ide H, Fukushima T, Tabata M, Sekine F, Kobayashi K, Negishi

M, Niwa Y (1988) Antioxidant activity of synovial fluid, hyaluronic acid and two sub-components of hyaluronic acid. *Arthritis Rheum* 31: 63–71

23 Goebel KM, Storck U, Neurath F (1981) Intrasynovial orgotein therapy in rheumatoid arthritis. *Lancet* i: 1015–1017

24 Situnayake RD, Thurnham DI, Kootahep S, Chirico S, Lunec J, Davis M, McConkey B (1991) Chain breaking antioxidant status in rheumatoid arthritis: clinical and laboratory correlates. *Ann Rheum Dis* 50: 81–86

25 Lunec J and Blake DR (1985) The determination of dehydroascorbic acid and ascorbic acid in the serum and synovial fluid of patients with rheumatoid arthritis. *Free Rad Res Comm* 1: 31–39

26 Honkanen V, Konttinen YT, Mussalo-Rauhamaaa H (1989) Vitamins A and E, retinol binding protein and zinc in rheumatoid arthritis. *Clin Exp Rheumatol* 7: 465–469

27 Honkanen V, Pelkonen P, Konttinen YT, Mussalo-Rauhamaa H, Lehto J, Coestermarck T (1990) Serum cholesterol and vitamins A and E in juvenile chronic arthritis. *Clin Exp Rheumatol* 8: 187–191

28 Fairburn K, Grootveld M, Ward RJ, Abiuka C, Kus M, Williams RB, Winyard PG, Blake DR (1992) α-tocopherol, lipids and lipoproteins in knee-joint synovial fluid and serum from patients with inflammatory joint disease. *Clin Sci* 83: 657–664

29 Heliövaara M, Knekt P, Aho K, Aaran R-K, Alfthan G, Aromaa A (1994) Serum antioxidants and risk of rheumatoid arthritis. *Ann Rheum Dis* 53: 51–53

30 Comstock GW, Burke AE, Hoffman SC, Helzlsouer KJ, Bendich A, Masi AT, Norkus EP, Malamet RL, Gershwin ME (1997) Serum concentrations of a tocopherol, β-carotene, and retinol preceding the diagnosis of rheumatoid arthritis and systemic lupus erythematosus. *Ann Rheum Dis* 56: 323–325

31 Jensen HP , Spuler H (1962) Neuralgien und Vitamin E. *Kapsel* 2

32 Fischer J, Seuss J (1985) Antioxidans-therapierheumatische Erkrankungen. *Heilkunst* 3: 145–148

33 Machtey I (1969) Mefanamic acid in osteoarthritis. *Harefuah* 76: 280

34 Machtey I, Quaknine L (1978) Tocopherol in osteoarthritis. *J Am Geriatr Soc* 26: 328–329

35 Blankenhorn G (1986) Klinische Wirksamkeit von Spondyvit (Vitamin E) bei aktivierten Arthrosen. *Z Orthop* 124: 340–343

36 Klein KG, Blankenhorn G (1987) Vergleich der Klinischen Wirksamkeit von Vitamin E und Diclofenac-Natrium bei *Spondylitis ankylosans* (Morbus Bechterew). *Vita Min Spur* 3: 137–142

37 Sperling RI, Weinblatt M, Robin J-L, Ravalese J, Hoover RL, House F, Coblyn JS, Fraser PA, Spur BW, Robinson DR et al (1987) Effects of dietary supplementation with marine fish oils on leukocyte lipid mediator generation and function in rheumatoid arthritis. *Arthritis Rheum* 30: 988–997

38 van der Tempel H, Tulleken JE, Limburg PC, Muskiet FAJ, van Rijswijk MH (1990) Effects of fish oil supplementation in rheumatoid arthritis. *Ann Rheum Dis* 49: 76–80

39 Cleland LG, French JK, Betts WH, Murphy GA, Elliott MJ (1988) Clinical and bio-

chemical effects of dietary fish oil supplement in rheumatoid arthritis. *J Rheumatol* 15: 1471–1475

40 Tulleken JE, Limburg PC, Muskiet FAJ, van Rijswijk MH (1990) Vitamin E status during dietary fish oil supplementation in rheumatoid arthritis. *Arthritis Rheum* 33: 1416–1419

41 Kolarz G, Scherak O, Shohoumi MEL, Blankenhorn G (1990) Hochdosiertes Vitamin E bei Chronischer Polyarthritis. *Akt Rheumatol* 15: 233–237

42 Edmonds SE, Winyard PG, Guo R, Kidd B, Merry P, Langrish-Smith A, Hansen C, Ramm S, Blake DR (1997) Putative analgesic activity of repeated oral doses of vitamin E in the treatment of rheumatoid arthritis Results of a prospective placebo controlled double blind trial. *Ann Rheum Dis* 56: 649–655

43 Coderre TJ, Yashpal K (1994) Intracellular messengers contributing to persistent nociception and hyperalgesia induced by L-glutamate and substance P in the rat formalin pain model. *Eur J Neurosci* 6: 1328–1334

44 Niedbala B, Sanchez A, Feria M (1995) Nitric oxide mediates neuropathic pain behaviour in peripherally denervated rats. *Neurosci Lett* 188: 57–60

45 de Groot H, Hegi U, Sies H (1993) Loss of α-tocopherol upon exposure to nitric oxide or the sydnonimine SIN-1. *FEBS Lett* 315: 139–142

46 Hattori S, Hattori Y, Barba N, Kasai K, Shimoda S (1995) Pentamethyl hydroxychromone, vitamin E derivative, inhibits induction of nitric oxide synthase by bacterial lipopolysaccharide. *Biochem Mol Biol Int* 35: 177–183

47 Hoyos B, Ballard DW, BohnleinE, SiekevityM, GreeneWC (1989) Kappa-B specific DNA binding proteins: Role in the regulation of human interleukin-2 gene expression. *Science* 244: 457–460

48 Liberman TA and Baltimore D (1990) Activation of interleukin-6 gene expression through the NFkB transcription factor. *Mol Cell Biol* 10: 2327–2334

49 Shakhov AN, Collart MA, Vassilli P, Nedospasov SA, Jongeneel CV (1990) κB-type enhancers are involved in lipopolysaccharide-mediated transcriptional activation of the tumor necrosis factor a gene in primary macrophages. *J Exp Med* 171: 35–47

50 Collins T, Read MA, Neish AS, Whitley MZ, Thanos D, Maniatis T (1995) Transcriptional regulation of endothelial cell adhesion molecules: NFκB and cytokine-inducible enhancers. *FASEB J* 9: 899–909

51 Uden S, Bilton D, Guyan PM, Kay PM, Braganza JM (1990) Rationale for antioxidant therapy in pancreatitis and cystic fibrosis. *Adv Exp Med Biol* 264: 555–572

52 Lauritsen K, Laursen LS, Bukhave K, Rask-Madsen J (1987) Does vitamin E supplementation modulate *in vivo* arachidonate metabolism in human inflammation? *Pharmacol Toxicol* 61: 246–249

53 Hoffenberg EJ, Deutsch J, Smith S, Sokol RJ (1997) Circulating antioxidant concentrations in children with inflammatory bowel disease. *Am J Clin Nutr* 65: 1482–1488

54 Buffinton GD and Doe WF (1995) Depleted mucosal antioxidant defences in inflammatory bowel disease. *Free Rad Biol Med* 19: 911–918

55 Millar AD, Rampton DS, Chander CL, Claxson AW, Blades S, Coumbe A, Panetta J,

Morris CJ, Blake DR (1996) Evaluating the antioxidant potential of new treatments for inflammatory bowel disease using a rat model of colitis. *Gut* 39: 407–415

56   Houglum K, Venkataramani A, Lyche K, Chojkier M (1997) A pilot study of the effects of d-alpha-tocopherol on hepatic stellate cell activation in chronic hepatitis C. *Gastroenterology* 113: 1069–1073

57   Packer JE, Slater TF, Willson RL (1979) Direct observation of a free radical interaction between vitamin E and vitamin C. *Nature* 278: 737–738

58   Burton GW, Wronska U, Stone L, Foster DO, Ingold KU (1990) Biokenetics of dietary RRR-α-tocopherol in the male guinea pig at three dietary levels of vitamin C and two dietary levels of vitamin E Evidence that vitamin C does not "spare" vitamin E *in vivo*. *Lipids* 25: 199–210

59   Bowry VW, Stocker R (1993) Tocopherol-mediated peroxidation. The prooxidant effect of vitamin E on the radical-initiated oxidation of human low-density lipoprotein. *J Am Chem Soc* 115: 6029–6044

60   Bowry VW, Ingold KU, Stocker R (1992) Vitamin E in human low-density lipoprotein When and how this antioxidant becomes a pro-oxidant. *Biochem J* 288: 341–344

61   Demling R, LaLonde C, Ikegami K, Picard L, Nayak U (1995) Alpha-tocopherol attenuates lung edema and lipid peroxidation caused by acute zymosan-induced peritonitis. *Surgery* 117: 226–231

62   Alpha-tocopherol, Beta-carotene Cancer Prevention Study Group (1994) The effect of vitamin E and beta carotene on the incidence of lung cancer and other cancers in male smokers. *N Engl J Med* 330: 1029–1035

63   Roberts HJ (1994) *Mega vitamin E. Is it safe?* Sunshine Sentinel Press, Inc West Palm Beach, Florida

Index

cancer metastasis 121

Candida albicans 57

caries 55

carotenoid 226

carotid body cell 38

cartilage 91, 155, 157, 158, 161-163

caspase 213

catalase 15

CD11/CD18 102

CD28-responsive complex 87

cell 34

cell adhesion molecule (CAM) 121

cell free system 30

c-*fos* 88, 89, 139

chemiluminescence detector 55

3-chlorotyrosine 226

5-chlorocytosine 232

chondrocyte 36, 91, 136, 155, 158, 161, 162

chronic granulomatous disease (CGD) 21, 23

chronic granulomatous disease (CGD) patient 30, 34

chronic inflammation 1, 221

citrulline 50

c-*jun* 88, 139

Clostridium botulinum 57

collagen 155, 161

collagenase 48, 89

collagen-induced arthritis 158, 159

conjugated diene 226

copper 49

copper ion 222

COX-2 90, 91

creatinine 228

Cu/Zn superoxide dismutase (SOD) 17

cyclic guanosine monophosphate (cGMP) 48

cyclooxygenase 12, 87

cysteine residue 85, 88

cytochrome b558 22

cytochrome P450 224

cytochrome P450 reductase 51

cytokine 52, 99, 138, 156, 157, 171, 189

decosahexaenoic acid (DHA) 228

demolybdo xanthine oxireductase (demolybdo XOR) 71

desulpho xanthine oxireductase (desulpho XOR) 72, 73

diacylglycerol (DAG) 31

3,5-dibromo-4-nitrobenzenesulphonic acid (DBNBS) 224

2,3-dihydroxybenzoate 224

2,5-dihydroxybenzoate 224

5,5-dimethylpyrroline-N-oxide 224

2,4-dinitrophenylalanine (DNPH) 230

diphenyl iodonium (IDP) 35, 37

diphenylene iodonium (DPI) 33, 38, 87

dityrosine 230

DNA 221

DNA damage 185, 231

DNA repair 186

E. coli 57

E. coli 0157 57

eicosapentaenoic acid (EPA) 228

electrochemical detection (HPLC-e.c.d.) 231

electron spin resonance (ESR) 223

electron-transport chain 209

electrophoretic mobility shift assay (EMSA) 90

emphysema 21

endothelial cell 37, 66, 73-75

endothelial cell adhesion molecule (ECAM) 99

endothelium derived relaxing factor (EDRF) 13, 47

eosinophil 21, 34, 221

epithelial cell 74

Epstein-Barr virus (EBV) 34

Epstein-Barr virus (EBV)-transformed B lymphocyte (EBVL) 31

erythropoietin 38

E-selectin 101, 103

ethan 229

F_2-isoprostane 228

facultative anaerobe 54